Sports Performance and Health

Sports Performance and Health

Editors

Matej Supej
Jörg Spörri

MDPI • Basel • Beijing • Wuhan • Barcelona • Belgrade • Manchester • Tokyo • Cluj • Tianjin

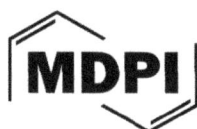

Editors
Matej Supej
University of Ljubljana
Slovenia
Mid Sweden University
Sweden

Jörg Spörri
University of Zurich
Switzerland

Editorial Office
MDPI
St. Alban-Anlage 66
4052 Basel, Switzerland

This is a reprint of articles from the Special Issue published online in the open access journal *Applied Sciences* (ISSN 2076-3417) (available at: https://www.mdpi.com/journal/applsci/special_issues/Sports_Performance_Health).

For citation purposes, cite each article independently as indicated on the article page online and as indicated below:

LastName, A.A.; LastName, B.B.; LastName, C.C. Article Title. *Journal Name* **Year**, *Volume Number*, Page Range.

ISBN 978-3-0365-1258-7 (Hbk)
ISBN 978-3-0365-1259-4 (PDF)

Cover image courtesy of Aleš Fevžer.

© 2021 by the authors. Articles in this book are Open Access and distributed under the Creative Commons Attribution (CC BY) license, which allows users to download, copy and build upon published articles, as long as the author and publisher are properly credited, which ensures maximum dissemination and a wider impact of our publications.
The book as a whole is distributed by MDPI under the terms and conditions of the Creative Commons license CC BY-NC-ND.

Contents

About the Editors vii

Matej Supej and Jörg Spörri
Special Issue on "Sports Performance and Health"
Reprinted from: *Appl. Sci.* **2021**, *11*, 2755, doi:10.3390/app11062755 1

Yanyan Du and Yubo Fan
Changes in the Kinematic and Kinetic Characteristics of Lunge Footwork during the Fatiguing Process
Reprinted from: *Appl. Sci.* **2020**, *10*, 8703, doi:10.3390/app10238703 7

Martin Zorko, Karmen Hirsch, Nejc Šarabon and Matej Supej
The Influence of Ski Waist-Width and Fatigue on Knee-Joint Stability and Skier's Balance
Reprinted from: *Appl. Sci.* **2020**, *10*, 7766, doi:10.3390/app10217766 19

Filip Ujaković and Nejc Šarabon
Change of Direction Performance Is Influenced by Asymmetries in Jumping Ability and Hip and Trunk Strength in Elite Basketball Players
Reprinted from: *Appl. Sci.* **2020**, *10*, 6984, doi:10.3390/app10196984 33

Matej Supej, Jan Ogrin, Nejc Šarabon and Hans-Christer Holmberg
Asymmetries in the Technique and Ground Reaction Forces of Elite Alpine Skiers Influence Their Slalom Performance
Reprinted from: *Appl. Sci.* **2020**, *10*, 7288, doi:10.3390/app10207288 47

Jacek Stodółka, Wieslaw Blach, Janez Vodicar and Krzysztof Maćkała
The Characteristics of Feet Center of Pressure Trajectory during Quiet Standing
Reprinted from: *Appl. Sci.* **2020**, *10*, 2940, doi:10.3390/app10082940 63

Darjan Smajla, Žiga Kozinc and Nejc Šarabon
Elbow Extensors and Volar Flexors Strength Capacity and Its Relation to Shooting Performance in Basketball Players—A Pilot Study
Reprinted from: *Appl. Sci.* **2020**, *10*, 8206, doi:10.3390/app10228206 73

Jeton Havolli, Abedin Bahtiri, Tim Kambič, Kemal Idrizović, Duško Bjelica and Primož Pori
Anthropometric Characteristics, Maximal Isokinetic Strength and Selected Handball Power Indicators Are Specific to Playing Positions in Elite Kosovan Handball Players
Reprinted from: *Appl. Sci.* **2020**, *10*, 6774, doi:10.3390/app10196774 85

Carson Patterson and Christian Raschner
Supramaximal Eccentric Training for Alpine Ski Racing—Strength Training with the Lifter
Reprinted from: *Appl. Sci.* **2020**, *10*, 8831, doi:10.3390/app10248831 97

Olga Bugaj, Krzysztof Kusy, Adam Kantanista, Paweł Korman, Dariusz Wieliński and Jacek Zieliński
The Effect of a 7-Week Training Period on Changes in Skin NADH Fluorescence in Highly Trained Athletes
Reprinted from: *Appl. Sci.* **2020**, *10*, 5133, doi:10.3390/app10155133 111

Goichi Hagiwara, Hirotoshi Mankyu, Takaaki Tsunokawa, Masaru Matsumoto and Hirokazu Funamori
Effectiveness of Positive and Negative Ions for Elite Japanese Swimmers' Physical Training: Subjective and Biological Emotional Evaluations
Reprinted from: *Appl. Sci.* **2020**, *10*, 4198, doi:10.3390/app10124198 123

Bernardino J Sánchez-Alcaraz, Diego Muñoz, Francisco Pradas, Jesús Ramón-Llin, Jerónimo Cañas and Alejandro Sánchez-Pay
Analysis of Serve and Serve-Return Strategies in Elite Male and Female Padel
Reprinted from: *Appl. Sci.* **2020**, *10*, 6693, doi:10.3390/app10196693 133

Milan Čoh, Nejc Bončina, Stanko Štuhec and Krzysztof Mackala
Comparative Biomechanical Analysis of the Hurdle Clearance Technique of Colin Jackson and Dayron Robles: Key Studies
Reprinted from: *Appl. Sci.* **2020**, *10*, 3302, doi:10.3390/app10093302 145

Duo Wai-Chi Wong, Winson Chiu-Chun Lee and Wing-Kai Lam
Biomechanics of Table Tennis: A Systematic Scoping Review of Playing Levels and Maneuvers
Reprinted from: *Appl. Sci.* **2020**, *10*, 5203, doi:10.3390/app10155203 155

Attilio Carraro, Martina Gnech, Fabio Sarto, Diego Sarto, Jörg Spörri and Stefano Masiero
Lower Back Complaints in Adolescent Competitive Alpine Skiers: A Cross-Sectional Study
Reprinted from: *Appl. Sci.* **2020**, *10*, 7408, doi:10.3390/app10217408 177

Yali Liu, Ligang Qiang, Qiuzhi Song, Mingsheng Zhao and Xinyu Guan
Effects of Backpack Loads on Leg Muscle Activation during Slope Walking
Reprinted from: *Appl. Sci.* **2020**, *10*, 4890, doi:10.3390/app10144890 187

Carlos Romero-Morales, Carlos López-Nuevo, Carlos Fort-Novoa, Patricia Palomo-López, David Rodríguez-Sanz, Daniel López-López, César Calvo-Lobo and Blanca De-la-Cruz-Torres
Ankle Taping Effectiveness for the Decreasing Dorsiflexion Range of Motion in Elite Soccer and Basketball Players U18 in a Single Training Session: A Cross-Sectional Pilot Study
Reprinted from: *Appl. Sci.* **2020**, *10*, 3759, doi:10.3390/app10113759 199

Duo Wai-Chi Wong, Wing-Kai Lam, Tony Lin-Wei Chen, Qitao Tan, Yan Wang and Ming Zhang
Effects of Upper-Limb, Lower-Limb, and Full-Body Compression Garments on Full Body Kinematics and Free-Throw Accuracy in Basketball Players
Reprinted from: *Appl. Sci.* **2020**, *10*, 3504, doi:10.3390/app10103504 209

Yunqi Tang, Zhikang Wang, Yifan Zhang, Shuqi Zhang, Shutao Wei, Jiahao Pan and Yu Liu
Effect of Football Shoe Collar Type on Ankle Biomechanics and Dynamic Stability during Anterior and Lateral Single-Leg Jump Landings
Reprinted from: *Appl. Sci.* **2020**, *10*, 3362, doi:10.3390/app10103362 219

Špela Bogataj, Maja Pajek, Slobodan Andrašić and Nebojša Trajković
Concurrent Validity and Reliability of My Jump 2 App for Measuring Vertical Jump Height in Recreationally Active Adults
Reprinted from: *Appl. Sci.* **2020**, *10*, 3805, doi:10.3390/app10113805 231

About the Editors

Matej Supej is Professor of Sport Sciences–Kinesiology and Head of the Laboratory of Biomechanics at the Faculty of Sport, University of Ljubljana and Guest Professor at the Department of Health Sciences at Mid-Sweden University. He received his Bs.C. in Physics, Ms.C. in Mechanical Engineering, and Ph.D. in Sports Sciences from the University of Ljubljana. His main research interests are biomechanics of sports and measurement techniques, especially for optimizing sports performance and reducing the risk of injury. He has received two awards for scientific excellence and won an international prize for innovation.

Jörg Spörri is Head of Sports Medical Research at Balgrist University Hospital, University of Zurich. His research focuses on the prevention and rehabilitation of sports injuries with special emphasis on epidemiology, load management, movement biomechanics, musculoskeletal imaging, and exercise physiology. In addition, his research group supports leading national/international sports associations and clubs in translating scientific knowledge on health and performance into clinical practice and sports.

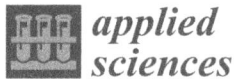

Editorial

Special Issue on "Sports Performance and Health"

Matej Supej [1,2,*] and Jörg Spörri [3,4]

1. Faculty of Sport, University of Ljubljana, 8008 Zurich, Slovenia
2. Swedish Winter Sports Research Centre, Mid Sweden University, SE-83140 Östersund, Sweden
3. Sports Medical Research Group, Department of Orthopaedics, Balgrist University Hospital, University of Zurich, 8008 Zurich, Switzerland; joerg.spoerri@balgrist.ch
4. University Centre for Prevention and Sports Medicine, Department of Orthopaedics, Balgrist University Hospital, University of Zurich, 8008 Zurich, Switzerland
* Correspondence: matej.supej@fsp.uni-lj.si; Tel.: +386-1-5207-762

Citation: Supej, M.; Spörri, J. Special Issue on "Sports Performance and Health". *Appl. Sci.* 2021, 11, 2755. https://doi.org/10.3390/app11062755

Academic Editor: Roger Narayan

Received: 15 March 2021
Accepted: 16 March 2021
Published: 19 March 2021

Publisher's Note: MDPI stays neutral with regard to jurisdictional claims in published maps and institutional affiliations.

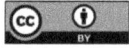

Copyright: © 2021 by the authors. Licensee MDPI, Basel, Switzerland. This article is an open access article distributed under the terms and conditions of the Creative Commons Attribution (CC BY) license (https://creativecommons.org/licenses/by/4.0/).

Sports performance is primarily perceived to be associated with elite sport, where athletes strive for a place on the podium, with the most prestigious result probably being an Olympic gold medal. On the other hand, recreational athletes are increasingly attempting to emulate top athletes by pushing their limits and setting their ambitions ever higher. As such, both elite and recreational athletes are seeking to optimize their performance.

Performance optimization is distinctly multidisciplinary. "Internal" performance optimization includes all of the athlete's technical to tactical skills, which depend heavily on the pillars of his or her physical and mental capabilities. "External" performance optimization, on the other hand, involves the development of innovative sports equipment and adjusting it to the athlete and the current conditions in which the equipment is used.

To improve both internal and/or external performance, optimized training concepts and incorporating state-of-the-art technologies are key. Besides a better understanding of human physical and mental performance and the possibilities to improve it, nowadays miniature and wearable sensors and advanced data processing approaches can also be supportive. Such technological advances can provide new real-time feedback opportunities and, when combined with artificial intelligence, may even allow the prediction/optimization of current performance enhancement strategies.

However, despite or even because of such possibilities for improvement, sports performance enhancement is in a permanent trade-off with the protection of athletes' health. Regardless of the well-known positive effects of physical activity on health, the prevention and management of sports injuries remain major challenges that need to be addressed. The treatment of sports injuries is often difficult, expensive and time-consuming, so preventive strategies and activities are justified for both medical and economic reasons. Moreover, improved physiological and psychological understanding of the factors influencing/protecting health, as well recent technological advances, could help to monitor and counteract injuries and their risk factors, and thus promote safe participation in sport.

Accordingly, this Special Issue on "Sports Performance and Health" was open (but not limited) to submissions from the following areas: (i) benefits of sport for health, (ii) tradeoffs between sports performance and health, (iii) optimization of sports performance by training, (iv) technique and/or tactics enhancements, prevention and management of sports injuries, (v) optimization of sports equipment to increase performance and/or decrease the risk of injury, and (vi) innovations for sports performance, health, and load monitoring. Covering such a wide range of sports performance and health-related aspects, this Special Issue contains 19 scientific contributions, 17 of which are original research papers, one review paper, and one commentary.

Two factors equally important to sports performance and health, and addressed by a total of five articles within this issue are fatigue and motion asymmetries. With respect to the first, the study by Du and Fan [1] investigated the effects of fatigue on the kinematics and kinetics of lunging maneuvers. Results showed that the initial contact angles, peak angles, moments, power, and time needed to reach the peak angles at the hip, knee, and ankle in the sagittal plane all decreased post-fatigue. Accordingly, with respect to preventing fatigue-induced injuries, the authors suggested focusing particularly on the muscular strengthening of the knee and hip extensors. A second study by Zorko et al. [2] examined the influence of fatigue and ski waist-width on knee-joint stability and skier's balance. They demonstrated that the skiers' knee-joint kinematics and balance were hampered in the state of fatigue, as well as when using skis with a large waist-width. They suggested avoiding the fatigue state and the use of skis with a large waist-width while skiing on hard surfaces to decrease the risk of injury.

Concerning motion asymmetries, two studies in this Special Issue examined potential relationships with performance. Ujakovič and Šarabon [3] reported asymmetries in jumping ability and hip and trunk strength to influence the change of direction performance in elite basketball players. Furthermore, as the magnitudes of asymmetry revealed to be highly dependent on the specific movement, test and parameter, the authors suggested not to use uniform asymmetry thresholds, such as <10%, when deciding on athletes' return to sport or when planning counteractive training interventions. Supej et al. [4] investigated whether asymmetries in the technique and acting ground reaction forces (GRF) associated with left and right turns influence the asymmetries in the performance of elite slalom skiers. They found that although slalom skiers moved their bodies in a quite symmetrical fashion, asymmetry in their skiing technique and GRF influenced variables related to asymmetries in performance. Finally, the third study on motion asymmetries by Stodółka et al. [5] investigated the asymmetry between the right and left foot center of pressure (COP) trajectory. Strong positive correlations were observed between the right and left foot anteroposterior COP displacement trajectory, while in the mediolateral direction, moderate to strong negative correlations were present. However, according to the authors, additional investigations are warranted to better understand the causes of COP asymmetry and to help clinicians with the diagnosis of posture-related pathologies.

Concerning the submission area (iii), i.e., the optimization of sports performance by training, technique and/or tactics enhancements, the study by Smajla et al. [6] investigated elbow extensors and volar flexors strength in basketball players, and demonstrated significant associations between strength and shooting performance, particularly for long-distance shooting. Havolli et al. [7] reported the anthropometric characteristics, maximal isokinetic strength and selected handball power as indicators that are specific to playing position in elite Kosovan handball players. In fact, the study found that shooting success is largely determined by the player's height, weight, muscle strength and power, while it seems that anthropometric characteristics and physical performance are closely related to the game demands of each playing position. A commentary by Patterson and Raschner [8] introduced an Intelligent Motion Lifter (IML) that allows safe supramaximal eccentric loads training with a free barbell and no spotters. The IML was suggested to be used for free barbell training: a spotter for normal training, eccentric only, concentric only, and squat jumps. Along with the introduction of the IML concept, the commentary addressed the necessity of eccentric training for elite alpine ski racers. The study by Bugaj et al. [9] explored the effects of a 7-week training period on changes in skin NADH Fluorescence in highly trained athletes and concluded that physical training results in an increase in the skin NADH fluorescence levels at rest and after exercise in athletes. The effect of the environment on training was investigated by Hagiwara et al. [10]. They examined the subjective and objective arousal of elite swimmers during physical training under positive and negative ion environments. Their analysis of the change in the arousal level at rest and during training revealed that both subjective and objective arousal levels were significantly higher in the positive and negative ion environments than in the control environment. Based on the fact that the average training performance scores were also significantly higher in the positive and negative ion environments, the authors concluded that such conditions have a positive effect on sports training.

Regarding the optimization of sports performance by technique and/or tactics enhancements Sánchez-Alcaraz et al. [11] analyzed the serve and return statistics in elite padel players regarding courtside and gender. They found female players to execute more backhand and cross-court returns and to use more lobs than men. The presented results appear particularly useful to develop appropriate game strategies and to design specific training exercises. The study by Čoh et al. [12] compared the biomechanical parameters of the hurdle clearance technique of the fifth hurdle in the 110 m hurdle race of Colin Jackson and Dayron Robles, two world record holders. The authors demonstrated differences in temporal parameters, as well as in the center-of-mass flight trajectory of the hurdle clearance. Finally, Wong et al. [13] conducted a systematic scoping review to present the available evidence on the biomechanics of table-tennis strokes. They summarized current trends, categorized research foci, and biomechanical outcomes regarding various movement maneuvers and playing levels. Most notably, their review uncovered that there is a lack of studies that investigated backspin maneuvers, longline maneuvers, strikes against sidespin, and pen-hold players. Meanwhile, higher-level players were found to be able to better utilize the joint power of the shoulder and wrist joints through the full-body kinetic chain.

With regard to the submission area (iv), i.e., prevention and management of sports injuries, the study by Carraro et al. [14] assessed the lower back complaints in adolescent competitive alpine skiers in view of sex, category, discipline preference, and training attributes. Particularly noteworthy is their finding that the characteristic pain intensity was found to be significantly related to the skiers' years of sports participation, the number of competitions/season, and the number of skiing days/season. Furthermore, this study showed a relatively high magnitude of lower back-related pain in adolescent competitive alpine skiers and that training attributes are a key driver for such complaints. In a second study addressing this submission area, Liu et al. [15] investigated the effects of backpack loads on leg muscle activation during slope walking. Their results implied that the hip and knee muscles play an important role during slope walking with loads. They interpreted their findings as being useful for designing assistant devices, such as exoskeleton robots, to enhance hikers' and soldiers' walking abilities.

The submission area (v) related to the optimization of sports equipment to increase performance and/or decrease the risk of injury was addressed by three papers. Romero-Morales et al. [16] investigated the effectiveness of ankle taping in elite soccer and basketball players and found a decrease in the ROM of ankle dorsiflexion as a reason why taping may be considered a useful prophylactic approach for the prevention of ankle sprain injuries. The study by Wong et al. [17] examined the effects of wearing upper-, lower- and full-body compression garments on basketball free-throw shooting accuracy, consistency and the range of motion of body joints. Overall, they demonstrated that upper-body or full-body compression garments constrained the range of motion and resulted in an improvement in shooting accuracy. In the context of football, Tang et al. [18] studied the effect of football shoe collar type on ankle biomechanics and dynamic stability during anterior and lateral single-leg jump landings. They found that medial-lateral stability was significantly improved with the high collar, compared to the low collar and that, during the lateral single-leg jump landing, ankle inversion ROM and total ankle frontal ROM were significantly smaller for the high collar, compared to the elastic collar. Accordingly, high collar shoes may be effective in decreasing the ROM and increasing dynamic stability, leading to high ankle joint stiffness. Overall, various equipment in sports can be used to improve performance or decrease the risk of injury. In this context, the designers, researchers and producing companies may still significantly contribute to the developments of sports and safety.

Last, but not least, one paper addressed the submission area (vi), i.e., innovations for sports performance, health, and load monitoring. Here, the study by Bogataj et al. [19] aimed to examine the reliability, validity, and usefulness of the smartphone-based application "My Jump 2". They showed that My Jump 2 is a valid, reliable, and useful tool for measuring vertical jump in recreationally active adults. Moreover, the authors concluded that, due to its simplicity and practicality, it can be used by practitioners, coaches, and recreationally active adults to measure vertical jump performance.

In summary, the current Special Issue provided several new insights and multidisciplinary perspectives on sports performance and health, and emphasized the ongoing challenges within this field. However, since the outbreak of the COVID 19 pandemic in early 2020, additional new issues emerged, such as the impact of COVID-19-related restrictions on performance and health in elite sports, the implications for mental and physical health in the general population, and the challenges related to the management of COVID-19 infection-related long-term sports performance and health consequences. Thus, there is an evident need to address such issues and fill our current large knowledge gaps through joint upcoming research efforts.

Author Contributions: Conceptualization, M.S. and J.S.; writing—original draft preparation, M.S. and J.S.; writing—review and editing, M.S. and J.S.; project administration, M.S. and J.S.; All authors have read and agreed to the published version of the manuscript.

Funding: This research was funded by Slovenian Research Agency, grant number P5-0147.

Conflicts of Interest: The authors declare no conflict of interest.

References

1. Du, Y.; Fan, Y. Changes in the Kinematic and Kinetic Characteristics of Lunge Footwork during the Fatiguing Process. *Appl. Sci.* **2020**, *10*, 8703. [CrossRef]
2. Zorko, M.; Hirsch, K.; Šarabon, N.; Supej, M. The Influence of Ski Waist-Width and Fatigue on Knee-Joint Stability and Skier's Balance. *Appl. Sci.* **2020**, *10*, 7766. [CrossRef]
3. Ujaković, F.; Šarabon, N. Change of Direction Performance Is Influenced by Asymmetries in Jumping Ability and Hip and Trunk Strength in Elite Basketball Players. *Appl. Sci.* **2020**, *10*, 6984. [CrossRef]
4. Supej, M.; Ogrin, J.; Šarabon, N.; Holmberg, H.-C. Asymmetries in the Technique and Ground Reaction Forces of Elite Alpine Skiers Influence Their Slalom Performance. *Appl. Sci.* **2020**, *10*, 7288. [CrossRef]
5. Stodółka, J.; Blach, W.; Vodicar, J.; Maćkała, K. The Characteristics of Feet Center of Pressure Trajectory during Quiet Standing. *Appl. Sci.* **2020**, *10*, 2940. [CrossRef]
6. Smajla, D.; Kozinc, Ž.; Šarabon, N. Elbow Extensors and Volar Flexors Strength Capacity and Its Relation to Shooting Performance in Basketball Players—A Pilot Study. *Appl. Sci.* **2020**, *10*, 8206. [CrossRef]
7. Havolli, J.; Bahtiri, A.; Kambič, T.; Idrizović, K.; Bjelica, D.; Pori, P. Anthropometric Characteristics, Maximal Isokinetic Strength and Selected Handball Power Indicators Are Specific to Playing Positions in Elite Kosovan Handball Players. *Appl. Sci.* **2020**, *10*, 6774. [CrossRef]
8. Patterson, C.; Raschner, C. Supramaximal Eccentric Training for Alpine Ski Racing—Strength Training with the Lifter. *Appl. Sci.* **2020**, *10*, 8831. [CrossRef]
9. Bugaj, O.; Kusy, K.; Kantanista, A.; Korman, P.; Wieliński, D.; Zieliński, J. The Effect of a 7-Week Training Period on Changes in Skin NADH Fluorescence in Highly Trained Athletes. *Appl. Sci.* **2020**, *10*, 5133. [CrossRef]
10. Hagiwara, G.; Mankyu, H.; Tsunokawa, T.; Matsumoto, M.; Funamori, H. Effectiveness of Positive and Negative Ions for Elite Japanese Swimmers' Physical Training: Subjective and Biological Emotional Evaluations. *Appl. Sci.* **2020**, *10*, 4198. [CrossRef]
11. Sánchez-Alcaraz, B.J.; Muñoz, D.; Pradas, F.; Ramón-Llin, J.; Cañas, J.; Sánchez-Pay, A. Analysis of Serve and Serve-Return Strategies in Elite Male and Female Padel. *Appl. Sci.* **2020**, *10*, 6693. [CrossRef]
12. Čoh, M.; Bončina, N.; Štuhec, S.; Mackala, K. Comparative Biomechanical Analysis of the Hurdle Clearance Technique of Colin Jackson and Dayron Robles: Key Studies. *Appl. Sci.* **2020**, *10*, 3302. [CrossRef]
13. Wong, D.W.-C.; Lee, W.C.-C.; Lam, W.-K. Biomechanics of Table Tennis: A Systematic Scoping Review of Playing Levels and Maneuvers. *Appl. Sci.* **2020**, *10*, 5203. [CrossRef]
14. Carraro, A.; Gnech, M.; Sarto, F.; Sarto, D.; Spörri, J.; Masiero, S. Lower Back Complaints in Adolescent Competitive Alpine Skiers: A Cross-Sectional Study. *Appl. Sci.* **2020**, *10*, 7408. [CrossRef]
15. Liu, Y.; Qiang, L.; Song, Q.; Zhao, M.; Guan, X. Effects of Backpack Loads on Leg Muscle Activation during Slope Walking. *Appl. Sci.* **2020**, *10*, 4890. [CrossRef]
16. Romero-Morales, C.; López-Nuevo, C.; Fort-Novoa, C.; Palomo-López, P.; Rodríguez-Sanz, D.; López-López, D.; Calvo-Lobo, C.; De-la-Cruz-Torres, B. Ankle Taping Effectiveness for the Decreasing Dorsiflexion Range of Motion in Elite Soccer and Basketball Players U18 in a Single Training Session: A Cross-Sectional Pilot Study. *Appl. Sci.* **2020**, *10*, 3759. [CrossRef]
17. Wong, D.W.-C.; Lam, W.-K.; Chen, T.L.-W.; Tan, Q.; Wang, Y.; Zhang, M. Effects of Upper-Limb, Lower-Limb, and Full-Body Compression Garments on Full Body Kinematics and Free-Throw Accuracy in Basketball Players. *Appl. Sci.* **2020**, *10*, 3504. [CrossRef]

18. Tang, Y.; Wang, Z.; Zhang, Y.; Zhang, S.; Wei, S.; Pan, J.; Liu, Y. Effect of Football Shoe Collar Type on Ankle Biomechanics and Dynamic Stability during Anterior and Lateral Single-Leg Jump Landings. *Appl. Sci.* **2020**, *10*, 3362. [CrossRef]
19. Bogataj, Š.; Pajek, M.; Andrašić, S.; Trajković, N. Concurrent Validity and Reliability of My Jump 2 App for Measuring Vertical Jump Height in Recreationally Active Adults. *Appl. Sci.* **2020**, *10*, 3805. [CrossRef]

Article

Changes in the Kinematic and Kinetic Characteristics of Lunge Footwork during the Fatiguing Process

Yanyan Du [1,2] and Yubo Fan [1,3,*]

[1] Key Laboratory for Biomechanics and Mechanobiology of Ministry of Education, Beijing Advanced Innovation Centre for Biomedical Engineering, School of Biological Science and Medical Engineering, Beihang University, Beijing 100083, China; duyanyan@cupes.edu.cn
[2] Beijing Key Laboratory of Sports Function Assessment and Technical Analysis, Capital University of Physical Education and Sports, Beijing 100191, China
[3] School of Medical Science and Engineering, Beihang University, Beijing 100083, China
* Correspondence: yubofan@buaa.edu.cn; Tel.: +86-10-82339428

Received: 29 September 2020; Accepted: 2 December 2020; Published: 4 December 2020

Featured Application: 1. The kinematic and kinetic characteristics of the lunge maneuver were gradually impaired in the fatiguing process. 2. Period IV (pre-drive-off) of the stance phase showed the most significant fatigue response. 3. Improving the strength of the knee extensor is important for the lunge maneuver, particularly in period IV. 4. It is important to improve the strength of hip extensors for the lunge maneuver. 5. The analysis of waveform data is more useful for the assessment of weak areas of the body and periods of motion.

Abstract: Fatigue is a major injury risk factor. The aim of this study was to investigate the effects of fatigue on lunging during the fatiguing process. The lower extremity joint kinematics and kinetics of fifteen male collegiate badminton players were simultaneously recorded by optical motion-capture and force plate systems during lunging. In addition to statistical analyses of discrete variables, one-dimensional statistical parametric mapping (SPM (1D)) was used to analyze the waveform data. The hypotheses were that the biomechanics of lunging maneuvers would change during the fatiguing process, and the fatigue effects would differ in different periods (I–V) of the stance phase and in different joints. Results showed that the initial contact angles, peak angles, moments, power, and time needed to reach the peak angles at the hip, knee, and ankle in the sagittal plane all decreased post-fatigue. A continuous decreasing tendency was reflected in the moments and power of hip and, in particular, knee joints (mostly $p < 0.001$). Period IV showed a significant fatigue response. In conclusion, both discrete and waveform data illustrated the effects of fatigue, however, the results of SPM (1D) analysis showed both the key period and body segments affected by the fatigue response.

Keywords: badminton; knee joint; injury; one-dimensional statistical parametric mapping

1. Introduction

Badminton, one of the most popular sports globally [1–4], is the fastest non-contact racket sport, and requires a combination of strength, speed, and stamina. While playing this sport, players must repetitively lunge, jump, and quickly change direction from a wide variety of positions. A previous epidemiology study conducted in Ireland reported that badminton was the sport with the most injuries [5]. Lower extremity injuries accounted for 43 to 86% of all injuries regardless of the nationality [6], and overuse is considered the major reason [7,8]. Ankles and knees are the most injured sites [1,7,9], particularly the knee joint [7,8]. Patellar tendinopathy [7] is the most common type of knee injury. As a specific and often-used example of footwork [10,11], the repetitive lunge is a likely cause of patellar tendinopathy, particularly for teenager players [3,12].

Moreover, epidemiology studies have also shown that a higher badminton injury rate was found at the end of a match or training [13], and higher rates have been found during training [7,14]. This could be explained by a higher intensity of training routine [7], which may induce fatigue. Because fatigue reduces the capacity of muscles to generate force, it may be an important factor causing injury. In badminton, increased ankle sprain injuries were found to occur at the end of a training or match session due to the accumulation of fatigue [6]. Due to fatigue caused by repeating the forward lunge, the activity of the vastus lateralis, vastus medialis, and biceps femoris showed a significant change [15], and knee injury risk was increased [16].

A number of studies [10,17–21] have investigated the biomechanical characteristics of the lunge, particularly its stance phase, which is defined as the period of time from initial contact to final lift-off from the ground by the dominant limb [10]. Ankle sprain [6] and patellar tendinopathy [14] may occur during the stance phase. However, the relationship between the repetitive lunge and injury is still not clear. A previous study examined the lunge under the condition of exhaustion to investigate the fatigue effect on the knee [16]. A limitation of this study is that the changes of lunge motion during the fatiguing process were ignored. Injury usually occurs at a certain time, instantaneously, and the factors inducing injury are prolonged. However, we are unaware of any studies that have investigated the biomechanical changes during the fatiguing process in badminton. Therefore, there is a lack of objective data on lower joint kinematics and kinetics of the lunge during the fatiguing process, which may provide essential insight into the understanding of the mechanism of injury.

Additionally, discrete data (related, for example, to the peak angle) has traditionally been used for statistical analysis to confirm the differences outlined above. However, it is worth noting that all kinematic and kinetic variables are continuous variables with time. Furthermore, as mentioned above, injury occurs partly due to the accumulation of changes. Thus, continuous data analysis may provide other useful information. In recent years, one-dimensional statistical parametric mapping (SPM (1D)) has been accepted as an effective method to analyze waveform data [22]. Kinematic waveform data of hip, knee, and ankle joints in three planes, measured in players with different levels, have been analyzed by SPM (1D) [18,19]. However, to the best of the authors' knowledge, no research has investigated the fatigue response by analyzing the biomechanics waveform data of the lunge.

Consequently, the purpose of this study was to investigate the changes of lunge biomechanical characteristics during the fatiguing process, from normal to fatigued states. To achieve this objective, a repetitive forehand forward lunge to exhaustion was proposed as the fatigue protocol. The fatiguing process was divided into sub-stages. In addition to the discrete data (ground reaction force (GRF), lower extremity joint angles, range of motion (RoM), moments, and power), waveform data (GRF and lower extremity joint angles, moments, and power) were also analyzed during different fatiguing stages. The hypotheses are (i) both discrete and waveform data of lunge biomechanical characteristics change significantly during the fatiguing process, especially post-fatigue; (ii) effects of fatigue vary with different periods of the stance phase; and (iii) the lower limb joints have different fatigue responses.

2. Materials and Methods

2.1. Participants

Fifteen male collegiate badminton players (age: 21.1 ± 2.2 years; height: 1.81 ± 0.04 m; weight: 72.5 ± 8.4 kg; years of badminton training: 8.9 ± 3.5 years) were recruited for the study. All participants were free from any injuries within the previous 3 months and did not take part in any high-intensity training or competitions during the two days prior to the experiment. All participants were informed of the procedures and requirements of the test, and written informed consent was obtained from each participant. In addition, a questionnaire about anthropometrics, health status, injury history, and physical activity level was completed. To minimize the potential effect of footwear, participants wore badminton shoes and socks of the same brand and series. The study was approved by the ethics committee of Beihang University (No. BM201900077).

2.2. Experimental Protocol

The test was conducted on a simulated badminton court of the biomechanics laboratory. Prior to the test, participants performed a familiarization of the forehand forward lunge and the study protocol, which included 10 min warm-up; tests of heart rate (HR), blood lactate (BL), and Borg 6–20 rating of perceived exertion (RPE); and a fatigue protocol. Considering the dependency of fatigue on the task being undertaken [23,24] and the aim of this study, repeating the forehand forward lunge until participants reached the state of exhaustion was proposed as the fatigue protocol [16]. More specifically, a forehand forward lunge cycle was defined as lunging from the starting position using the dominate limb with a sliding step, landing on the force plate positioned at the right front, hitting one shuttlecock, and then moving backward to the starting position. The degree of fatigue was estimated by values of HR [15], BL, and RPE [25], which were measured before (pre) and immediately after (post) the fatigue protocol.

A system of 9 optoelectronic cameras (Oqus 300+ Series, Qualisys AB®, Gothenburg, Sweden) and a Kistler mobile multi-component force plate (Type 9286A, Kistler, Kistler Instrument AG, Winterthur, Switzerland), integrated into the walkway, were used to record the marker position and ground reaction forces, and synchronized at 200 and 1000 Hz, respectively. According to the color atlas of skeletal (CAST) landmark definitions of the lower leg [26], twenty-eight reflective markers (diameter: 18 mm) were attached to the lower extremity for dynamic motion capture. The locations included anterior superior iliac spines, posterior superior iliac spines, thigh (markers cluster), shank (markers cluster), calcaneus, hallux, and 2nd and 5th metatarsal head of the left and right lower extremity. The markers on calcaneus, hallux, and 2nd and 5th metatarsal head were placed on the corresponding anatomical location of the badminton shoes.

2.3. Data Analysis

The kinematic and force data were obtained by the optical motion-capture system and then exported and saved as c3d files. Then, the hip, knee, and ankle joint angles, moments, power, and ground reaction force (GRF) were calculated using visual 3D software (V5, C-Motion, Bethesda, MD, USA). The raw kinematic data were filtered with a low-pass (Butterworth) filter with frequency of 20 Hz [10]. The threshold of the vertical ground reaction force (vGRF) data was set as 10 N.

The stance phase, from initial contact (heel strike) to final lift-off from the force-plate by the dominant limb, was determined by the vGRF value. During this phase, there were three vGRF peaks, namely, the initial impact peak (PF1) for heel strike transient, the secondary impact peak (PF2) for impact loading, and the third impact peak (PF3) for drive-off. Based on the classification of previous studies [10,20,21], five periods can be clearly identified in the stance phase: (I) initial contact (from heel strike to PF1); (II) impact loading (from PF1 to PF2); (III) weight acceptance (from PF2 to peak knee joint flexion angle (PAK)); (IV) pre drive-off (from PAK to PF3); and (V) drive-off (from PF3 to lift-off from ground). In addition, the fatiguing process was divided into four stages according to the slope of the HR–time curve. Six continuous lunging motions were assessed at the end of each stage, and the kinematic and kinetic data of three lunge motions were then averaged and normalized for further statistical analysis.

During the stance phase, the motion of lower extremity joints, particularly the knee, occurs primarily in the sagittal plane. This contributes to the major knee joint biomechanical characteristics in badminton research [10,21]. Based on the previous literature linked to the lunge in badminton [10,17–21,27], we analyzed the impact peak; duration of five sub-stance phases; hip, knee, and ankle joint initial contact angles; durations to peak angle; ranges of motion (RoM); peak angles; moments; and power in the sagittal plane.

2.4. Statistical Analysis

All variables of the fatiguing process were calculated during four sub-stages. The kinetic data were normalized by body weight. All discrete variables were reported as mean ± standard deviation (SD), and examined for normality using a Shapiro–Wilk test prior to statistical analysis. One-way repeated measures ANOVA was used for the analysis of the influence of fatigue on the related parameters and discrete biomechanical data. Paired t-tests were performed to identify the differences. All statistical procedures were performed with SPSS 25 (IBM SPSS Statistics for Window, IBM Corp., NY, USA). Additionally, the waveform data of joint angles, moments, and power in the sagittal plane were analyzed (paired t-test) and plotted using one-dimensional statistical parametric mapping (SPM (1D)) (https://spm1d.org/)) in MATLAB (R2014b, Mathworks, Inc., Natick, MA, USA). In addition, prior to statistical analysis, normality tests were performed for the waveform data with SPM (1D). The statistical significance level was set at 0.05.

3. Results

3.1. Fatigue Protocol

After the fatigue protocol, the mean values of HR, BL, and RPE were greater than 185 beats/min, 14 mmol/L, and a score of 18, respectively. Results of repeated measurement indicated that HR, BL, and RPE were all affected by the fatigue protocol (partial η^2: 0.99, 0.876, and 0.994 respectively), and the p values were all less than 0.001 (Table 1).

Figure 1 illustrates the HR–time curve (mean) of four participants throughout the fatigue protocol. To divide the fatigue protocol into stages, time was normalized, the slope of the HR–time curve was calculated, and four stages were distinguished, namely, P1 (0–10% duration of fatiguing process (D)), P2 (10–30%D), P3 (30–60%D) and P4 (60–100%D).

Table 1. Values of heart rate (HR), blood lactate acid (BL), and rating of perceived exertion (RPE) pre- and post-fatigue protocol (mean ± SD).

	Mean ± SD			95% CI of the Difference			
	Pre	Post	η_p^2	Lower	Upper	t	p
HR (beats/min)	78.2 ± 9.4	185.8 ± 9.1	0.99	−115.013	−100.32	−32.256	<0.001
BL (mmol/L)	3 ± 2.4	14.3 ± 3.1	0.876	−14.241	−8.543	−8.801	<0.001
RPE	6 ± 0	18.4 ± 1	0.994	−13.05	−11.784	−43.176	<0.001

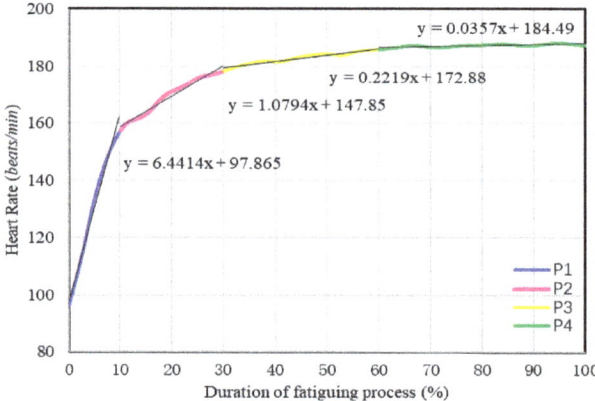

Figure 1. Heart rate (HR) of four participants during the fatiguing process (mean). According to the slope of the HR–time curve, the overall duration of the fatiguing process was divided into four stages, that is, P1, P2, P3, and P4. Duration of fatiguing process (%) vs. heart rate (beats/min).

3.2. Kinematics of Lower Extremity Joints

In the sagittal plane, Table 2 shows that the hip, knee, and ankle initial contact angle (CAH, CAK, CAA, respectively), peak angle (PAH, PAK, PAA, respectively), time to peak angle, and range of motion (RoM) all decreased during the process of the fatigue protocol (from P1 to P4).

Table 2. Kinematics variables in the four stages of fatiguing process (P1–P4) from pre- to post-fatigue protocol in the sagittal plane (mean ± SD).

	P1	P2	P3	P4	p
Joint angle at initial contact (°)					
CAH	46.08 ± 12.7	46.12 ± 10.32	42.2 ± 11.77	42.17 ± 11.77	c, d*, e*
CAK	13.11 ± 7.43	9.65 ± 7.55	7.82 ± 6.78	7.87 ± 6.09	a, b, c*
CAA	10.35 ± 8.05	6.81 ± 8.25	8 ± 8.47	6.42 ± 9.11	
Peak joint angle (°)					
PAH	74.08 ± 11.94	73.3 ± 9.93	67.34 ± 11.74	67.84 ± 12.78	
PAK	69.46 ± 8.77	65.43 ± 9.44	64.17 ± 10.26	62.46 ± 8.84	a*, b, c*
PAA	−20.84 ± 5.7	−18.74 ± 5.2	−18.4 ± 4.9	−18.19 ± 6.55	
Time to peak joint angle (%)					
PAH	41.63 ± 6.59	42.13 ± 8.79	38.88 ± 7.55	36.75 ± 6.94	
PAK	45.88 ± 6.51	38.63 ± 9.12	37.25 ± 10.44	33.63 ± 9.43	c*, f
PAA	14.13 ± 2.95	12.75 ± 2.82	12.38 ± 3.42	11.25 ± 2.71	a, b, c
Range of Motion (°)					
Hip joint	44.57 ± 10.44	39.16 ± 5.09	34.54 ± 6.85	38.67 ± 10.8	
Knee joint	59.32 ± 7.31	56.63 ± 6.84	56.74 ± 7.95	55.07 ± 6.28	a, c
Ankle joint	34.11 ± 8.09	29.82 ± 9.46	34.92 ± 9.68	31.98 ± 8.23	

Notes: CAH, CAK, and CAA: initial contact angle of hip, knee, and ankle joint, respectively; PAH, PAK, and PAA: peak joint angle of hip, knee, and ankle joint, respectively. P1–P4: the 1st, 2nd, 3rd, and 4th stages of the fatiguing process, respectively. a, a^*: significant differences between P1 and P2 at 0.05 and 0.01 levels, respectively; b: significant differences between P1 and P3 at 0.05 level; c: significant differences between P1 and P4 at 0.05 level; d^*: significant differences between P2 and P3 at 0.01 level; e^*: significant differences between P2 and P4 at 0.01 level; f: significant differences between P3 and P4 at 0.05 level.

At initial contact, a significant decrease was found for hip flexion (P1 vs. P4, $p = 0.044$; P2 vs. P3, $p = 0.009$; P2 vs. P4, $p = 0.003$) and knee flexion (P1 vs. P2, $p = 0.028$; P1 vs. P3, $p = 0.037$; P1 vs. P4, $p = 0.004$). Hip, knee, and ankle joints were all flexed (plantar-flexed) to the peak joint angle in less time. There were statistically significant differences in the time to peak value for the knee joint (P1 vs. P4, $p = 0.009$; P3 vs. P4, $p = 0.012$) and the ankle joint (P1 vs. P2, $p = 0.036$; P1 vs. P3, $p = 0.021$; P1 vs. P4, $p = 0.001$). The significance values (p) of the knee joint RoM were 0.013 (P1 vs. P2) and 0.048 (P1 vs. P4).

3.3. Five Sub-Phases of the Stance Phase

Table 3 shows that significant differences existed in the duration of the sub-stance phases II, III, IV, and V during the fatiguing process: durations were shorter for II (P1 vs. P3: $p = 0.012$), III (P1 vs. P4: $p = 0.041$; P3 vs. P4: $p = 0.005$), and V (P1 vs. P3: $p = 0.021$; P1 vs. P4: $p = 0.005$), and longer for IV (P1 vs. P2: $p = 0.022$; P1 vs. P3: $p = 0.024$; P1 vs. P4: $p = 0.002$; P2 vs. P4: $p = 0.002$; P3 vs. P4: $p = 0.036$).

3.4. Kinetics of Lower Extremity Joints

For the mean moments and power at the hip, knee, and ankle joints in the sagittal plane. Significant differences were found for moments at the hip (the 1st peak, P1 vs. P4: $p = 0.03$; the 2nd peak, P1 vs. P4: $p = 0.01$) and the knee (the 1st peak, P1 vs. P4: $p < 0.001$; the 2nd peak, P1 vs. P4: $p = 0.01$); power generation at the hip (P1 vs. P3: $p = 0.025$; P1 vs. P4: $p = 0.014$) and knee (P1 vs. P2, P1 vs. P3, P1 vs. P4: $p < 0.001$); and power consumption at the knee (P1 vs. P2: $p = 0.029$; P1 vs. P3: $p = 0.009$ and P1 vs. P4: $p < 0.001$) (details in Figure 4a).

3.5. SPM (1D) of Kinematics of Lower Extremity Joints

For the four stages of the fatiguing process (P1–P4), Figure 2a illustrates the joint angle–time curves in the sagittal plane (mean ± SD). SPM (1D) analysis results with significant differences are illustrated in Figure 2b. At the hip, significant differences exist in the initial contact (I), impact loading (II), weight acceptance (III), and pre-drive-off (IV) phases (P2 vs. P3 (I and II: $p = 0.01$; III and IV:

$p < 0.001$); P2 vs. P4 (I–IV: $p < 0.001$)). At the knee, significant differences were found mainly in the weight acceptance and pre-drive-off phases (P1 vs. P2 and P1 vs. P4: $p < 0.001$).

Table 3. Duration of five sub-phases (%) (mean ± SD).

	P1	P2	P3	P4	p
Duration of Five Sub-Phases (%)					
I (0-PF1)	3.88 ± 0.64	4 ± 0.93	4 ± 0.76	3.75 ± 0.71	
II (PF1-PF2)	11.13 ± 2.75	8.63 ± 4.44	8 ± 3.55	8.88 ± 3.31	b
III (PF2-PAK)	30.88 ± 6.03	26 ± 7.11	25.25 ± 9.25	21 ± 9.3	c, f^*
IV (PAK-PF3)	27.25 ± 10.69	36.5 ± 14.32	39.25 ± 17.17	43.38 ± 15.24	a, b, c^*, e^*, f
V (PF3-FO)	26.88 ± 5.57	24.88 ± 7.24	23.5 ± 7.23	23 ± 6.68	b, c^*

Notes: PF1: initial impact peak (the 1st peak vertical ground reaction force, vGRF); PF2: secondary impact peak (the 2nd peak vGRF); PF3: third impact peak (the 3rd peak vGRF); PAK: peak knee joint flexion angle. FO: foot off. The stance phase was divided into five sub-phases (I–V) according to impact peak and PAK. P1–P4: the 1st, 2nd, 3rd, and 4th stages of the fatiguing process, respectively. a, a^*: significant differences between P1 and P2 at 0.05 and 0.01 levels, respectively; b: significant differences between P1 and P3 at 0.05 level; c, c^*: significant differences between P1 and P4 at 0.05 and 0.01 levels, respectively; e^*: significant differences between P2 and P4 at 0.01 level; f, f^*: significant differences between P3 and P4 at 0.05 and 0.01 levels, respectively.

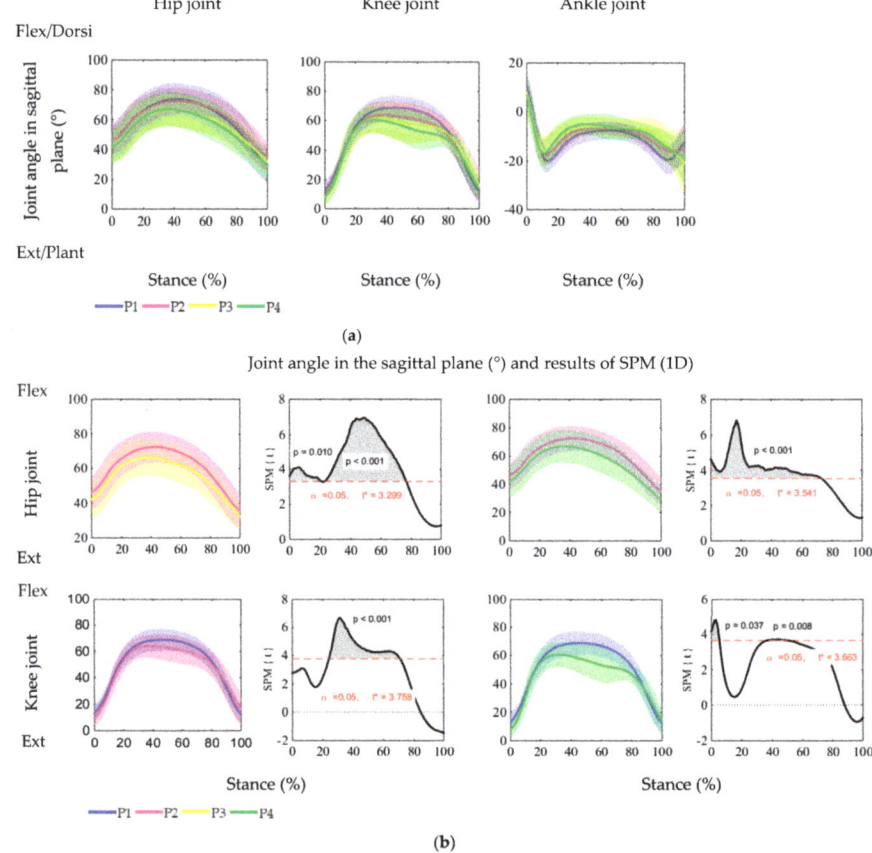

Figure 2. (**a**) Summary of the joint angles (mean ± SD) of lower limbs in the sagittal plane. (**b**) Results with significant differences of one-dimensional statistical parametric mapping (SPM (1D)) for hip and knee joint angles. Positive angles represent hip and knee flexion and ankle dorsi-flexion. P1–P4: the 1st, 2nd, 3rd, and 4th stages of the fatiguing process, respectively.

3.6. SPM (1D) of Kinetics of Lower Extremity Joints

Figure 3 illustrates the vGRF waveform data of P1, P2, P3, and P4, and the results of SPM (1D) analysis with significant differences, which are shown mainly in the pre-drive-off phases between P1 and P4 ($p < 0.001$).

Figure 4a illustrates the waveform data of the hip, knee, and ankle joint moments and power in the sagittal plane (mean ± SD) in P1, P2, P3, and P4. SPM (1D) analysis results of moments and power with significant differences are illustrated in Figure 4b,c, respectively. For hip and knee moments, significant differences exist in the partial period of the pre-drive-off phase (IV) between P1 and P3 ($p < 0.001$), and in the IV phase between P1 and P4 ($p < 0.001$). Moreover, Figure 4c illustrates that significant differences exist in the partial IV and drive-off (V) phases for hip power (P1 vs. P4: $p < 0.05$) and knee power (P1 vs. P3: $p < 0.001$; P1 vs. P4: $p < 0.001$).

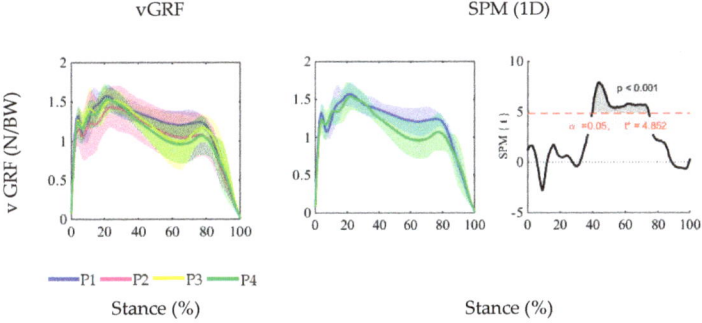

Figure 3. Vertical ground reaction force (vGRF) and results with significant differences of one-dimensional statistical parametric mapping (SPM (1D)). P1–P4: the 1st, 2nd, 3rd, and 4th stages of the fatiguing process, respectively.

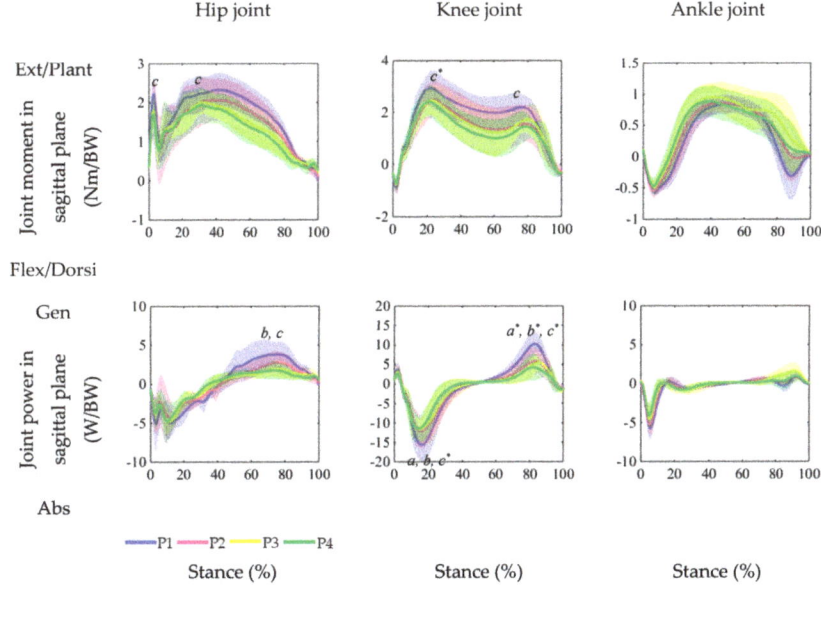

(**a**)

Figure 4. *Cont.*

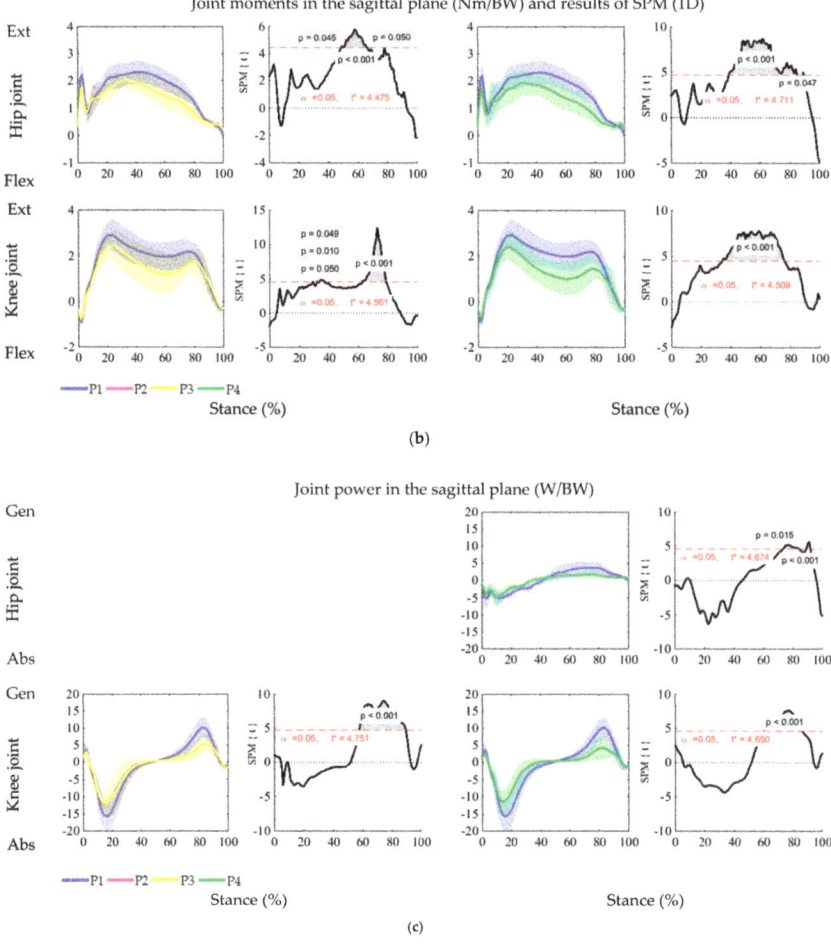

Figure 4. (**a**) Summary of joint moments and power (mean ± SD) of lower extremities in the sagittal plane during the lunge. (**b**) Results with significant differences of one-dimensional statistical parametric mapping (SPM (1D)) for hip and knee joint moments. (**c**) Results with significant differences of SPM (1D) for hip and knee joint power. Positive moments represent hip and knee extensor and ankle plantar flexor moments, and positive joint power indicates periods of power generation. P1–P4: the 1st, 2nd, 3rd, and 4th stages of the fatiguing process, respectively. a, a*: significant differences between P1 and P2 at 0.05 and 0.01 levels, respectively; b: significant differences between P1 and P3 at 0.05 level; c, c*: significant differences between P1 and P4 at 0.05 and 0.01 levels, respectively.

4. Discussion

An increasing number of people now play badminton. Both athletes and recreational players attempt to optimize their performance, thus increasing the risk of injury. Prevention of sports-related injuries is an important challenge. Fatigue is a major factor causing injury. Consequently, this study investigated the fatigue effects on a specific movement in badminton, i.e., the footwork associated with the lunge, which is one of the most used and integral movements [10,11].

Considering the task dependency of fatigue, a repeated forehand forward lunge, until reaching exhaustion, was proposed as the fatigue protocol, which was subdivided into four stages (P1, P2, P3, and P4) according to the slope of the heart rate (HR)–time curve. After the protocol, the mean values of HR, blood lactate (BL), and rating of perceived exertion (RPE) increased significantly at the significance level of 0.001; in particular, the mean HR was greater than 185 beats/min, the mean BL value was greater than 14 mmol/L, and the mean RPE score was greater than 18, indicating that all participants were fatigued. At P1, the first stage of the fatigue protocol, all participants were in a pre-fatigue state and, at P4, the final stage of the fatigue protocol, they were fatigued. In addition, according to previous studies [10,20,21], the first, second, and third impact peak (PF1, PF2, and PF3) and knee flexion peak angle (PAK) were used to subdivide the lunge stance phase into initial contact (I: 0-PF1)), impact loading (II: PF1-PF2), weight acceptance (III: PF2-PAK), pre drive-off (IV: PAK-PF3), and drive-off (V: PF3-end) periods. Then, statistical analyses were undertaken for both discrete and waveform kinematic and kinetic data in the sagittal plane, in which the largest movements occurred, comparing not only the pre- and post-fatigue states, but also the four stages of the fatiguing process.

The results supported the hypothesis that the biomechanical characteristics of the lunge change significantly during the fatiguing process. At the initial contact time, participants exhibited a more "erect" posture for the lunge, which is usually observed by coaches, and was shown as less hip and knee flexion, and ankle dorsi-flexion. Less dorsi-flexion at the foot strike has been found for recreational players with a relative lack of muscle power compared to national-level badminton athletes [19]. In the lateral jump performed in badminton, Herbaut et al. [27] found a decreased plantar-flexion angle at the foot strike post-fatigue. These changes may be induced by muscle fatigue caused by repeated stretch-shortening. Furthermore, the range of motion (RoM) of hip, knee, and ankle joints was decreased due to the fatiguing process.

Smaller peak joint angles were found at hip, knee, and ankle joints in the sagittal plane, particularly at the knee joint (with significant differences between P1 and the other three stages of the fatiguing process). After fatigue, a decrease in the knee peak angle was also found by Valldecabres et al. [16], however, no significant difference was found. The discrepancy may be due to the participant's sports level [24]. The decrease in the peak angle could be explained by the decrease in joint moments (details in Figure 4). There were significant differences in peak joint moments at the hip and knee extensor (P1 vs. P4: hip ($p = 0.03$), knee ($p < 0.001$)). A similar relationship was illustrated by Fu et al. [19] between professional and amateur badminton players; that is, professional players with greater muscle strength and better performance showed higher knee and ankle joint moments. Additionally, a shorter time was taken to flex to the peak angle, with significant decreases in time shown at the knee and ankle. This may be caused by impaired control due to fatigue. This can also be explained in this study by the decrease in joint moments and power.

In addition to the angles, the durations of the four sub-stance phases (II–V) changed during the process of the fatigue protocol. The shorter durations of II and III indicate that less time was taken to reach PF2 and PAK, respectively; that is, due to the fatiguing process, the participant placed his foot flat and flexed his knee more quickly. This is consistent with the increased ankle plantar flexor and knee flexor moments in the present study (Figure 4a), and with the opinion that fatigue reduces the capacity of muscles to generate force. The most significant increase was found in the IV phase (pre-drive-off), increasing from 27.25 ± 10.69% stance to 43.38 ± 15.24% stance. Significantly decreased hip and knee peak power in this phase provided sufficient support for this change. Less power was generated for players for the drive-off. Kuntz et al. [10] indicated that a hop style lunge generates higher peak vertical force during loading. In this study, three participants used the hop style at the final stage of the fatigue protocol. The change of lunge style may be a strategy to generate more power for driving-off and returning to the starting position [14].

Furthermore, considering the time continuity of biomechanical variables of the lunge motion, one-dimensional statistical parametric mapping SPM (1D) was used to analyze the biomechanical waveform data in the sagittal plane. Most of the joint angle, moment, and power waveforms decreased consistently during the process of the fatigue protocol (among P1, P2, P3, and P4). Significant differences were found in the hip and knee joint angles, mainly in the pre-drive-off phase (IV) (most p values were less than 0.001). The results support the hypothesis that the fatigue effects were different in the five periods of the lunge. Moreover, these results support the view that lunge characteristics change due to fatigue.

Taking into account the joint moments, both the hip and knee joints showed a significant response to the fatigue protocol. Significant differences were found between P1 and P3 in part of the period of IV, and between P1 and P4 in IV. The hip moments had a larger effective scope. However, there were only significant differences in the hip power between P1 and P4. For knee power, the significant differences were seen between P1 and P3, and also between P1 and P4, with a larger effective scope of the period. This indicates that the significant decrease in joint power occurred earlier and was mostly evident at the knee; that is, the fatigue responses manifested mostly at the knee joint. This result is consistent with a previous epidemiology study that reviewed musculoskeletal injuries among Malaysian badminton players, which reported that the majority of injuries sustained by players were due to overuse, primarily of the knee [7]. Another study [28] suggested that the rapidly changing eccentric/concentric work of the quadriceps in the varying degree of knee flexion was probably associated with patellar tendon injury. This may be why patellar tendinopathy is the most common injury of lower limbs among badminton players, and this result also supports our third hypothesis. Coaches and players should pay more attention to the training of the knee, and particularly the knee extensors.

Additionally, a comparison indicates that the discrete and waveform results are consistent. There are significant differences in CAH (P2 vs. P3), CAK (P2 vs. P4), PAK (P1 vs. P2; P1 vs. P4), knee peak moment (P1 vs. P4), hip peak power (P1 vs. P4), and knee peak power (P1 vs. P3; P1 vs. P4). In addition, significant differences were shown in these periods of stance phase in the discrete data. The results of SPM (1D) analysis clearly provided more information, indicating the period rather than a point of time in the fatigue response. This is also helpful in identifying the key body segments affected by fatigue. Thus, it is important for coaches and players to design a corresponding training program to improve the technique and muscle strength. Moreover, the results of SPM (1D) can provide support for monitoring of training.

Considering the key findings of this study, a few limitations should be noted when interpreting the results. First, the participants were male badminton players with at least 8 years of special badminton training. Results may differ for players of different levels, ages, and gender, thus studies of players with a range of abilities and ages, including female players, should be considered. Second, all tests were conducted on a simulated badminton court. Third, the sample size was limited. Fourth, the changing slope of the HR–time curve was used to subdivide the fatiguing process. However, it is not sufficient to explain the status of fatigue. Electromyography (EMG) data might be more suitable and could be used in future work. Finally, although joint moments and power allow further assessment of the functional contribution of the joints, EMG and musculoskeletal system simulations would help understand movement changes during the fatiguing process.

5. Conclusions

This study investigated the changes in the kinematic and kinetic characteristics of lunge footwork during the fatiguing process. To the best of our knowledge, this study was the first to subdivide the fatiguing process and analyze the changes among different sub-stages. It was also the first study to use one-dimensional statistical parametric mapping (SPM (1D)) to analyze the effect of fatigue on the lunge footwork in badminton. Statistically significant differences were found in both the discrete and waveform data. Moreover, these differences were shown not only between pre- and post-fatigue, but also among other sub-stages.

Overall, the results presented in this study confirm that period IV of the stance phase is more sensitive to fatigue than the other periods. In addition, the training program should focus on muscular strengthening of the knee extensor, particularly in period IV. It is also important to improve the strength of hip extensors. Furthermore, although the results show consistent changes between the discrete and waveform data, findings from this study highlight that results of SPM (1D) are more useful for the assessment of weak areas of the body and periods of motion. This information may contribute to the future design and development of training plans and to the monitoring of training.

Author Contributions: Y.D. designed, carried out the experiments, analyzed the data and wrote the paper, Y.F. designed the experiments, reviewed and revised the paper. All authors have read and agreed to the published version of the manuscript.

Funding: This study was supported by the National Natural Science Foundation of China (NSFC), grant number 11421202.

Acknowledgments: We thank Changhao Jiang from Capital University of Physical Education and Sports and Huijuan Tian from Tianjin Polytechnic University for giving suggestions for the analysis. We thank all the participants in this study.

Conflicts of Interest: The authors have no conflict of interest concerning this manuscript.

References

1. Krøner, K.; Schmidt, S.A.; Nielsen, A.; Yde, J.; Jakobsen, B.W.; Møller-Madsen, B.; Jensen, J. Badminton injuries. *Br. J. Sports Med.* **1990**, *24*, 169–172. [CrossRef] [PubMed]
2. Fahlstrom, M.; Bjornstig, U.; Lorentzon, R. Acute badminton injuries. *Scand. J. Med. Sci. Sports* **1998**, *8*, 145–148. [CrossRef] [PubMed]
3. Yung, P.S.; Chan, R.H.; Wong, F.C.; Cheuk, P.W.; Fong, D.T. Epidemiology of injuries in Hongkong elite badminton athletes. *Res. Sports Med.* **2007**, *15*, 133–146. [CrossRef] [PubMed]
4. Badminton World Federation. Players Worldwide. In Badminton World Federation [Online]. Available online: http://smj.sma.org.sg/5011/5011a10.pdf (accessed on 25 June 2009).
5. Weir, M.A.; Watson, A.W. A twelve month study of sports injuries in one Irish school. *Irish J. Med. Sci.* **1996**, *165*, 165–169. [CrossRef] [PubMed]
6. Herbaut, A.; Delannoy, J.; Foissac, M. Injuries in French and Chinese regular badminton players. *Sci. Sport* **2018**, *33*, 145–151. [CrossRef]
7. Shariff, A.H.; George, J.; Ramlan, A.A. Musculoskeletal injuries among Malaysian badminton players. *Singap. Med. J.* **2009**, *50*, 1095–1097.
8. Goh, S.L.; Mokhtar, A.H.; Mohamad Ali, M.R. Badminton injuries in youth competitive players. *J. Sports Med. Phys. Fit.* **2013**, *53*, 65–70.
9. Hensley, L.D.; Paup, D.C. A survey of badminton injuries. *Brit. J. Sports Med.* **1979**, *13*, 156–160. [CrossRef]
10. Kuntze, G.; Mansfield, N.; Sellers, W. A biomechanical analysis of common lunge tasks in badminton. *J. Sports Sci.* **2010**, *28*, 183–191. [CrossRef]
11. Phomsoupha, M.; Laffaye, G. The science of badminton: Game characteristics, anthropometry, physiology, visual fitness and biomechanics. *Sports Med.* **2015**, *45*, 473–495. [CrossRef]
12. Muttalib, A.; Zaidi, M.; Khoo, C. A survey on common injuries in recreational badminton players. *Malays. Orthop. J.* **2009**, *3*, 8–11. [CrossRef]
13. Kondric, M.; Matković, B.R.; Furjan-Mandić, G.; Hadzić, V.; Dervisević, E. Injuries in racket sports among Slovenian players. *Coll Antropol.* **2011**, *35*, 413–417. [PubMed]
14. Jørgensen, U.J.; Winge, S.J. Injuries in Badminton. *Sports Med.* **1990**, *10*, 59–64. [CrossRef] [PubMed]
15. Pincivero, D.M.; Aldworth, C.; Dickerson, T.; Petry, C.; Shultz, T. Quadriceps-hamstring EMG activity during functional, closed kinetic chain exercise to fatigue. *Eur. J. Appl. Physiol.* **2000**, *81*, 504–509. [CrossRef] [PubMed]
16. Valldecabres, R.; De Benito, A.M.; Littler, G.; Richards, J. An exploration of the effect of proprioceptive knee bracing on biomechanics during a badminton lunge to the net, and the implications to injury mechanisms. *Peer J.* **2018**, *6*, e6033. [CrossRef]
17. Hong, Y.; Wang, S.J.; Lam, W.K.; Cheung, J.T.M. Kinetics of badminton lunges in four directions. *J. Appl. Biomech.* **2014**, *30*, 113–118. [CrossRef]
18. Mei, Q.; Gu, Y.; Fu, F.; Fernandez, J. A biomechanical investigation of right-forward lunging step among badminton players. *J. Sports Sci.* **2017**, *35*, 457–462. [CrossRef]
19. Fu, L.; Ren, F.; Baker, J.S. Comparison of joint loading in badminton lunging between professional and amateur badminton players. *Appl. Bionics Biomech.* **2017**, *2017*, 5397656. [CrossRef]

20. Lees, A.; Hurley, C. Forces in a badminton lunge movement. In *Science and Racket Sports*; Reilly, T., Hughes, M., Lees, A., Eds.; E & FN Spon: London, UK, 1994; pp. 249–256.
21. Lam, W.K.; Ding, R.; Qu, Y. Ground reaction forces and knee kinetics during single and repeated badminton lunges. *J. Sports Sci.* **2017**, *35*, 587–592. [CrossRef]
22. Pataky, T.C. Generalized n-dimensional biomechanical field analysis using statistical parametric mappin. *J. Biomech.* **2010**, *43*, 1976–1982. [CrossRef]
23. Barber-Westin, S.D.; Noyes, F.R. Effect of fatigue protocols on lower limb neuromuscular function and implications for anterior cruciate ligament injury prevention training: A systematic review. *Am. J. Sports Med.* **2017**, *45*, 3388–3396. [CrossRef] [PubMed]
24. Roth, R.; Donath, L.; Zahner, L.; Faude, O. Acute leg and trunk muscle fatigue differentially affect strength, sprint, agility, and balance in young adults. *J. Strength Cond. Res.* **2019**. [CrossRef] [PubMed]
25. Borg, G.A.V. Psychophysical bases of perceived exertion. *Med. Sci. Sports Exerc.* **1982**, *14*, 377–381. [CrossRef] [PubMed]
26. Cappozzo, A.; Catani, F.; Della Croce, U.; Leardini, A. Position and orientation in space of bones during movement: Anatomical frame definition and determination. *Clin. Biomech.* **1995**, *10*, 171–178. [CrossRef]
27. Herbaut, A.; Delannoy, J. Fatigue increases ankle sprain risk in badminton players: A biomechanical study. *J. Sports Sci.* **2020**, *38*, 1560–1565. [CrossRef]
28. Peers, K.H.; Lysens, R.J. Patellar tendinopathy in athletes: Current diagnostic and therapeutic recommendations. *Sports Med.* **2005**, *35*, 71–87. [CrossRef]

Publisher's Note: MDPI stays neutral with regard to jurisdictional claims in published maps and institutional affiliations.

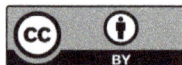

© 2020 by the authors. Licensee MDPI, Basel, Switzerland. This article is an open access article distributed under the terms and conditions of the Creative Commons Attribution (CC BY) license (http://creativecommons.org/licenses/by/4.0/).

Article

The Influence of Ski Waist-Width and Fatigue on Knee-Joint Stability and Skier's Balance

Martin Zorko [1,*], Karmen Hirsch [2], Nejc Šarabon [3,*] and Matej Supej [2,*]

1. Clinical Institute of Occupational, Traffic and Sports Medicine, University Medical Centre Ljubljana, 1000 Ljubljana, Slovenia
2. Faculty of Sport, University of Ljubljana, 1000 Ljubljana, Slovenia; laksmipria@gmail.com
3. Faculty of Health Sciences, University of Primorska, Polje 42, 6310 Izola, Slovenia
* Correspondence: zorkom@gmail.com (M.Z.); nejc.sarabon@fvz.upr.si (N.Š.); matej.supej@fsp.uni-lj.si (M.S.)

Received: 23 September 2020; Accepted: 30 October 2020; Published: 3 November 2020

Abstract: Alpine skiing is a complex sport that demands a high level of motor control and balance. In general, skiers are prone to deterioration in the state of fatigue due to using inappropriate equipment. As a consequence, the risk of injury might increase. This study aimed to examine the influence of fatigue and ski waist-width on knee-joint stability and skier's balance. A laboratory skiing simulation in a quasistatic ski-turning position was conducted where the lower-limb kinematics was recorded using an optical system, and the balance-determining parameters were captured using a force plate. It was demonstrated that the knee-joint kinematics and skier's balance were hampered in the state of fatigue, as well as when using skis with a large waist-width. The results of the study suggest avoiding the fatigue state and the use of skis having a large waist-width while skiing on hard surfaces to decrease the risk of injury.

Keywords: skiing simulation; optical motion capture; tensiometer; ski waist-width; balance; knee injury

1. Introduction

Competitive alpine skiing is a physically demanding sport that requires a combination of strength, strength endurance, postural balance, and coordination [1,2]. It comprises a sequence of high-intensity isometric and concentric-eccentric contractions [3]. Recreational skiing is also considered a very intense activity, especially when viewing a recreational skier in terms of their physical abilities. In alpine skiing, the ground reaction force and, thus, the body load is the greatest in the steering phase of the turn after passing the fall line [4,5]. That is when the eccentric work of the muscles also occurs [3]. In competitive skiing, fatigue reduces the skiing speed, increases the turning radius [3], and debilitates the ability to maintain balance, which can result in a loss of skiing control, fall, or injury [6,7]. Indeed, alpine skiing is a sport with a high risk of injury, having an overall injury rate of approximately 2–4 injuries per 1000 skier-days in recreational skiing [8–10] and ~10 per 1000 runs in World Cup competitive skiing [11].

Fatigue may occur in the muscle itself (local or peripheral fatigue) and on the level of the nervous system (central fatigue). Local fatigue is related to the impaired transmission of an action potential, an impaired association between muscle stimulation and contraction, and inhibition of the contractile process [6], while central fatigue is connected to reduced initiation or transmission of motoneuron electrical activity [12]. The development of peripheral fatigue is progressive and depends on the duration of the activity and its intensity. Peripheral muscle fatigue is considered short-lived when it largely ends within 1 min, with phosphocreatine and strength recovery, and it is long-term when the effects of fatigue remain for at least 30 min after activity [13].

Static equilibrium is defined as the ability to maintain the center of mass (CoM) above the support surface [14]. When the center of pressure (CoP) of the ground reaction force is outside the support surface, the body loses balance or an appropriate human action (e.g., a step) occurs in order to maintain or restore equilibrium [15]. In upright standing, the body uses two main strategies to compensate for challenged balance. In anterior–posterior disturbances, an ankle strategy occurs in which most compensatory movements are performed by the ankle and foot [16]. In disturbances that act in the medial–lateral direction, the body responds with a hip strategy, in which more complex movements occur, especially in the hip joint and torso [16,17]. The contribution of the hip increases with a reduced support surface and with larger and faster disturbances. In skiing, the strategy of the ankle is not expressed because the ankle joint is in a stiff ski-boot and, therefore, does not possess much freedom of movement. Thus, the skier uses predominantly knee and hip joint movements to maintain balance and to regulate the angle of the ski against the snow, from which the turning radius is determined (and, consequently, radial forces) in connection with carved turns [18].

Recently, skis have appeared on the market that are much wider than ordinary skis in the part under the ski boot (waist-width above 100 mm compared to 60 mm on classic skis). Such skis were originally designed for skiing off-piste. However, current skis with waist-widths between 80 and 90 mm are considered "allride skis" for on- and off-piste skiing, consequently often being used on hard or icy snow. In powder (off-piste) skiing, such skis have a wider support base and better flow on the snow. When wide skis are being used on icy/hard snow conditions, the outside and more loaded ski's point of application of the ground reaction force is farther away from the middle of the foot and shifted medially compared to when using narrower skis [19]. It was found that the knee-joint kinematics is consequently different on wider skis than on narrower ones, with knee rotation being more affected than knee abduction/adduction. In a study that simulated a quasi-static equilibrium position in a ski turn, it was found that the kinematic changes in the knee were such that the torque in the joint remained unchanged, regardless of the width of the ski [20]. The possible explanation for this was that, by keeping the external torques relatively low, there was also less muscle effort.

From studies analyzing human gait, it is known that, as the antigravity muscles get fatigued, the total speed of movement of the CoM, the amplitude of movement in the mediolateral and anteroposterior directions, and the total range of motion of the CoM increase [21,22]. The purpose of the current research was to investigate the functional stability of the knee joint and balance in a quasi-static simulation of a ski turn when using skis of different waist-widths in connection with fatigue, as the lower-limb muscle fatigue might be an injury risk factor in skiing [23]. In a broader context, the study examined hitherto unknown factors that could affect knee-joint injury, which was proven to be the most commonly injured joint in both recreational and competitive skiing [24,25].

The following hypotheses were set:

Hypotheses H1a. *Fatigue causes a statistically significant increase in external tibial rotation and knee abduction/valgus compared to prefatigue values.*

Hypotheses H1b. *The fatigue-induced change in the position of the knee joint (external rotation and abduction/valgus of the knee) is statistically significantly more pronounced in connection with wider skis compared to narrower ones.*

Hypotheses H2a. *Fatigue results in a statistically significant increase in the movement of the center of pressure on the ground (CoP) compared to prefatigue values.*

Hypotheses H2b. *The fatigue-induced increase in the movement of the CoP is statistically significantly more pronounced with wider skis compared to narrower ones and, consequently, the body balance and the knee-joint stability in the fatigue state are hampered more when using wide skis compared to narrow ones.*

2. Materials and Methods

Fifteen healthy male participants were included in the study (age 33.4 ± 8.6 years; height: 176.9 ± 7.9 cm; weight: 77.3 ± 13.2 kg). They were all physically fit and they were all skiers. None of them had any injury in the last year and no serious injury of any body part at any time in their life span. The study was approved by the responsible Ethics Committee at the University of Ljubljana (No. 1327/2017) and informed consent following the Declaration of Helsinki was obtained from all subjects.

2.1. Measurement System

For three-dimensional photogrammetry, 11 reflective optical markers were placed in accordance with a standardized protocol [26]: six on the outer lower limb, two on the ski boot, and three on the movable plate of the simulator (Figure 1). The reflective markers were recorded using an optical kinematic system (Optitrack V120: Trio, Natural Point, USA), consisting of three calibrated infrared cameras (sampling rate: 120 Hz). With the manufacturer's software (Motive, version 1.5.0.), we obtained real-time information on the position of body segments and standard Euler's angles in the knee joint in three anatomical planes [27].

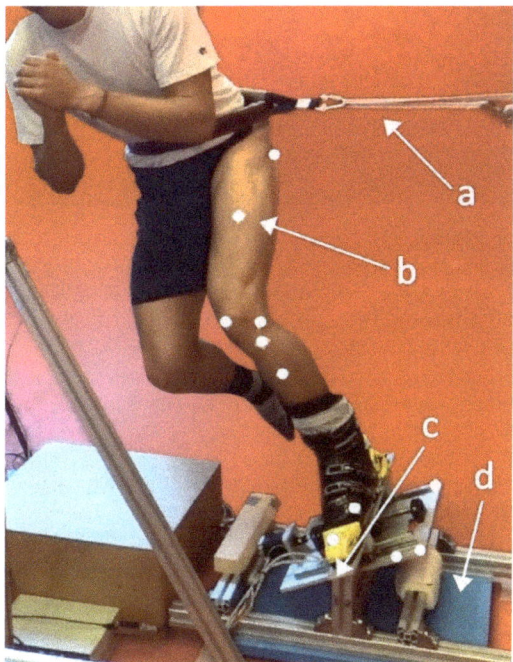

Figure 1. A ski turn simulator with a participant: (**a**) lateral supporting strap with pressure/tensile force gauge; (**b**) optical marker; (**c**) axis of rotation; (**d**) force plate.

The same ski simulator as in a previous study [20] consisted of a metal plate that was attached to the frame such that the plate could be tilted around the sagittal axis (Figure 1). With the help of three optical markers mounted on the simulator's plate, the ski-binding-boot (lower shell of the ski boot) coordinate system was determined. This coordinate system was used to calculate the Euler angles in the knee joint (flexion–abduction–rotation). The ski binding for fastening the ski boot moved freely in the plane of the plate transverse to the axis of rotation with the help of a stepper electric motor controlled by a computer. The ski waist-width was simulated by the displacement of the ski-binding-boot from the axis of rotation (imaginary ski-edge) as shown in Figure 2. The starting position, i.e., ski width = 0, was defined when the mid-sole of the ski-boot was aligned with the axis of rotation (nonrealistic ski width) and, thereafter, two realistic waist widths were simulated: narrow ski = 60 mm and wide ski = 120 mm.

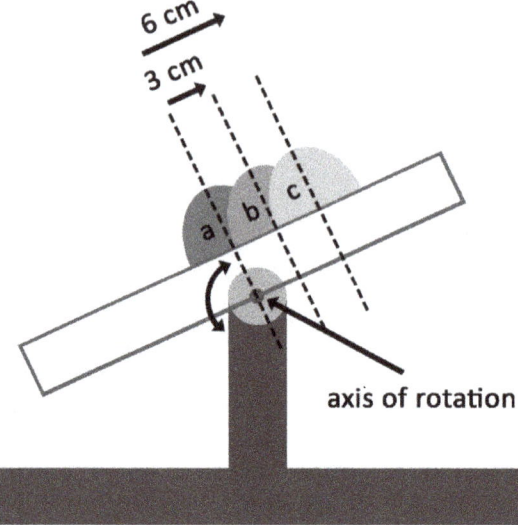

Figure 2. A frontal-plane schematic of the apparatus that enabled simulating different ski waist-widths. The elliptic shapes represent the left/outside ski-boot in the simulated right ski-turn. The axis of rotation (pointed by the arrow) represents the inner edge of the left (outside) ski. The simulated width of the ski is equal to the doubled distance between the axis of the rotation (ski edge) and the mid of the boot. The positions "b" and "c" simulated the 60 and 120 mm ski waist-widths, respectively. The position "a" is nonrealistic and was used only to collect reference values. The computer-guided electromotor (not shown on the schema) moved the platform with the ski-boot-binding system between the presented positions.

The participant was strapped to the side via a pressure/tensile force gauge (HBM model: S9M/2 kN, Hottinger Baldwin Messtechnik GmbH, Darmstadt, Germany). The force gauge was connected to an analog-to-digital converter (DEWE 43, Dewesoft d.o.o., Trbovlje, Slovenia). With the help of the Dewesoft X program and the appropriate length of the rope, it was initially ensured that the radial force always represented approximately the same proportion of the force of gravity and, thus, the angle of inclination of the entire body was quasi-statically determined.

Data on the magnitude and direction of the ground reaction force were captured using the Kistler 5691 force plate (Kistler, Winterthur, Switzerland) on which the ski simulator was placed and the accompanying Kistler MARS software (Kistler, Winterthur, Switzerland).

2.2. Measurement Protocol

The subject was bonded to a robotic ski simulator with his left ski-boot, while the other ski-boot was lifted from the ground throughout the measurement (simulation as if all the weight is on one leg during the turn). The computer-controlled system randomly changed the position of the ground reaction force four times every 10 s, simulating three ski waist-widths: 0 mm (used as a reference value), 60 mm ("narrow ski"), and 120 mm ("wide ski"). The subject had to maintain 60° of flexion in the knee joint and 25° inclination of the plate for 10 s after each ski-width change on the simulator. These predefined values of knee flexion and ski inclination were set to avoid other influences on knee kinematics and to focus only on ski width, as well as to enable a skiing-like body position and ground reaction forces [20]. Both knee flexion and ski inclination conditions were monitored in real time using on-screen visual feedback. Sets lasting 40 s were repeated three times with a 2 min resting interval. This was followed by a fatigue protocol, during which the subject performed three series of one-legged squats in a ski-boot to a knee flexion angle of 70°. The knee angle during squats was monitored on the screen in real time by the participant. The participants were loudly encouraged to perform the squats until failure, i.e., until no additional squat could be performed, which enabled us to meet one of the most common definitions of muscle fatigue: "the exercise-induced decrease in the ability to produce force" [28]. During each series of squats, the subject had 30 s of rest. The fatigue phase was followed by three additional 40 s random "waist-width" load sequences on the simulator: the first immediately after fatigue, the second 2 min after fatigue, and the third 4 min after fatigue.

2.3. Data Processing

For each 10 s measurement on the simulator under different simulated waist-widths, data from the last 5 s before the new waist-width position occurred were used. Thus, the subject had sufficient time for each simulated waist-width to occupy a quasi-static balanced position.

From the kinematics system, flexion, abduction, and rotation in the knee joint [27] were obtained. The force transducer enabled monitoring the magnitude of the radial force in the simulated turn. From the force plate, the following data were obtained:

1. CoP velocity, defined as the common length of the trajectory of the CoP sway calculated as a sum of the point-to-point Euclidian distance divided by the measurement time (total velocity; V_{tot}), or the total length of the trajectory of the CoP sway only in the anteroposterior (V_{AP}) or mediolateral (V_{ML}) direction, divided by the measurement time.
2. CoP amplitude, defined as the average amount of the CoP sway in anteroposterior (A_{AP}) and mediolateral (A_{ML}) direction, calculated as the total length of the trajectory of the CoP sway only in the given direction divided by the number of changes.
3. CoP area (AR), defined as the area swayed by the CoP trajectory with respect to the central stance point (i.e., a product of mean anteroposterior and mediolateral values).

The mean frequency (MF) of the power spectrum of CoP in both directions (anteroposterior: MF_{AP}, mediolateral: MF_{ML}), defined as the frequency of the oscillations of the CoP calculated as the mean frequency of the power spectrum in a given direction. The peak frequency (PF) of the power spectrum of motion CoP in both directions (anteroposterior: PF_{AP}, mediolateral: PF_{ML}), calculated as the peak frequency of the power spectrum in a given direction.

Frequency was calculated as CoP changes in a direction (i.e., signal local extremes or peaks) divided by the measurement time (FP) for both directions (anteroposterior: FP_{AP}, mediolateral: FP_{ML}).

First, the baseline value of the parameters was determined by calculating the average of the first three measurements for all CoP parameters at a reference waist-width of 0 mm. In the next step, these CoP prefatigue reference values were compared with the values obtained immediately after fatigue, 2 min after fatigue, and 4 min after fatigue on simulated skis of different widths.

2.4. Statistical Analysis

SPSS.20 (IBM Corporation, New York, NY, USA) and MS Excel 2013 were used for statistical analysis. Data were presented as mean and standard deviation.

The normality of the distribution was first tested using Kolmogorov–Smirnov test and then the homogeneity of variances was tested using the Leven test. Analysis of variance for repeated measurements was used to test the differences between the dependent variables. In the post hoc analysis, the difference between individual pairs was tested with paired-sample *t*-tests.

A two-way analysis of variance for repeated measurements (measurement time (4) × ski waist-width (3)) was used to determine whether there were statistically significant differences in parameters at the measurement time factor (before fatigue, immediately after fatigue, 2 min after fatigue, and 4 min after fatigue), with the ski waist-width factor (neutral, narrow, and wide) and with the interaction of both factors (measurement time × ski waist-width). To separately determine whether the groups differ from each other, in terms of ski waist-width (narrow vs. wide ski) and in terms of measurement time, a one-way analysis of variance was performed. Effect sizes were calculated as η2 for variance analysis, as well as for pairwise comparisons using the Cohen's d measure [29]. The level of statistical significance was determined at $p < 0.05$.

3. Results

The knee flexion angle was predetermined and monitored in real time for all measurements on the ski simulator, and the results revealed that there were no statistically significant differences in knee flexion parameters. There were also no statistically significant differences in knee rotation parameters, whether with the ski waist-width parameter or with time before or after fatigue (Figure 3).

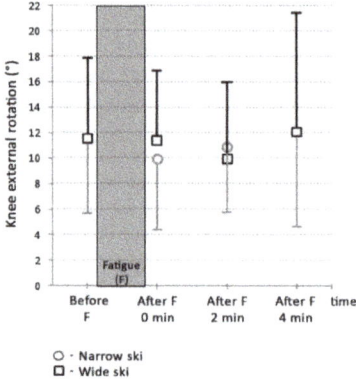

Figure 3. External tibial rotation in a prefatigued state (before F) and at different times after fatigue (after F) with two different ski waist-widths.

The knee abduction was significantly larger in connection with the wide skis (Figure 4) compared to the narrow ones ($t = -5.1$; $p < 0.01$; $d = 0.46$).

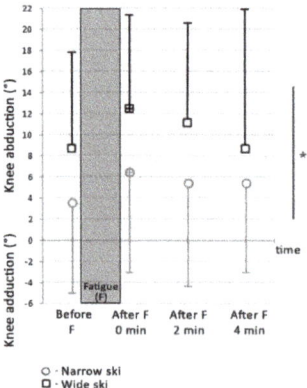

Figure 4. Knee abduction/adduction in a prefatigued state (before F) and at different times after fatigue (after F) with two different ski waist-widths. + depicts statistically significant difference compared to prefatigued state ($p < 0.05$); * depicts statistically significant difference between all-narrow against all-wide waist-width measurements.

After fatigue, there was significant increase in knee abduction with narrow skis ($t = -2.16$; $p = 0.05$; $d = 0.31$), as well as with the wide ones ($t = -2.39$; $p < 0.05$; $d = 0.41$).

Significant differences were observed in V_{AP} with wide skis compared to narrow ones (F = 3.78; $p < 0.05$; $\eta^2 = 0.27$) (Figure 5).

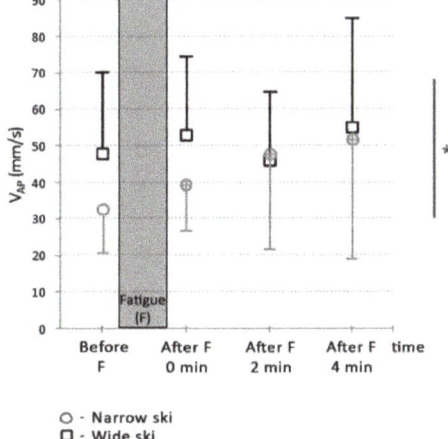

Figure 5. Center of pressure (CoP) velocity in anteroposterior direction (V_{AP}) in a prefatigued state (before F) and at different times after fatigue (after F) with two different ski waist-widths. + depicts statistically significant difference compared to prefatigued state ($p < 0.05$); * depicts statistically significant difference between all-narrow against all-wide waist-width measurements.

The V_{AP} value for wide skis was significantly higher compared to that for narrow ones ($t = -3.44$; $p < 0.01$; $d = 0.52$). With narrow skis, all three after fatigue V_{AP} values were significantly higher compared to the prefatigue value with the immediate after fatigue value being the highest ($t = -2.70$; $p < 0.05$; $d = 0.42$).

There were significantly higher V_{ML} values with wide skis (F = 19.94; $p < 0.01$; $\eta^2 = 0.67$) compared to narrow ones ($t = -4.87$; $p < 0.01$; $d = 0.70$) (Figure 6).

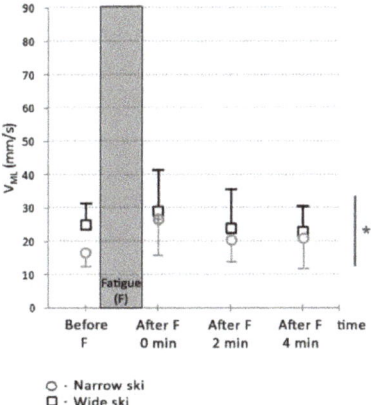

Figure 6. CoP velocity in mediolateral direction (V_{ML}) in a prefatigued state (before F) and at different times after fatigue (after F) with two different ski waist-widths. + depicts statistically significant difference compared to prefatigued state ($p < 0.05$); * depicts statistically significant difference between all-narrow against all-wide waist-width measurements.

The effect of time was statistically significant for narrow skis only (F = 4.42; $p < 0.01$; $\eta^2 = 0.29$). Specifically, there was an increment in V_{ML} immediately after fatigue compared to the prefatigue state with narrow skis ($t = -3.73$; $p < 0.01$; $d = 0.56$).

The results demonstrated significant differences in A_{ap} values between different ski widths (F = 4.89; $p < 0.05$; $\eta^2 = 0.31$) (Figure 7).

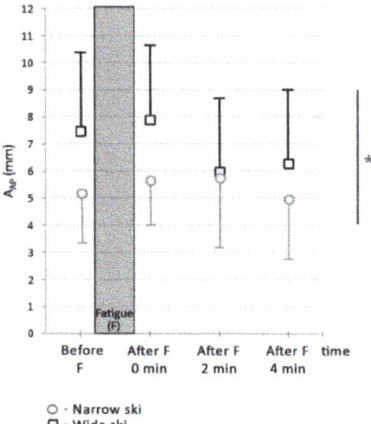

Figure 7. CoP amplitude in anteroposterior direction (A_{AP}) in a prefatigued state (before F) and at different times after fatigue (after F) with two different ski waist-widths. * depicts statistically significant difference between all-narrow against all-wide waist-width measurements.

The A_{AP} values were significantly higher with wide skis compared to narrow ones ($t = 2.23$; $p < 0.05$; $d = 0.31$). The differences between pre and after fatigue times were significant with wide skis only (F = 4.28; $p < 0.05$; $\eta^2 = 0.28$). There was a decrement in A_{AP} value 2 min after fatigue compared to the state immediately after fatigue ($t = 2.92$; $p < 0.05$; $d = 0.38$).

There were significant differences in A_{ML} values between different ski widths (F = 20.36; $p < 0.01$; $\eta^2 = 0.63$). The A_{ML} values were significantly higher with wide skis compared to narrow ones ($t = -5.18$; $p < 0.01$; $d = 0.69$) (Figure 8).

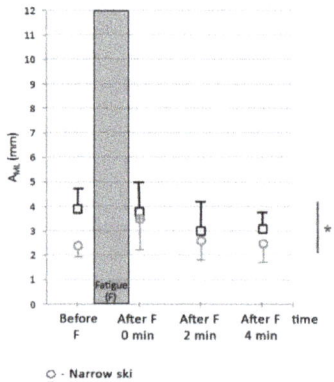

Figure 8. CoP amplitude in mediolateral direction (A_{ML}) in a prefatigued state (before F) and at different times after fatigue (after F) with two different ski waist-widths. + depicts statistically significant difference compared to prefatigued state ($p < 0.05$); * depicts statistically significant difference between all-narrow against all-wide waist-width measurements.

The effect of time of measurement was statistically significant for narrow skis only (F = 5.00; $p < 0.01$; $\eta^2 = 0.31$) and A_{ML} was significantly higher only immediately after fatigue ($t = -3.44$; $p < 0.01$; $d = 0.52$).

Significant differences were observed in MF_{AP} with different ski widths (F = 5.93; $p < 0.01$; $\eta^2 = 0.37$). The MF_{AP} value was significantly lower with wide skis compared to the narrow ones ($t = 2.86$; $p < 0.05$; $d = 0.43$) (Figure 9).

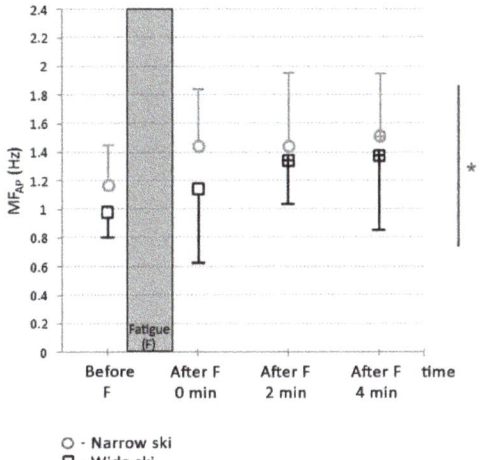

Figure 9. The mean frequency of the power spectrum of CoP in the anteroposterior direction (MF_{AP}) in a prefatigued state (before F) and at different times after fatiguing (after F) with two different ski waist-widths. + depicts statistically significant difference compared to prefatigued state ($p < 0.05$); * depicts statistically significant difference between all-narrow against all-wide waist-width measurements.

The differences between different times of measurement were significant with wide skis only (F = 3.38; $p < 0.05$; $\eta^2 = 0.30$) and MF_{AP} was significantly higher 2 min after fatiguing compared to the prefatigue value ($t = -4.17$; $p < 0.01$; $d = 0.66$), as well as 4 min after fatigue compared to the prefatigue value ($t = -3.32$; $p < 0.01$; $d = 0.50$). With narrow skis, there was a significant increment in MF_{AP} value only at 4 min after fatigue compared to the prefatigue value ($t = -3.5$; $p < 0.01$; $d = 0.53$).

There were significant differences in MF_{ML} values with time of measurement (F = 3.96; $p < 0.05$; $\eta^2 = 0.36$), as well as with different ski widths (F = 3.70; $p < 0.05$; $\eta^2 = 0.35$) (Figure 10).

MF_{ML} was significantly lower with wide skis compared to narrow ones ($t = 2.33$; $p < 0.05$; $d = 0.31$). With narrow skis, there was a significant increment in MF_{ML} values 4 min after fatigue compared to the prefatigue state ($t = -3.85$; $p < 0.01$; $d = 0.55$), as well as 4 min after fatigue compared to immediately after fatigue ($t = -2.73$; $p < 0.05$; $d = 0.40$). With wide skis, there was significant difference in MF_{ML} value only 4 min after fatigue compared to values 2 min after fatigue ($t = -2.33$; $p < 0.05$; $d = 0.31$).

With AR values, there were significant differences with different times of measurement (F = 5.36; $p < 0.01$; $\eta^2 = 0.52$), as well as with different ski widths (F = 4.33; $p < 0.05$; $\eta^2 = 0.46$). There were significantly higher AR values with wide skis compared to narrow ones ($t = -3.67$; $p < 0.01$; $d = 0.53$). With respect to different measurement times, there were significant differences in AR value with narrow skis only (F = 5.58; $p < 0.01$; $\eta^2 = 0.34$) with all the after fatigue values being significantly higher compared to the prefatigue state.

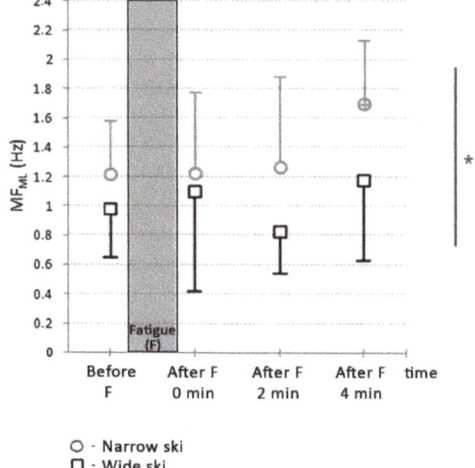

Figure 10. The mean frequency of the power spectrum of CoP in the mediolateral direction (MF_{ML}) in a prefatigued state (before F) and at different times after fatigue (after F) with two different ski waist-widths. + depicts statistically significant difference compared to prefatigued state ($p < 0.05$); * depicts statistically significant difference between all-narrow against all-wide waist-width measurements.

4. Discussion

The main findings of the study were, firstly, that knee joint stability (kinematics) was affected by the waist-width of the ski, as well as by the level of fatigue. Secondly, hypotheses H1a and H1b were only partly confirmed as only knee abduction increased with the ski waist-width and with the level of fatigue but not the knee rotation. Concerning the comparison of the functional stability in the simulated skiing position using different ski waist-widths, it was demonstrated that the fatigue caused a significant deterioration in knee stability with wide skis compared to narrow ones. Thirdly, fatigue resulted in an increase in CoP movement compared to prefatigue values, confirming hypothesis H2a. The fatigue effect on balance deterioration was significantly more influential with narrow skis compared to wide ones. Thus, hypothesis H2b was not confirmed. With most CoP parameters, it was shown that the effect of fatigue on balance was in accordance with previous studies [21,22,30].

Previous on-snow [19] and laboratory [20] studies demonstrated that knee rotation was the primary adaptation mechanism to avoid an increase in knee-joint torque when using wide skis. The knee abduction was independent of the ski waist-width [20]. In the present investigation, where the muscular fatigue effect was studied, knee abduction increased in the fatigue state with both ski widths, while rotation remained unchanged or there was even a trend of diminishing external rotation. One possible explanation is that, in a state of fatigue, abduction took on the role of minimizing torque in the knee joint instead of external rotation in combination with flexion, as found in a previous study. However, the knee-joint abduction that presently occurred imposes an additional strain on the medial collateral ligament [31]. The stiffness of this ligament is increased by lower-limb muscle activation [32], which is considered as an additional mediolateral knee stabilizer. This additional active stabilization mechanism could be hampered in the state of muscle fatigue. Thus, the knee abducted/valgus position becomes more pronounced and nearer to the ligamentous limitation of the end range of the knee valgus position, which might represent the risk of acute medial collateral injury in the case of additional sudden external valgus thrust [31], which may occur during skiing.

It is known from other biomechanical studies that knee-joint malalignment predisposes the knee joint to degenerative changes [33] via the local overload of joint surfaces. In our study, it was shown that, in the state of fatigue, and even more so in connection with wide skis, the knee is forced to the pronounced valgus position in the simulated ski turn. It can be assumed that, in such cases, the lateral knee compartment might be notably more loaded or, in the worst case, even overloaded. Nevertheless, knowing that ground reaction forces in recreational skiing are as high as two body weights [34] and in competitive skiing as high as 4.2 body weights [4,5], in combination with vibrations [35–37], this may increase the risk of chronic joint conditions. This especially applies to competitive and advanced recreational skiers/ski instructors because of their high number of ski runs/turns per season.

With most CoP movement parameters, the fatigue effect was most significantly expressed immediately after the fatigue procedure, in accordance with a previous study conducted on an isokinetic dynamometer [12]. Some of the parameters (V_{AP}, MF_{AP}, MF_{ML} with narrow ski, and MF_{AP} with wide ski) did not return to baseline even at the time of the last measurement (4 min after fatigue). Therefore, typical short breaks along the descent appear not to be sufficient to level out fatigue effects. These results in terms of skiing safety put into question long chair lifts or gondolas when skiers are not taking long enough breaks during their descents. In other studies that investigated the fatigue effect on the deterioration of muscle force production [12,38] and CoP movement [30], most of the force-producing functions and the balance returned to normal after 6 to 10 min. Such longer resting periods typically only occur in alpine skiing between runs, waiting for lifts, and travelling (back) up the mountain/slope. Nevertheless, previous studies reported that the body sway increased proportionally to the developing fatigue when the subjects ran on a treadmill [39]. In contrast, Bryanton and Bilodeau [40] observed that CoP movement started to increase with but plateaued or possibly even decreased during their fatigue protocol, consisting of a sit–stand exercise. It remains unknown how repeated bouts of high-intensity skiing throughout the training session/skiing day affect postural control. For future research, the effect of additional repetitive fatiguing should be examined to elucidate what is expected to happen with postural stability on a typical skiing day consisting of several consecutive runs.

The main limitation of this study was probably that it simulated skiing and was not conducted during on-snow skiing. On the other hand, in this way, the experiment was significantly more controlled. Moreover, forceful fatigue, applied in this study, would most likely pose a high risk of injury during experiments if it were to be performed in real skiing. Undoubtedly, such measurements should be performed in situations to minimize the risk of injury, and this was provided by the fatigue and skiing simulation in the laboratory. Future research incorporating less forceful (to decrease the risk of injury during the experiment) but repetitive fatigue followed by a resting period would further elucidate the effects of real skiing fatigue on balance and knee-joint stability.

5. Conclusions

The present study showed that the knee joint adapted to the fatigue state with an increase in knee abduction/valgus, with the effect being stronger with wide skis. Furthermore, the balance also deteriorated with fatigue using either ski width. The balance-hampering effect was more pronounced with the narrow skis. However, the stability parameters that were shown to be worse even before fatigue in connection with the wide skis compared to the narrow ones further deteriorated in the fatigue state and remained worse compared to the narrow skis throughout all after fatigue experiments. The study elucidates the fact that fatigue is an injury risk factor in skiing [6,7] from an additional point of view and exposes the further risk of using skis with a large waist-width, especially on hard frozen surfaces, as simulated in the study. Considering fatigue and ski waist-width related to balance deterioration, it is obvious that the injury risk for the whole body and not only the knee joint can be compromised. More specifically, the possible mechanisms of acute and chronic knee-joint injury were suggested. The medial collateral ligament tension and the uneven joint pressure distribution while turning in the fatigue state are potential biomechanical injury risk factors. Consequently, apart from using skis with a narrower waist-width, it might also be suggested to regularly interrupt "long" skiing runs/descents with long enough breaks to decrease the risk of injury.

Author Contributions: Conceptualization, M.S. and N.Š.; methodology, K.H.; formal analysis, K.H.; resources, M.S. and N.Š.; data curation, K.H. and M.Z.; writing—original draft preparation, M.Z. and K.H.; writing—review and editing, M.S., N.Š., and M.Z; visualization, M.Z. and M.S.; supervision, M.S. and N.Š.; project administration, N.Š. and M.S.; funding acquisition, N.Š. and M.S. All authors have read and agreed to the published version of the manuscript.

Funding: This research was funded by the Slovenian Research Agency (L5-1845, L54142, and P5-0147).

Acknowledgments: The authors would like to sincerely thank all participants for their involvement, as well as Bojan Nemec, Zlatko Matjačič, and Andrej Olenšek for development of the skiing simulator.

Conflicts of Interest: The authors declare no conflict of interest.

References

1. Raschner, C.; Hildebrandt, C.; Mohr, J.; Müller, L. Sex Differences in Balance among Alpine Ski Racers: Cross-Sectional Age Comparisons. *Percept. Motor Skills* **2017**, *124*, 1134–1150. [CrossRef]
2. Gilgien, M.; Reid, R.; Raschner, C.; Supej, M.; Holmberg, H.-C. The Training of Olympic Alpine Ski Racers. *Front. Physiol.* **2018**, *9*, 1772. [CrossRef] [PubMed]
3. Klimek, A. Physiological Background of Muscular Pain during Skiing and Delayed Muscle Soreness after Skiing. *J. Hum. Kinet.* **2010**, *23*, 55–61. [CrossRef]
4. Supej, M.; Kugovnik, O.; Nemec, B. Modelling and simulation of two competition slalom techniques. *Kinesiol. Int. J. Fundam. Appl. Kinesiol.* **2004**, *36*, 206–212.
5. Supej, M.; Holmberg, H.C. How gate setup and turn radii influence energy dissipation in slalom ski racing. *J. Appl. Biomech.* **2010**, *26*, 454–464. [CrossRef] [PubMed]
6. Ferguson, R. Limitations to performance during alpine skiing. *Exp. Physiol.* **2009**, *95*, 404–410. [CrossRef] [PubMed]
7. Spörri, J.; Kröll, J.; Schwameder, H.; Müller, E. Turn Characteristics of a Top World Class Athlete in Giant Slalom: A Case Study Assessing Current Performance Prediction Concepts. *Int. J. Sports Sci. Coach.* **2012**, *7*, 647–659. [CrossRef]
8. Bergstrøm, K.A.; Ekeland, A. Effect of trail design and grooming on the incidence of injuries at alpine ski areas. *Br. J. Sports Med.* **2004**, *38*, 264–268. [CrossRef] [PubMed]
9. Langran, M.; Sivasubramaniam, S. Snow sports injuries in Scotland. *Br. J. Sports Med.* **2002**, *36*, 135–140. [CrossRef] [PubMed]
10. Warda, L.J.; Yanchar, N.L. Skiing and snowboarding injury prevention. *Paediatr. Child Health* **2012**, *17*, 35–38. [CrossRef]
11. Flørenes, T.W.; Bere, T.; Nordsletten, L.; Heir, S.; Bahr, R. Injuries among male and female World Cup alpine skiers. *Br. J. Sports Med.* **2009**, *43*, 973–978. [CrossRef] [PubMed]
12. Froyd, C.; Millet, G.Y.; Noakes, T.D. The development of peripheral fatigue and short-term recovery during self-paced high-intensity exercise. *J. Physiol.* **2013**, *591*, 1339–1346. [CrossRef] [PubMed]
13. Smith, I.C.; Newham, D.J. Fatigue and functional performance of human biceps muscle following concentric or eccentric contractions. *J. Appl. Physiol.* **2007**, *102*, 207–213. [CrossRef]
14. Sarabon, N.; Kern, H.; Löfler, S.; Rosker, J. Selection of body sway parameters according to their sensitivity and repeatability. *Eur. J. Transl. Myol.* **2010**, *20*, 5–12. [CrossRef]
15. Kinzey, S.J.; Armstrong, C.W. The reliability of the star-excursion test in assessing dynamic balance. *J. Orthop. Sports Phys. Ther.* **1998**, *27*, 356–360. [CrossRef] [PubMed]
16. Winter, D.A. Human balance and posture control during standing and walking. *Gait Posture* **1995**, *3*, 193–214. [CrossRef]
17. Horak, F.B.; Nashner, L.M.; Diener, H.C. Postural strategies associated with somatosensory and vestibular loss. *Exp. Brain Res.* **1990**, *82*, 167–177. [CrossRef]
18. Howe, J. *The New Skiing Mechanics: Including the Technology of Short Radius Carved Turn Skiing and the Claw® Ski*; Waterford: McIntire, VA, USA, 2001.
19. Zorko, M.; Nemec, B.; Babi, J.; Lfanik, B.; Supej, M. The Waist Width of Skis Influences the Kinematics of the Knee Joint in Alpine Skiing. *J. Sports Sci. Med.* **2015**, *14*, 606–619.
20. Zorko, M.; Nemec, B.; Matjačić, Z.; Olenšek, A.; Tomazin, K.; Supej, M. Wide Skis as a Potential Knee Injury Risk Factor in Alpine Skiing. *Front. Sports Act. Living* **2020**, *2*, 1–9. [CrossRef]

21. Thedon, T.; Mandrick, K.; Foissac, M.; Mottet, D.; Perrey, S. Degraded postural performance after muscle fatigue can be compensated by skin stimulation. *Gait Posture* **2011**, *33*, 686–689. [CrossRef]
22. Simoneau, M.; Bégin, F.; Teasdale, N. The effects of moderate fatigue on dynamic balance control and attentional demands. *J. Neuroeng. Rehabil.* **2006**, *3*, 22. [CrossRef]
23. Koller, A.; Fuchs, B.; Leichtfried, V.; Schobersberger, W. Decrease in eccentric quadriceps and hamstring strength in recreational alpine skiers after prolonged skiing. *BMJ Open Sport Exerc. Med.* **2015**, *1*. [CrossRef]
24. Brucker, P.U.; Katzmaier, P.; Olvermann, M.; Huber, A.; Waibel, K.; Imhoff, A.B.; Spitzenpfeil, P. [Recreational and competitive alpine skiing. Typical injury patterns and possibilities for prevention]. *Der Unf.* **2014**, *117*, 24–32. [CrossRef]
25. Haaland, B.; Steenstrup, S.E.; Bere, T.; Bahr, R.; Nordsletten, L. Injury rate and injury patterns in FIS World Cup Alpine skiing (2006–2015): Have the new ski regulations made an impact? *Br. J. Sports Med.* **2016**, *50*, 32–36. [CrossRef] [PubMed]
26. Breen, D.; Zordan, V.; Horst, N. Mapping Optical Motion Capture Data to Skeletal Motion Using a Physical Model. In Proceedings of the 2003 ACM SIGGRAPH/Eurographics Symposium on Computer Animation, San Diego, CA, USA, 26–27 July 2003.
27. Grood, E.S.; Suntay, W.J. A joint coordinate system for the clinical description of three-dimensional motions: Application to the knee. *J. Biomech. Eng.* **1983**, *105*, 136–144. [CrossRef] [PubMed]
28. Wan, J.J.; Qin, Z.; Wang, P.Y.; Sun, Y.; Liu, X. Muscle fatigue: General understanding and treatment. *Exp. Mol. Med.* **2017**, *49*, e384. [CrossRef]
29. Fritz, C.O.; Morris, P.E.; Richler, J.J. Effect size estimates: Current use, calculations, and interpretation. *J. Exp. Psychol. Gen.* **2012**, *141*, 2–18. [CrossRef]
30. Harkins, K.; Mattacola, C.; Uhl, T.; Malone, T. Effects of 2 Ankle Fatigue Models on the Duration of Postural Stability Dysfunction. *J. Athl. Train.* **2005**, *40*, 191–194. [PubMed]
31. Heitmann, M.; Preiss, A.; Giannakos, A.; Frosch, K.-H. [Acute medial collateral ligament injuries of the knee: Diagnostics and therapy.]. *Der Unf.* **2013**, *116*, 497–503.
32. Juneja, P.; Hubbard, J.B. Anatomy, Bony Pelvis and Lower Limb, Knee Medial Collateral Ligament. In *StatPearls*; StatPearls Publishing LLC.: Treasure Island, FL, USA, 2020.
33. Sharma, L.; Song, J.; Felson, D.T.; Cahue, S.; Shamiyeh, E.; Dunlop, D.D. The role of knee alignment in disease progression and functional decline in knee osteoarthritis. *JAMA* **2001**, *286*, 188–195. [CrossRef]
34. Nakazato, K.; Scheiber, P.; Müller, E. A Comparison of Ground Reaction Forces Determined by Portable Force-Plate and Pressure-Insole Systems in Alpine Skiing. *J. Sports Sci. Med.* **2011**, *10*, 754–762.
35. Supej, M.; Ogrin, J.; Holmberg, H.C. Whole-Body Vibrations Associated with Alpine Skiing: A Risk Factor for Low Back Pain? *Front. Physiol.* **2018**, *9*, 204. [CrossRef]
36. Supej, M.; Ogrin, J. Transmissibility of whole-body vibrations and injury risk in alpine skiing. *J. Sci. Med. Sport* **2019**, *22* (Suppl. 1), S71–S77. [CrossRef]
37. Spörri, J.; Kröll, J.; Fasel, B.; Aminian, K.; Müller, E. The Use of Body Worn Sensors for Detecting the Vibrations Acting on the Lower Back in Alpine Ski Racing. *Front. Physiol.* **2017**, *8*, 522. [CrossRef] [PubMed]
38. Cortes, N.; Quammen, D.; Lucci, S.; Greska, E.; Onate, J. A functional agility short-term fatigue protocol changes lower extremity mechanics. *J. Sports Sci.* **2012**, *30*, 797–805. [CrossRef] [PubMed]
39. Beurskens, R.; Haeger, M.; Kliegl, R.; Roecker, K.; Granacher, U. Postural Control in Dual-Task Situations: Does Whole-Body Fatigue Matter? *PLoS ONE* **2016**, *11*, e0147392. [CrossRef]
40. Bryanton, M.A.; Bilodeau, M. Postural stability with exhaustive repetitive sit-to-stand exercise in young adults. *Hum. Mov. Sci.* **2016**, *49*, 47–53. [CrossRef] [PubMed]

Publisher's Note: MDPI stays neutral with regard to jurisdictional claims in published maps and institutional affiliations.

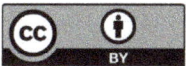

© 2020 by the authors. Licensee MDPI, Basel, Switzerland. This article is an open access article distributed under the terms and conditions of the Creative Commons Attribution (CC BY) license (http://creativecommons.org/licenses/by/4.0/).

 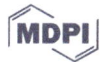

Article

Change of Direction Performance Is Influenced by Asymmetries in Jumping Ability and Hip and Trunk Strength in Elite Basketball Players

Filip Ujaković [1,2] and Nejc Šarabon [3,4,*]

1. Faculty of Kinesiology, University of Zagreb, 10110 Zagreb, Croatia; fujakovic@gmail.com
2. Basketball Club Cedevita Olimpija Ljubljana, 1000 Ljubljana, Slovenia
3. Faculty of Health Sciences, University of Primorska, 6310 Izola, Slovenia
4. S2P, Science to Practice, Ltd., Laboratory for Motor Control and Motor Behavior, 1000 Ljubljana, Slovenia
* Correspondence: nejc.sarabon@fvz.upr.si

Received: 8 September 2020; Accepted: 3 October 2020; Published: 6 October 2020

Abstract: Change of direction (COD) ability is essential for sport performance in high level team sports such as basketball, however, the influence of asymmetries on COD ability is relatively unknown. Forty-three junior and senior level elite basketball players performed isometric hip and trunk strength testing, passive hip and trunk range of motion testing, and unilateral horizontal and vertical jumps, as well as the T-test to measure COD performance. Mean asymmetry values ranged from 0.76% for functional leg length up to 40.35% for rate of torque development during hip flexion. A six-variable regression model explained 48% ($R^2 = 0.48$; $p < 0.001$) of variation in COD performance. The model included left hip internal/external rotation strength ratio, and inter-limb asymmetries in hip abduction rate of torque development, hip flexion range of motion, functional leg length, single leg triple jump distance, and peak torque during trunk lateral flexion. Results suggest that the magnitude of asymmetries is dependent of task and parameter, and using universal asymmetry thresholds, such as <10 %, is not optimal. The regression model showed the relationship between asymmetries and COD performance. None of tests were sufficient to explain a complex variable like COD performance.

Keywords: asymmetry; agility; basketball; strength; power; inter-limb asymmetry

1. Introduction

Inter-limb asymmetry has been mostly researched from the aspect of sports injury risk, especially in view of athletes returning to sport after anterior cruciate ligament reconstruction [1–4]. Only recently, the relationship between inter-limb asymmetry and sports performance has been a popular topic of investigation [5,6]. Inter-limb asymmetry is found to be a normal adaptation in many sports that involve unilateral movements (e.g., cricket) [7], but further research in team sports is needed to elucidate whether asymmetries influence performance or injury risk [5,6]. Lately researchers are trying to elucidate whether asymmetries (and which particular type of asymmetry) influence performance [8]. Inter-limb asymmetry may present at the level of different motor abilities (e.g., strength, power, and range of motion) and can be measured locally (e.g., one joint) and globally (e.g., within a complex movement, such as vertical jump). Therefore, various methods have been used for its quantification [9], however, many studies used local knee isokinetic dynamometry [10,11], isometric mid-thigh pull (IMTP) [12,13] or vertical jump tests [14–18]. Further, Sheppard and Young´s [19] model of change of direction (COD) determinants showed that asymmetries could negatively affect COD performance. However, supporting evidence is inconsistent.

Two studies investigated the relationship between local inter-limb knee strength asymmetry and performance in COD. Lockie et al. [10] showed mostly positive correlation between different parameters and speed of isokinetic strength asymmetries during knee flexion and extension and T-test performance ($r = 0.638, 0.669, p < 0.01$). Exception was one negative correlation ($r = −568, p < 0.01$) between peak torque during knee extension (240°/s) and T-test performance. Similarly, Coratella et al. [11] observed that the same local asymmetries negatively impact COD performance (T-test and 180° turn test) ($r = 0.397–0.614, p < 0.05$). As the mentioned studies measured local strength asymmetries in the knee joint, they demonstrate the need to study proximal body parts like hip and trunk.

When it comes to the relationship between global asymmetries and performance in COD, results are less consistent. Many studies, using different tests for assessing asymmetries and COD performance, did not detect a relationship between global asymmetries and COD performance. Chiang [12] investigated the relationship between peak torque asymmetry during IMTP and COD ability (assessed as 180° turn test) and reported no significant correlation. However, he used bilateral IMTP to quantify asymmetry, which may have influenced methodological validity. While this methodological shortcoming was corrected by Dos Santos et al. [13], who used unilateral IMTP test, they have not found any significant correlation between inter-limb asymmetry in various parameters related to unilateral IMTP and COD performance ($r ≤ 0.35, p ≥ 0.380$). Hoffman et al. [14] have not found any significant correlation between asymmetry in single-leg countermovement jump (SLCMJ) height and COD ability (three-cone drill). Although reporting high average asymmetry in jump height and length (up to 10.2%), Lockie et al. [15], have not found any significant correlation between these asymmetries and COD (505 and T-test) performance ($r = 0.00–0.018, p = 0.31–0.99$). Similarly, Dos Santos et al. [16] found no significant correlations between asymmetries in horizontal jumping tasks and performance in two COD tasks ($r ≤ 0.35, p > 0.05$). Furthermore, Fort-Vanmeerhaeghe et al. [20] have not found a relationship between asymmetry in jump height during SLCMJ and V-cut COD test ($r = 0.10, p > 0.05$). Finally, Loturco et al. [18], have found no significant correlation between asymmetries in different parameters during single leg vertical jumps and performance in zig-zag test.

By contrast, few studies have found a significant correlation between global asymmetry in jumping tests and COD performance. Studying female soccer players, Bishop et al. [21] found a significant positive correlation between inter-limb asymmetry in single-leg depth jump height and performance in 505 COD test on left ($r = 0.66, p < 0.01$) and right ($r = 0.52, p < 0.05$) side. Another study that reported a relationship between asymmetry and performance was of Maloney et al. [22], that explained 63% ($p < 0.001$) of variance of COD performance with leg stiffness and height asymmetry during vertical depth jump.

The reason for inconsistent findings could lay in discrepancies among populations, methods of asymmetry calculation, and COD tests, as well as in low asymmetry values, that are not large enough to influence performance. Taking that into consideration, Sarabon et al. [23] found that explosive strength parameters like rate of torque development (RTD) are more sensitive to detect inter-limb asymmetries compared to maximal strength outcomes like peak force or peak torque during maximal voluntary contractions (MVC), which were used in previous research. Also, local inter-limb asymmetries were assessed only for the knee joint, while proximal regions of hip and trunk were overlooked. Moreover, asymmetries in range of motion were not previously researched in relation to performance. A substantial portion of asymmetry studies was done on amateur athletes and soccer players, which does not give enough insight into the functioning of elite athletes and other team sports, such as basketball. Basketball is characterized by many high intensity changes of direction (COD) [24], indicating that COD ability plays a critical role in basketball performance.

Therefore, the aim of this study is two-fold: (a) to profile elite basketball players in different local strength and range of motion asymmetries of hip and trunk region, and global power asymmetries in horizontal and vertical jumping and (b) to quantify the relationship of those asymmetries with COD performance. We hypothesized that these asymmetries could predict COD performance.

2. Materials and Methods

2.1. Subjects

Forty-three (17 senior and 26 junior) male elite basketball players (age = 20.54 ± 6 years; height = 194.48 ± 7.19 cm; body mass = 86.77 ± 10.13 kg) from three different professional basketball clubs (Adriatic basketball association league (all three clubs); Liga Nova KBM, Slovenia (one club), and Premier Croatian basketball league (two clubs)) volunteered to participate in the study. A minimum sample size of 18 participants was determined from an a priori power analysis (G*Power 3.1, Heinrich-Heine-Universität, Düsseldorf, Germany) based upon an estimated squared multiple correlation of 0.45 and a power of 0.8 [25]. Subjects were in training program from 18 to 24 h per week, had at least one-year experience in resistance training and reported no previous (within the last 12 months) or present lower-limb injuries. All subjects provided informed consent to participate in the study. For the underage subjects their parents or guardians signed consent prior to their participation. This study was a part of TELASI–PREVENT (Body asymmetries as a risk factor in musculoskeletal injury development: studying etiological mechanisms and designing corrective interventions for primary and tertiary preventive care—L5-1845) project which was approved by Slovenian Medical Ethics committee.

2.2. Procedures

The study was conducted in February of 2019, in the middle of the 2018/2019 basketball season. Testing was performed in each of the clubs playing/training courts. All tests were performed during a single testing session lasting approximately 180 min per participant. Participants attended the sessions in larger groups and rotated between the testing sessions (see below). The subjects were instructed to refrain from any physical activity for at least 24 hours before testing. Testing started with anthropometric measurements, after which the subjects performed a warm-up (5 min of low intensity running, 8 repetitions of dynamic stretching and body weight activation exercises). After the warm-up, subjects were randomized into 4 groups to complete four testing stations in a random order: (i) jumping, (ii) COD, (iii) hip and trunk dynamometry; and (iv) hip and trunk range of motion (ROM). There was a 5-minute rest between the testing stations. Each test began after the subject reported that they felt comfortable with the task (no more than 3 practice trials were taken by a player).

2.2.1. Functional Leg Length

Functional leg length was defined as the distance between anterior-superior iliac spine (ASIS) and the ground, and was measured with laser distance meter (LD 420, Stabila, Hungary). The subjects were instructed to stand with their bare feet on the ground, heels next to the wall, with feet separated hip distance apart. During left leg measurement subjects were instructed to put their left hand on the right shoulder and vice versa. Three measurements on each leg were performed and the mean from these three repetitions was taken for further analysis.

2.2.2. Single-Leg Countermovement Jump

SLCMJ was performed on a force platform (Type 9260AA, Kistler, Winterthur, Switzerland). Subjects were informed to step on the force platform with their testing leg and hands on their hips. The opposite leg was slightly flexed at the knee, but was not touching the shin of the tested leg. Swinging with the opposite leg during jumping was not allowed. The subjects were instructed to jump as high as possible, with the countermovement depth being self-selected, land on two legs and a hold balanced position for 3 s. The jump would be accepted if all of the above-mentioned instructions were met. Three trials on left and right leg were performed with 30 s of rest between each trial. Peak force (N), peak power (W), and highest jump height (m) for each leg was taken for further analysis.

2.2.3. Single-Leg Horizontal Jump

Tape measure was used to measure Single leg horizontal jump (SLHJ), which was performed on the basketball court sufficing the standards of international basketball federation (FIBA). Subjects were informed to put their testing leg with toe at the starting line and hands on the hips. Subjects performed a countermovement to self-selected depth before pushing themselves into the horizontal jump, landing onto both legs and holding a balanced position for 3 s. Three trials on each leg were performed with 30 s of rest between each trial. The distance (m) was measured to the nearest 0.01 m with a tape measure. The longest jump from each leg was taken for further analysis.

2.2.4. Single-Leg Triple Jump

Single leg triple jump (SLTJ) was measured similarly to SLHJ. Subject performed three consecutive horizontal jumps in which they landed onto both legs and held a balanced position for 3 s. The jump would be accepted for if all of the above-mentioned instructions were met. As with the SLHJ, the longest of the three jumps was taken for further analysis for each leg.

2.2.5. Single-Leg Lateral Jump

Tape measure was used to measure Single leg lateral jump (SLLJ). Subjects were informed to put the inner (i.e., medial) edge of their feet at the starting line and hands on their hips. When a subject was ready, he performed a countermovement to self-selected depth before pushing himself into lateral jump landing onto both legs and holding a balanced position for 3 s. Three trials on left and right leg were performed with 30 s of rest between each trial. Distance (m) was measured to the nearest 0.01 m with a tape measure. Longest jump from each leg was taken for further analysis.

2.2.6. Trunk Strength

Trunk strength assessment was done according to Markovic et al. [26] protocol. A trunk dynamometer (S2P Ltd., Ljubljana, Slovenia) with a bending beam load cell (model 1-Z6FC3/200 kg, HBM, Darmstadt, Germany) was used to measure trunk flexion, extension, and lateral flexion isometric strength. Isometric strength was measured as peak torque (Nm/kg) of the best one second interval during maximal voluntary contraction. All of the output variables were normalized with subject's body mass. During trunk extension measurement, subjects were standing with back turned towards the dynamometer with sensors on level of scapular spine and hands crossed on their shoulders. During trunk flexion measurement, subjects were standing turned face towards dynamometer with sensors on the same level as during extension and arms floating in the air to prevent their contribution. During trunk lateral flexion, subjects were standing sideways to the dynamometer, positioned so that their spine was in neutral position. The hand closer to the sensor was placed on their opposite shoulder and the other one was placed on opposite hip. During all trunk strength measurements, subjects were in their training shoes, standing with feet hip width distance apart, while a rigid strap was tightly fastened across pelvic girdle to achieve good fixation. During every trial subject was verbally encouraged to reach his best performance and hold it for 3–5 s. Each task was done three times with 60 s of rest in between. The best result for each task was taken for further analysis.

2.2.7. Hip Strength

Hip strength assessment was modeled based on Markovic et al. [27] protocol. A multipurpose dynamometer (Muscleboard, S2P Ltd., Ljubljana, Slovenija) was used to measure hip flexion, extension, abduction, adduction, internal and external rotation strength. Peak force values were multiplied by lever arm (leg length, in meter) to calculate hip torque. Isometric strength was measured as peak torque (PT) (Nm/kg) during one second interval of maximal voluntary contraction and rate of torque development (RTD) (Nm/ms) was measured in 100 ms interval as Δ torque/Δ time value. During all of the measurements, the offset of the sensor was performed with the relaxed leg, but with the subject having minimal contact with sensor (~5% MVC). Then, the subject was instructed to reach MVC as fast as possible. During all measured actions (except hip rotations), the distance between the mid-part of the aluminum brace of sensor and medial malleoli was set to 5 cm and a rigid strap was tightly fastened across pelvic girdle to achieve good fixation. Hip flexion and extension were measured unilaterally while the remaining tasks were performed bilaterally. During hip flexion (Figure 1A) subject was sitting on dynamometer with hands on the ground and the tested leg extended in knee with hip flexion (~30°), while the non-tested leg was on the ground with knee flexion of ~90°. During hip extension (Figure 1B) subject was laying prone on elbows on the ground, with the tested leg extended, non-tested leg was in the 90° knee flexion, resting on dynamometer surface. During abduction and adduction (Figure 1C) subject was sitting with legs hip apart, knees fully extended and hip in ~30° flexion. During hip internal and external (Figure 1D) rotation, the subject was kneeling on all fours with knees and hip in 90° flexion with knees hip apart. The best out of three results from each movement was taken for further analysis.

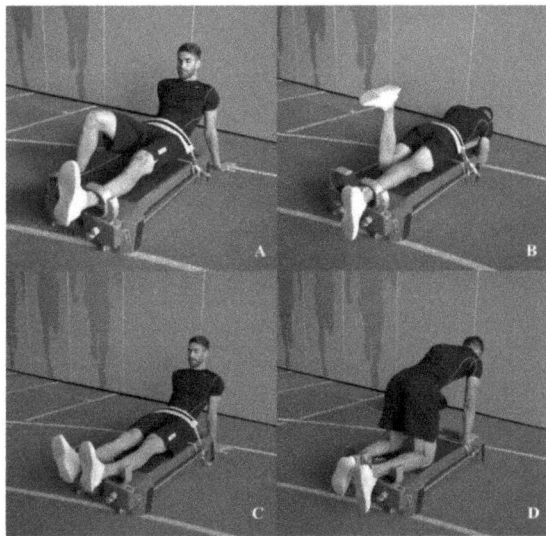

Figure 1. Position of subjects during isometric hip strength testing. (**A**) flexion; (**B**) extension; (**C**) abduction/adduction; and (**D**) internal/external rotation.

2.2.8. Range of Motion

Passive hip range of motion (ROM) during flexion, extension and internal/external rotation was measured with a digital inclinometer (Baseline, Fabrication Enterprises Inc., White Plains, NY, USA) and abduction/adduction with a handheld goniometer (Baseline, Fabrication Enterprises Inc., White Plains, NY, USA). All of the measurements were performed by the same measurer to minimize error. For flexion and extension, the inclinometer was aligned between the tested side femur trochanter major and lateral condyle. Hip flexion ROM was measured with the subject in supine position (the non-tested leg was extended in knee and hip fixated) and the knee of the tested leg in extended position. The tested leg was then moved and kept extended during whole movement until first pelvic movement. During hip extension ROM, subject was in prone position, and tested leg was kept in knee flexion (~90°) during whole movement until first pelvic movement. Hip internal/external rotation ROM was measured with the inclinometer located in the center of vertically positioned (with pendulum) tibia with the subject in pronated position and knee in 90° flexion. Internal and external rotation were performed until the first pelvic movement, with hand-stabilization on the pelvis. Hip abduction and adduction ROM were measured with goniometer with stationary arm pointed toward the opposite anterior superior iliac spine and the movable arm pointed toward the patella of the tested leg. During abduction, the subject was laying supine with both legs in neutral position (start) from which the tested leg was moved into abduction until first pelvic movement (finish). During adduction, the subject was supine with non-tested leg laying from table in ~30° abduction and tested leg in neutral position (start) from which leg was moved into adduction until first pelvic movement (finish). Mean result from three attempts on each leg was taken for further analysis with all of the results expressed in degrees (°).

For the trunk lateral flexion ROM, the subject was standing barefoot with feet hip width distance apart with his back and heels touching the wall. Starting position was measured with a tape as distance between the middle finger (hand on the wall) and the floor. Subjects performed lateral flexion, sliding downwards with the hands without breaking contact with the wall and lifting their heels of the ground. At the end of movement, the end position was measured, and the difference between starting and end position was calculated. Mean result from three attempts on each side was taken for further analysis with all of the results expressed in meters (m).

2.2.9. Change of Direction

For COD performance, the T-test (Figure 2) was used, as outlined by Semenik [28]. All of the COD testing was done on the basketball court sufficing the standards of international basketball federation (FIBA) using photocells timing gates (Brower Timing Systems; Draper, Utah). At the beginning of test, the subject was standing 30 cm behind the start/finish line where photocells were placed. Subject was instructed to sprint (filled line up in Figure 2) from the start to the first cone, touch the tip with one hand, shuffle (dashed lines in Figure 2) to the cone opposite of the touching hand and touch the tip of the lateral cone, then shuffle to the third cone and touch it with the first hand, shuffle back to the middle cone touching the tip with the second hand and then pedal back (filled line down in Figure 2) to the finish line. One-minute recovery was given between each trial. The best out of three trials was taken for further analysis.

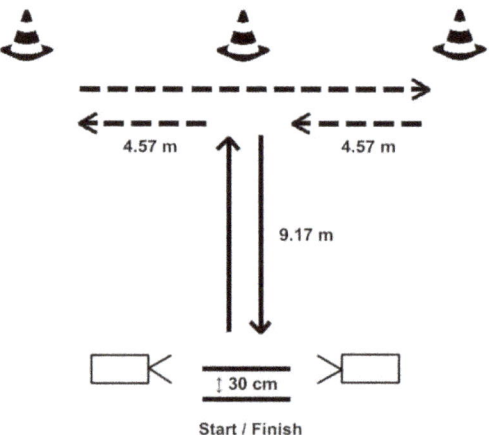

Figure 2. Schematic representation of the T-test.

2.3. Statistical Analyses

Due to the unknown reliability of the strength assessment with a novel MuscleBoard device (S2P Ltd., Ljubljana, Slovenia), particularly in view of RTD, we checked the intra-session reliability of the strength outcome measures that were used as potential predictors for COD performance. We used (a) intra-class coefficient correlation to assess relative reliability, (b) absolute typical error and relative typical error (expressed as coefficient of variation) to assess absolute reliability, and (c) paired-sample two-tailed T-tests to check for systematic bias. We used the data from our larger study involving 115 basketball players, who had completed the exact same protocol for strength assessment, the only difference was the lower number of repetitions (2 compared to 3 in our study) for each task. We used guidelines of Koo and Li [29] for reporting Intraclass Correlation Coefficient (ICC). Based on the 95% confident interval of ICC estimate values < 0.5 = poor, 0.5–0.75 = moderate, 0.75–0.90 = good, and > 0.90 = excellent reliability.

We used multiple regression analysis to model prediction of COD performance (dependent variable) with asymmetries (independent variable). Independent variables were grouped into five categories of asymmetries (anthropometric asymmetries, lateral hip and trunk strength asymmetries, hip and trunk strength ratios, hip and trunk ROM asymmetries and jumping asymmetries)—a total of 33 potential independent variables.

Inter-limb asymmetry was calculated with the following equation [30]:

$$Asymmetry\ (\%) = \left(\frac{stronger - weaker}{stronger}\right) \times 100$$

Shapiro–Wilks tests were performed to assess the normality of distribution of independent variables; only 24 % (8/33) were considered to be normally distributed given an alpha level of $p > 0.05$. Step-wise regression analysis was performed for overall CODS performance using all independent variables. An analysis of standard residuals was carried out, which showed that the data contained no outliers (s standardized residuals minimum: −1.71, standardized residuals maximum: 2.51). A collinearity test indicated that multicollinearity was not a concern (minimum tolerance: 0.75, maximum VIF:1.33). The data met the assumption of independent errors (Durbin–Watson value: 2.26). Also, Breuch–Pagan (10.43, $p > 0.05$) and Koenker (8.32, $p > 0.05$) test indicated the homoscedasticity of the model. Statistical significance was set at alpha level of $p \leq 0.05$ and all statistical procedures were conducted using the Statistical Package for the Social Sciences for Windows (v.26.0; SPSS Inc., Chicago, IL, USA). Mann–Whitney U test was used to for testing statistical significance in difference between hip PT and RTD, and left and right leg strength ratios.

3. Results

The results regarding reliability analyses are summarized in Table 1. No systematic bias was present for any of the outcome measures. Relative reliability was good to excellent for the peak torque measures (ICC > 0.80) and acceptable for RTD measures (ICC = 0.5–0.8). Typical errors, expressed as coefficient of variation were low for peak torque measurements for adduction, abduction, and internal rotation, but higher (>10%) for external rotation, flexion, and extension, and for all RTD outcomes. This suggests that the predictive strength of the parameters related to hip strength in this study can be used on the level of a sample with high confidence, while the generalizability to an individual must be done with high caution.

Inter-limb asymmetry values ranged from 0.76% for functional leg length up to 40.35% for RTD during hip flexion (Table 2). Inter-limb asymmetries of hip peak torque were lower (except for internal rotation) than the rate of torque development (3.68–11.52% vs. 10.72–40.35%, $p < 0.05$) (Table 3). Hip extension/flexion (1.32 ± 0.33; 1.30 ± 0.25), abduction/adduction (1.08 ± 0.19; 1.07 ± 0.20) and internal/external rotation (1.13 ± 0.27; 1.18 ± 0.26) ratios were similar ($p > 0.05$) for the left and right side (Table 4). Mean inter-limb asymmetry in peak torque during trunk lateral flexion exceeded the 10% threshold (12.48 ± 9.61 %). Mean inter-limb asymmetry in hip ROM (5.91–13.54%), was above the 10% threshold for extension and internal/external rotations, while the trunk lateral flexion showed good symmetry (2.01 ± 1.27%). Asymmetries in horizontal jumps showed lower results (3.48–4.60%) than various parameters of SLCMJ (4.77–11.12%).

Table 1. Reliability results for outcome measures.

Outcome/Task		Repetition 1		Repetition 2		Systematic Bias		Relative Reliability			Absolute Reliability			
		Mean	SD	Mean	SD	T	P	ICC	95% CI for ICC	TE	CV	95% CI for CV		
Peak torques at the hip (Nm)	Hip Abduction—Left	73.1	18.8	72.9	19.8	0.908	0.365	0.97	0.96	0.98	3.4	4.65	4.59	4.74
	Hip Abduction—Right	71.9	18.6	71.5	19.4	1.384	0.168	0.97	0.96	0.98	3.3	4.54	4.49	4.63
	Hip Adduction—Left	70.4	19.5	71.2	19.7	−1.695	0.092	0.93	0.91	0.95	5.0	7.09	6.90	7.43
	Hip Adduction—Right	69.0	19.1	69.8	19.3	−1.435	0.153	0.93	0.91	0.95	5.0	7.16	6.96	7.50
	Hip Internal rotation—Left	73.1	21.7	72.6	20.7	0.617	0.538	0.92	0.89	0.94	5.9	8.06	7.82	8.51
	Hip Internal rotation—Right	74.8	20.9	74.6	19.9	−0.592	0.555	0.93	0.90	0.95	5.4	7.26	7.06	7.63
	Hip External rotation—Left	62.5	32.2	64.5	16.8	0.172	0.872	0.85	0.80	0.88	10.2	16.06	15.07	17.69
	Hip External rotation—Right	63.8	16.6	63.7	16.3	−0.263	0.793	0.86	0.81	0.90	11.5	17.99	17.01	19.83
	Hip Flexion—Left	139.8	45.9	138.8	39.8	−0.554	0.712	0.94	0.91	0.96	20.6	14.77	14.33	15.53
	Hip Flexion—Right	146.1	42.7	146.8	42.7	−0.114	0.909	0.96	0.94	0.97	18.2	12.41	12.19	12.79
	Hip Extension—Left	163.3	71.5	160.9	55.2	1.195	0.234	0.84	0.78	0.88	27.8	17.13	15.99	19.30
	Hip Extension—Right	169.4	53.0	169.4	50.6	−0.721	0.472	0.91	0.87	0.93	16.6	9.83	9.45	10.51
Peak force at the trunk (N)	Trunk extension	534.5	199.2	560.3	190.7	−3.506	0.001	0.88	0.83	0.91	65.3	11.82	9.64	13.32
	Trunk flexion	415.5	144.2	431.0	144.9	−4.106	0.000	0.94	0.91	0.96	33.5	7.91	5.42	9.11
	Trunk lat. flexion—Left	395.4	121.2	393.9	125.3	0.114	0.910	0.88	0.84	0.91	51.8	13.1	10.02	15.89
	Trunk lat. flexion—Right	395.3	129.8	405.5	129.8	−2.474	0.014	0.92	0.88	0.94	36.8	9.22	7.88	11.76
Hip RTD (Nm/s)	Hip Abduction—Left	268.2	138.9	278.8	145.1	−0.836	0.404	0.50	0.37	0.61	102.6	37.52	27.61	62.50
	Hip Abduction—Right	257.0	132.8	269.2	136.1	−1.266	0.208	0.51	0.38	0.62	94.4	35.89	26.83	58.25
	Hip Adduction—Left	285.9	157.2	299.2	170.8	−1.375	0.171	0.61	0.50	0.71	101.4	34.67	28.16	49.22
	Hip Adduction—Right	276.6	157.7	285.4	163.4	−1.167	0.245	0.62	0.51	0.71	97.1	34.55	28.19	48.71
	Hip Internal rotation—Left	209.1	117.3	219.7	121.8	−1.441	0.152	0.62	0.51	0.71	72.8	33.95	28.03	47.11
	Hip Internal rotation—Right	215.9	119.5	221.0	119.6	−0.784	0.434	0.56	0.43	0.66	79.2	36.24	28.28	54.91
	Hip External rotation—Left	244.5	257.8	229.8	123.7	1.112	0.264	0.72	0.61	0.79	77.7	32.78	27.78	42.33
	Hip External rotation—Right	236.9	129.1	225.3	122.1	1.425	0.156	0.69	0.60	0.76	79.6	34.46	29.86	44.02
	Hip Flexion—Left	418.9	283.9	427.7	289.9	−0.799	0.426	0.58	0.45	0.69	193.5	45.70	35.38	69.83
	Hip Flexion—Right	444.1	290.6	446.4	283.1	0.343	0.732	0.67	0.56	0.76	170.0	38.18	31.90	51.54
	Hip Extension—Left	460.3	321.9	487.9	289.1	−1.421	0.158	0.53	0.40	0.64	207.0	43.67	33.10	69.40
	Hip Extension—Right	534.9	303.3	518.1	313.4	0.271	0.786	0.63	0.51	0.72	191.4	36.34	29.70	51.05

SD—standard deviation; t—T-test statistics; p—statistical significance; CI—confidence interval; TE—typical error; CV—coefficient of variation; RTD—rate of torque development

Table 2. Descriptive and normality analysis of asymmetry variables.

Asymmetry (%)	Mean	SD	S-W
Functional leg length	0.76	0.62	0.002
Single-leg Countermovement Jump— height	11.12	8.36	0.005
Single-leg Countermovement Jump— PF	4.77	4.40	0.000
Single-leg Countermovement Jump—PP	7.06	5.98	0.001
Single-leg Horizontal Jump—distance	4.60	3.19	0.051
Single-leg Lateral Jump—distance	4.82	3.70	0.001
Single-leg Triple Jump—distance	3.48	2.67	0.005
Hip Abduction—PT	3.68	3.15	0.001
Hip Abduction—RTD	11.23	9.67	0.000
Hip Adduction—PT	5.59	4.77	0.001
Hip Adduction—RTD	10.72	10.34	0.000
Hip External Rotation—PT	7.90	5.82	0.000
Hip External Rotation—RTD	13.18	8.83	0.000
Hip Internal Rotation—PT	11.52	7.17	0.150
Hip Internal Rotation—RTD	13.17	9.55	0.020
Hip Extension—PT	11.01	8.92	0.000
Hip Extension—RTD	30.56	21.79	0.031
Hip Flexion—PT	9.86	8.36	0.000
Hip Flexion—RTD	40.35	20.42	0.619
Trunk Lateral Flexion—PT	12.81	9.61	0.013
Trunk Lateral Flexion—ROM	8.98	5.94	0.054
Hip Abduction—ROM	8.94	5.72	0.165
Hip Adduction—ROM	8.83	6.73	0.002
Hip Flexion—ROM	5.91	6.24	0.000
Hip Extension—ROM	12.80	10.95	0.000
Hip External Rotation—ROM	13.00	14.10	0.000
Hip Internal Rotation—ROM	13.54	10.57	0.002
Hip extension/flexion strength ratio (left leg)	1.32	0.33	0.183
Hip extension/flexion strength ratio (right leg)	1.30	0.25	0.011
Hip abduction/adduction strength ratio (left leg)	1.08	0.19	0.048
Hip abduction/adduction strength ratio (right leg)	1.07	0.20	0.010
Hip internal/external rotation strength ratio (left leg)	1.13	0.27	0.266
Hip internal/external rotation ratio (right leg)	1.18	0.26	0.279
Trunk extension/flexion strength ratio	1.27	0.27	0.331
T-test	9.10	0.50	0.013

SD = standard deviation, S-W = Shapiro–Wilks tests, PF = peak force, PP = peak power, RTD = rate of torque development, ROM = range of motion.

Table 3. Peak torque and Rate of torque development differences (Mann–Whitney U test).

Asymmetry (%)	PT Mean ± SD	RTD Mean ± SD	p-Value	Effect Size
Hip abduction	3.68 ± 3.15	11.23 ± 9.67	0.000	0.56
Hip adduction	5.59 ± 4.77	10.72 ± 10.34	0.002	0.23
Hip external rotation	7.90 ± 5.82	13.18 ± 8.83	0.001	0.27
Hip internal rotation	11.52 ± 7.17	13.17 ± 9.55	0.514	0.01
Hip extension	11.01 ± 8.92	30.56 ± 21.79	0.000	0.38
Hip flexion	9.86 ± 8.36	40.35 ± 20.42	0.000	1.00

PT = peak torque, RTD = rate of torque development; SD = standard deviation.

Table 4. Hip strength ratio differences between left and right leg (Mann–Whitney U test).

Hip Strength Ratio	Left Leg Mean ± SD	Right Leg Mean ± SD	p-Value	Effect Size
Extension/Flexion	1.32 ± 0.33	1.30 ± 0.25	0.779	0.00
Abduction/Adduction	1.08 ± 0.19	1.07 ± 0.20	0.826	0.00
Internal/External Rotation	1.13 ± 0.27	1.18 ± 0.26	0.218	0.03

SD = standard deviation

A six-variable regression model explained 48% ($R^2 = 0.48$; $p < 0.01$) of the variation in the T-test performance (Table 5). T-test time was predicted by left hip internal/external rotation strength ratio ($\beta = -0.58$; $p < 0.01$) and inter-limb asymmetries in hip abduction RTD ($\beta = -0.38$; $p = 0.01$), hip flexion ROM ($\beta = 0.32$; $p = 0.03$), functional leg length ($\beta = 0.31$; $p = 0.02$), SLTJ distance ($\beta = 0.29$; $p = 0.04$), and peak torque during trunk lateral flexion ($\beta = 0.27$; $p = 0.05$).

Table 5. Final regression model with six independent variables (dependent T-test).

Depended Variable	Independent Variable	B	Beta	R^2	p-Value
T-test (s)	-	-	-	0.48	<0.001
-	Left hip internal/external rotation strength ratio	−1.08	−0.58	-	0.00
-	Asymmetry in hip abduction RTD (%)	−0.02	−0.38	-	0.01
-	Asymmetry in hip flexion ROM (%)	0.03	0.32	-	0.03
-	Asymmetry in functional leg length (%)	0.25	0.31	-	0.02
-	Asymmetry in SLTJ (%)	0.06	0.29	-	0.04
-	Asymmetry in peak force during trunk lateral flexion (%)	0.01	0.27	-	0.05

RTD—rate of torque development; ROM—range of motion; SLTJ—single-leg triple jump.

4. Discussion

The aims of the present study were twofold: (a) to profile elite basketball players in different local strength and range of motion asymmetries of hip and trunk region, global power asymmetries in horizontal and vertical jumping and (b) to quantify the relationship of these asymmetries with COD performance. Results showed different magnitudes of asymmetries among tests, body regions, and parameters.

Regarding the magnitude of asymmetry scores reported in this study, largest asymmetries were found in hip RTD (10.72–40.35%), which were significantly larger (except internal rotation) than peak force asymmetries of different hip action (3.68–11.52%) (as shown in Table 2). Compared to local peak torque asymmetries, rate of torque development showed to be a more sensitive parameter for assessment of asymmetries. That is in accordance with findings of Sarabon et al. [23], who reported that the RTD showed larger magnitudes of asymmetries than peak torque during unilateral isometric knee flexion and extension.

To our knowledge, only one study profiled hip strength ratios in professional athletes using fixed point dynamometer [31]. Although study was done on Australian football players, it detected similar results in flexion/extension mean ratio (0.8) as our study (1.3). Moreover, their mean internal/external ratio was 1.15 which is in accordance to our values (1.13 and 1.18 for left and right leg).

They observed a hip adductor/abductor ratio of 1.05 which is much different from our abduction/adduction ratios (1.08 and 1.07), such differences can be attributed to sport specificity of ball kicking in Australian football.

Our results are also showing various magnitudes in hip range of motion asymmetries (5.91–13.54%), with largest being found for extension (12.80 ± 10.95%), internal rotation (13.54 ± 10.57%), and external rotation (13.00 ± 14.10%). Although some research indicates that there are significant differences in hip ROM between the dominant and non-dominant leg in football players [32], a direct comparison of results is limited because authors have not reported asymmetry indexes.

Mean asymmetry in functional leg length was 0.76 ± 0.62%. To our knowledge, studies that assessed asymmetries in anthropometry had not used the functional leg length to investigate the relationship with performance instead, they had utilized other anthropometric measurements, such as knee and ankle joint width [33] or lean mass asymmetry [34]. Although, there is no past research to compare our results with, a review of Knutson et al. [35] set a threshold of normal functional leg length discrepancy at 2 cm. The mean absolute asymmetry in our study was 0.9 cm, which is thus considered as normal leg length variation.

Inter-limb asymmetries in vertical jumping parameters (4.77–11.12%) showed larger values compared to horizontal jumps (3.48–4.60%), which is in accordance with research conducted by Lockie et al. [15], who reported SLCMJ mean inter-limb asymmetries at 10.4 % and only 5.4% and 3.3% for horizontal jumps (SLHJ and SLLJ). Similar results were reported by Bishop et al. [36] who found larger inter-limb asymmetries in SLCMJ (12.5%) compared to SLHJ (6.8%). Both of these studies were conducted on football players, which indicates that the variability between the testing methods might be substantially higher than the variability between the athletic populations. With that in mind, it can be suggested that vertical jumping is more sensitive for detecting asymmetries than horizontal jumping.

While all of our maximal strength measures showed an excellent reliability (displayed in Table 1), the explosive strength (rate of torque development) were only moderately reliable. As the structured strength and conditioning training as well as the experience level contribute to reliability of data [37], our data can be interpreted with confidence. In the past years, there has been a lot of debate about defining normal asymmetry threshold, most common one being 10%, but different authors suggested values from 5% to 20% [6]. Taking all that into consideration, variability of asymmetry results in our data shows that asymmetry magnitude is dependent on the specific movement, test and parameter which indicates that a unifying asymmetry threshold cannot be established.

Regression analysis revealed a relationship between asymmetries and performance: six variable model explained 49% of T-test performance variance. Independent variable Beta scores (0.27–0.58) show a small to medium individual relationship between different type of asymmetry and COD performance. Although several studies (including the present study) observed negative influence of asymmetries on COD performance, a number of studies identified contradicting evidence. Lockie et al. [10] showed negative influence ($r = 0.638, 0.669, p < 0.01$) of isokinetic concentric (60°/s, 180°/s, 240°/s) and eccentric (30°/s) knee strength asymmetries and COD performance (assessed with T-test). The study of Coratella et al. [11] reported similar results of association between knee strength asymmetries in slow (30°/s) and fast (300°/s) contractions and COD performance (T-test and 180° turn test). On the other hand, the relationship between COD performance (180° turn test) and strength asymmetries tested with the whole kinetic chain movements (e.g., IMTP) has not been detected [12,13]. This observation could be explained by local strength asymmetries show higher magnitudes. Negative influence of asymmetry in vertical drop jump height and COD performance (180° turn test) ($r = 0.66, p < 0.01$ and $0.52, p < 0.05$; depending on the side of the turn) was found by Bishop et al. [21]. Also, using horizontal jumps to assess asymmetries, Madruga-Parera et al. [38] found much lower correlations ($r = 0.32$ and 0.31, $p < 0.05$) between asymmetry in horizontal jumping length (SLLJ) and COD performance (V-cut and 180° turn test). Such a relationship was not found by Lockie et al. [15], who did not observe significant correlations between asymmetry in vertical (SLCMJ height) and horizontal (SLHJ and SLLJ distance) jumping and COD performance (T-test and 180° turn test). Similarly, Loturco et al. [18] suggested that asymmetry in various parameters during single-leg squat jump and CMJ do not influence COD performance (zig-zag test). The study conducted by Maloney et al. [22] is probably the most comparable to ours, it showed that stiffness and asymmetry in single-leg drop jump explained 63% variance of COD performance (2 × 90°cut test). However, they used just one type of asymmetry as the secondary predictor, while the stiffness during drop jump was main predictor in the model.

Our model consists of several independent variables, each representing a different type of asymmetry and together showing a significant relationship with COD performance. This is important because findings indicated an independent nature of asymmetry [39]. The most important finding of this study is the connection between asymmetry and COD performance, but also that testing large variety of asymmetry types is needed to gain a more complete understanding of athlete asymmetry and its relationship to performance.

Certain limitations of this study should be noted. The main limitation is the modest reliability of hip explosive strength measure, however, we find this acceptable as RTD is a highly variable parameter. Moreover, a slightly larger sample size would have been useful in the linear regression analyses, as the best model included a relatively large number of predictor variables.

5. Conclusions

This study was conducted to explore asymmetries in local strength, vertical jumping and ROM, and to investigate whether these asymmetries are related to COD performance in healthy elite-basketball players. A substantial variability among asymmetries in different tests was noted. This implies that coaches and physiotherapists should not rely exclusively on the <10 % threshold when they are deciding on the athletes return to play, or planning interventions for reducing asymmetries. In particular, it is expected for RTD asymmetries to be larger than maximal strength (i.e., peak torque) asymmetries. In the attempt to elucidate which asymmetries are more relevant for performance, specifically to the COD ability, we performed linear regressions which showed more than one type of asymmetry is should be considered in the analyses to sufficiently explain the COD performance. Notably, the best model for predicting COD performance included both maximal strength and RTD asymmetry, both hip and trunk asymmetry, one vertical jump asymmetry, one ROM asymmetry, as well as asymmetry in functional leg length. Therefore, interventions should likely target multiple types of asymmetries when trying to improve COD performance. We encourage practitioners to use a wide testing battery to test different aspects on local and global level of the body to obtain a clearer picture of athletes' asymmetries.

Author Contributions: Conceptualization, F.U. and N.Š.; Data curation, F.U.; Formal analysis, F.U.; Funding acquisition, N.Š.; Investigation, F.U.; Methodology, N.Š.; Project administration, N.Š.; Resources, N.Š.; Software, N.Š.; Supervision, N.Š.; Validation, F.U. and N.Š.; Writing—original draft, F.U. All authors have read and agreed to the published version of the manuscript.

Funding: The study was supported by the Slovenian Research Agency through the project TELASI-PREVENT [L5-1845] (Body asymmetries as a risk factor in musculoskeletal injury development: studying etiological mechanisms and designing corrective interventions for primary and tertiary preventive care).

Acknowledgments: The authors would like to thank the athletes and management from the basketball clubs participating in this study. Additionally, many thanks to the research assistants who helped at testing.

Conflicts of Interest: The authors declare no conflict of interest. The funders had no role in the design of the study; in the collection, analyses, or interpretation of data; in the writing of the manuscript; or in the decision to publish the results.

References

1. Bates, N.A.; Ford, K.R.; Myer, G.D.; Hewett, T.E. Impact differences in ground reaction force and center of mass between the first and second landing phases of a drop vertical jump and their implications for injury risk assessment. *J. Biomech.* **2013**, *46*, 1237–1241. [CrossRef]
2. Zwolski, C.; Thomas, S.; Schmitt, L.C.; Hewett, T.E.; Paterno, M.V. The Utility of Limb Symmetry Indices in Return-to-Sport Assessment in Patients With Bilateral Anterior Cruciate Ligament Reconstruction. *Am. J. Sports Med.* **2016**, *44*, 2030–2038. [CrossRef]
3. Mayer, S.W.; Queen, R.; Taylor, D.; Moorman, I.C.T.; Toth, A.P.; Garrett, J.W.E.; Butler, R. Functional Testing Differences in Anterior Cruciate Ligament Reconstruction Patients Released Versus Not Released to Return to Sport. *Am. J. Sports Med.* **2015**, *43*, 1648–1655. [CrossRef]
4. Paterno, M.V.; Ford, K.R.; Myer, G.D.; Heyl, R.; E Hewett, T. Limb Asymmetries in Landing and Jumping 2 Years Following Anterior Cruciate Ligament Reconstruction. *Clin. J. Sport Med.* **2007**, *17*, 258–262. [CrossRef] [PubMed]
5. Bishop, C.; Turner, A.; Read, P. Effects of inter-limb asymmetries on physical and sports performance: A systematic review. *J. Sports Sci.* **2017**, *36*, 1135–10144. [CrossRef] [PubMed]

6. McGrath, T.M.; Waddington, G.; Scarvell, J.M.; Ball, N.; Creer, R.; Woods, K.; Smith, D. The effect of limb dominance on lower limb functional performance – a systematic review. *J. Sports Sci.* **2015**, *34*, 289–302. [CrossRef] [PubMed]
7. Engstrom, C.M.; Walker, D.G.; Kippers, V.; Mehnert, A. Quadratus Lumborum Asymmetry and L4 Pars Injury in Fast Bowlers. *Med. Sci. Sports Exerc.* **2007**, *39*, 910–917. [CrossRef] [PubMed]
8. Bishop, C.; Read, P.; Bromley, T.; Brazier, J.; Jarvis, P.; Chavda, S.; Turner, A. The Association Between Interlimb Asymmetry and Athletic Performance Tasks. *J. Strength Cond. Res.* **2020**. [CrossRef]
9. Bishop, C.; Read, P.; Chavda, S.; Turner, A. Asymmetries of the Lower Limb. *Strength Cond. J.* **2016**, *38*, 27–32. [CrossRef]
10. Lockie, R.G.; Schultz, A.B.; Jeffriess, M.D.; Callaghan, S.J. The relationship between bilateral differences of knee flexor and extensor isokinetic strength and multi-directional speed. *Isokinet. Exerc. Sci.* **2012**, *20*, 211–219. [CrossRef]
11. Coratella, G.; Beato, M.; Schena, F. Correlation between quadriceps and hamstrings inter-limb strength asymmetry with change of direction and sprint in U21 elite soccer-players. *Hum. Mov. Sci.* **2018**, *59*, 81–87. [CrossRef] [PubMed]
12. Chiang, C.-Y. Lower Body Strength and Power Characteristics Influencing Change of Direction and Straight-Line Sprinting Performance in Division I Soccer Players: An Exploratory Study. Ph.D. Thesis, East Tennessee State University, Johnson City, TN USA, July 2014.
13. Dos'Santos, T.; Thomas, C.; Jones, P.A.; Comfort, P. Asymmetries in Isometric Force-Time Characteristics Are Not Detrimental to Change of Direction Speed. *J. Strength Cond. Res.* **2018**, *32*, 520–527. [CrossRef] [PubMed]
14. Hoffman, J.R.; Ratamess, N.A.; Klatt, M.; Faigenbaum, A.D.; Kang, J. Do Bilateral Power Deficits Influence Direction-Specific Movement Patterns? *Sport. Med.* **2007**, *15*(2), 125–132. [CrossRef] [PubMed]
15. Lockie, R.G.; Callaghan, S.J.; Berry, S.P.; Cooke, E.R.A.; Jordan, C.A.; Luczo, T.M.; Jeffriess, M.D. Relationship Between Unilateral Jumping Ability and Asymmetry on Multidirectional Speed in Team-Sport Athletes. *J. Strength Cond. Res.* **2014**, *28*, 3557–3566. [CrossRef] [PubMed]
16. Dos'Santos, T.; Thomas, C.; Jones, P.A.; Comfort, P. Asymmetries in single and triple hop are not detrimental to change of direction speed. *J. Trainology* **2017**, *6*, 35–41. [CrossRef]
17. Fort-Vanmeerhaeghe, A.; Montalvo, A.; Sitjà-Rabert, M.; Kiefer, A.W.; Myer, G.D.; Fort-Vanmeerhaeghe, A. Neuromuscular asymmetries in the lower limbs of elite female youth basketball players and the application of the skillful limb model of comparison. *Phys. Ther. Sport* **2015**, *16*, 317–323. [CrossRef]
18. Loturco, I.; Pereira, L.A.; Kobal, R.; Abad, C.C.C.; Rosseti, M.; Carpes, F.P.; Bishop, C. Do Asymmetry Scores Influence Speed and Power Performance in Elite Female Soccer Players? *Biol. Sport* **2019**, *36*, 209–216. [CrossRef]
19. Sheppard, J.M.; Young, W.B. Agility literature review: Classifications, training and testing. *J. Sports Sci.* **2006**, *24*, 919–932. [CrossRef]
20. Fort-Vanmeerhaeghe, A.; Bishop, C.; Buscà, B.; Aguilera-Castells, J.; Vicens-Bordas, J.; Gonzalo-Skok, O. Inter-limb asymmetries are associated with decrements in physical performance in youth elite team sports athletes. *PLoS ONE* **2020**, *15*, e0229440. [CrossRef]
21. Bishop, C.; Turner, A.; Maloney, S.J.; Lake, J.P.; LoTurco, I.; Bromley, T.; Read, P. Drop Jump Asymmetry is Associated with Reduced Sprint and Change-of-Direction Speed Performance in Adult Female Soccer Players. *Sports* **2019**, *7*, 29. [CrossRef]
22. Maloney, S.J.; Richards, J.; Nixon, D.G.D.; Harvey, L.J.; Fletcher, I.M. Do stiffness and asymmetries predict change of direction performance? *Sports Sci.* **2017**, *35*, 547–556. [CrossRef] [PubMed]
23. Sarabon, N.; Kozinc, Z.; Bishop, C.; Maffiuletti, N.A. Factors influencing bilateral deficit and inter-limb asymmetry of maximal and explosive strength: Motor task, outcome measure and muscle group. *Graefe's Arch. Clin. Exp. Ophthalmol.* **2020**, *120*, 1681–1688. [CrossRef] [PubMed]
24. Ben Abdelkrim, N.; Castagna, C.; Jabri, I.; Battikh, T.; El Fazaa, S.; El Ati, J. Activity Profile and Physiological Requirements of Junior Elite Basketball Players in Relation to Aerobic-Anaerobic Fitness. *J. Strength Cond. Res.* **2010**, *24*, 2330–2342. [CrossRef] [PubMed]
25. Beck, T.W. The Importance of A Priori Sample Size Estimation in Strength and Conditioning Research. *J. Strength Cond. Res.* **2013**, *27*, 2323–2337. [CrossRef] [PubMed]

26. Markovic, G.; Šarabon, N.; Greblo, Z.; Križanić, V. Effects of feedback-based balance and core resistance training vs. Pilates training on balance and muscle function in older women: A randomized-controlled trial. *Arch. Gerontol. Geriatr.* **2015**, *61*, 117–123. [CrossRef]
27. Markovic, G.; Šarabon, N.; Pausic, J.; Hadžić, V. Adductor Muscles Strength and Strength Asymmetry as Risk Factors for Groin Injuries among Professional Soccer Players: A Prospective Study. *Int. J. Environ. Res. Public Health* **2020**, *17*, 4946. [CrossRef]
28. Semenick, D. The T-Test. *NSCA J.* **1990**, *12*, 36–37.
29. Koo, T.K.; Li, M.Y. A Guideline of Selecting and Reporting Intraclass Correlation Coefficients for Reliability Research. *J. Chiropr. Med.* **2016**, *15*, 155–163. [CrossRef]
30. Bishop, C.; Read, P.; Lake, J.P.; Chavda, S.; Turner, A. Inter-Limb Asymmetries. *Strength Cond. J.* **2018**, *40*, 1. [CrossRef]
31. Althorpe, T.; Beales, D.; Skinner, A.; Caputi, N.; Mullings, G.; Stockden, M.; Boyle, J. Isometric hip strength and strength ratios in elite adolescent and senior Australian Rules Football players: An initial exploration using fixed-point dynamometry. *J. Sci. Med. Sport* **2018**, *21*, S81. [CrossRef]
32. Oliveira, A.; Barbieri, F.A.; Goncalves, M. Flexibility, torque and kick performance in soccer: Effect of dominance. *Sci. Sports* **2013**, *28*, e67–e70. [CrossRef]
33. Trivers, R.; Palestis, B.G.; Manning, J.T. The Symmetry of Children's Knees Is Linked to Their Adult Sprinting Speed and Their Willingness to Sprint in a Long-Term Jamaican Study. *PLoS ONE* **2013**, *8*, e72244. [CrossRef] [PubMed]
34. Bell, D.R.; Sanfilippo, J.L.; Binkley, N.; Heiderscheit, B.C. Lean Mass Asymmetry Influences Force and Power Asymmetry During Jumping in Collegiate Athletes. *J. Strength Cond. Res.* **2014**, *28*, 884–891. [CrossRef] [PubMed]
35. Knutson, G.A. Anatomic and functional leg-length inequality: A review and recommendation for clinical decision-making. Part I, anatomic leg-length inequality: Prevalence, magnitude, effects and clinical significance. *Chiropr. Osteopat.* **2005**, *13*, 11. [CrossRef]
36. Bishop, C.; Read, P.; McCubbine, J.; Turner, A. Vertical and Horizontal Asymmetries are Related to Slower Sprinting and Jump Performance in Elite Youth Female Soccer Players. *J. Strength Cond. Res.* **2018**. Available online: http://eprints.mdx.ac.uk/23569/ (accessed on 23 September 2020). [CrossRef]
37. Bishop, C.; Berney, J.; Lake, J.; LoTurco, I.; Blagrove, R.; Turner, A.; Read, P. Bilateral Deficit During Jumping Tasks. *J. Strength Cond. Res.* **2019**. Available online: http://eprints.chi.ac.uk/id/eprint/4183/ (accessed on 23 September 2020). [CrossRef]
38. Madruga-Parera, M.; Bishop, C.; Read, P.; Lake, J.; Brazier, J.; Romero-Rodriguez, D. Jumping-based Asymmetries are Negatively Associated with Jump, Change of Direction, and Repeated Sprint Performance, but not Linear Speed, in Adolescent Handball Athletes. *J. Hum. Kinet.* **2020**, *71*, 47–58. [CrossRef]
39. Raya-González, J.; Bishop, C.; Gómez-Piqueras, P.; Veiga, S.; Viejo-Romero, D.; Navandar, A. Strength, Jumping, and Change of Direction Speed Asymmetries Are Not Associated With Athletic Performance in Elite Academy Soccer Players. *Front. Psychol.* **2020**, *11*, 1. [CrossRef]

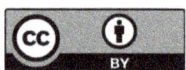

© 2020 by the authors. Licensee MDPI, Basel, Switzerland. This article is an open access article distributed under the terms and conditions of the Creative Commons Attribution (CC BY) license (http://creativecommons.org/licenses/by/4.0/).

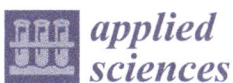 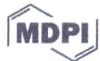

Article

Asymmetries in the Technique and Ground Reaction Forces of Elite Alpine Skiers Influence Their Slalom Performance

Matej Supej [1,*], Jan Ogrin [1], Nejc Šarabon [2] and Hans-Christer Holmberg [3,4]

1. Faculty of Sport, University of Ljubljana, 1000 Ljubljana, Slovenia; jan.ogrin@fsp.uni-lj.si
2. Faculty of Health Sciences, University of Primorska, Polje 42, 6310 Izola, Slovenia; nejc.sarabon@fvz.upr.si
3. Department of Physiology and Pharmacology, Biomedicum C5, Karolinska Institute, 171 77 Stockholm, Sweden; integrativephysiobiomech@gmail.com
4. China Institute of Sport and Health Science, Beijing Sport University, Beijing 100084, China
* Correspondence: matej.supej@fsp.uni-lj.si; +386-68-161-271

Received: 15 September 2020; Accepted: 15 October 2020; Published: 18 October 2020

Abstract: Background: Although many of the movements of skiers are asymmetric, little is presently known about how such asymmetry influences performance. Here, our aim was to examine whether asymmetries in technique and the ground reaction forces associated with left and right turns influence the asymmetries in the performance of elite slalom skiers. Methods: As nine elite skiers completed a 20-gate slalom course, their three-dimensional full-body kinematics and ground reaction forces (GRF) were monitored with a global navigation satellite and inertial motion capture systems, in combination with pressure insoles. For multivariable regression models, 26 predictor skiing techniques and GRF variables and 8 predicted skiing performance variables were assessed, all of them determining asymmetries in terms of symmetry and Jaccard indices. Results: Asymmetries in instantaneous and sectional performance were found to have the largest predictor coefficients associated with asymmetries in shank angle and hip flexion of the outside leg. Asymmetry for turn radius had the largest predictor coefficients associated with asymmetries in shank angle and GRF on the entire outside foot. Conclusions: Although slalom skiers were found to move their bodies in a quite symmetrical fashion, asymmetry in their skiing technique and GRF influenced variables related to asymmetries in performance.

Keywords: biomechanics; kinematics; kinetics; global navigation satellite system; GPS; IMU; inertial motion capture; pressure insoles; ski racing

1. Introduction

In connection with highly competitive elite alpine skiing, differences in finishing time are often very small [1]. Indeed, the overall finishing time is a major factor in determining a skier's FIS (International Ski Federation) ranking and it is therefore hardly surprising that analysis of gate-to-gate times has focused on determining where a skier loses or gains time in as much detail as possible [2,3]. However, although easy for coaches and athletes to understand [4], times on short sections of a course, such as from gate-to-gate, are not good direct indicators of either instantaneous or turning performance [5]. In this context, variables related to the dissipation of mechanical energy reflect kinetic performance more closely [5–7] and kinematic parameters related to the trajectory of the skis are also more reliable [8,9].

Although numerous descriptions of alpine skiing technique have been published, relatively little is yet known about the biomechanical factors that influence competitive performance [6]. One such factor is the start strategy, including the technique utilized and number of start-pushes [10]. Furthermore, the slalom skiing technique chosen exerts an impact on both ground reaction forces (GRF) and performance [11–13].

Thus, in the case of slalom, the larger the "attack angle" (i.e., the angle between the orientation of the skis and direction of skiing) when entering a turn, the more energy is dissipated [14], whereas with giant slalom, the choice of trajectory and smoothness of skiing during a turn are also major influences on energy loss and performance [7–9]. Furthermore, use of a more "dynamic" body posture reduces energy loss due to aerodynamic drag [15], although this is not a major determinant of the performance of elite giant slalom skiers [16]. Air drag is more important in super-G skiing and even more so when skiing downhill [17]. When skiing straight, the movement of the center of mass forwards and backwards does not affect skiing time, whereas the edge angle does [18].

Although the body movements of athletes, and especially those of left and right turns by elite alpine skiers, are often asymmetric, little is presently known about how these asymmetries influence performance [19]. Bell [20] and Hoffman [21] and co-workers have shown that asymmetries affect jump height, while Beck and colleagues [22] found that asymmetries in stride while running result in more consumption of energy. Although ski coaches are often concerned with eliminating such asymmetries (i.e., correcting "mistakes" made when performing the "worse" turn), to our knowledge, with respect to alpine skiing, only preferential usage of one of the legs is known to affect turning and the potential impact of asymmetry on overall performance remains to be determined [23].

Accordingly, our aim here was to examine whether asymmetries in technique and in the ground reaction forces associated with left and right turns influence the competitive performance of elite slalom skiers. Our hypothesis was that asymmetries in the performance of elite slalom skiers are influenced by asymmetries in their technique and in ground reaction forces.

2. Materials and Methods

2.1. Participants

Nine male slalom skiers, all members of the Swedish National Ski Team (age: 22.7 ± 3.4 y; height: 181.8 ± 6.9 cm; weight: 82.2 ± 5.6 kg; current SL FIS points: 24.9 ± 18.6 (means ± SD)), provided their written informed consent before participating in this study, which was conducted in accordance with the Declaration of Helsinki and pre-approved by the National Medical Ethics Committee (Approval ID: 0120-99/2018/5, Project ID: L5-1845).

2.2. Experimental Setup

Starting twice from the left and twice from the right side, in randomized order, each skier performed four runs on a corridor-shaped slalom course with 20 gates placed symmetrically at 12-m intervals and with a displacement of 4 m (Figure 1). To ensure that this course was set precisely, the gates were positioned using the Leica Geodetic Global Satellite Navigation System (GNSS) 1200 with its built-in Stake-Out application (Leica Geosystems AG, Heerbrugg, Switzerland). The terrain selected had an average incline of 16°, with a maximal tilt to either side of <1°, and was groomed on each day of testing. In light of the hard, icy snow and temperatures between −2 and 0 °C, the coaches and experimental team smoothed the course prior to each and every run in an attempt to standardize conditions for side-skidding.

As described previously [24,25], three-dimensional whole-body kinematics were monitored utilizing the MVN Biomech V2018 inertial system (Xsens Technologies B.V., Enschede, The Netherlands) and Leica Zeno GG04 plus Real-Time Kinematics RTK GNSS (Leica Geosystems AG, Heerbrugg, Switzerland). The inertial system (calibrated twice prior to each run) was worn under the skier's racing suit and the smart antenna (RTK GNSS) was integrated into the back protector and positioned at shoulder height to allow unobstructed satellite reception (Figure 2). Data collected by the inertial system were recorded on a memory card, while data from the GNSS RTK system were transmitted wirelessly to a handheld device (Conker NS6, Conker, Takeley, England). In connection with each measurement, the precise position of the smart antenna relative to the thoracic (T12) and cervical vertebrae (C7) was determined to allow reliable integration of these two sets of data.

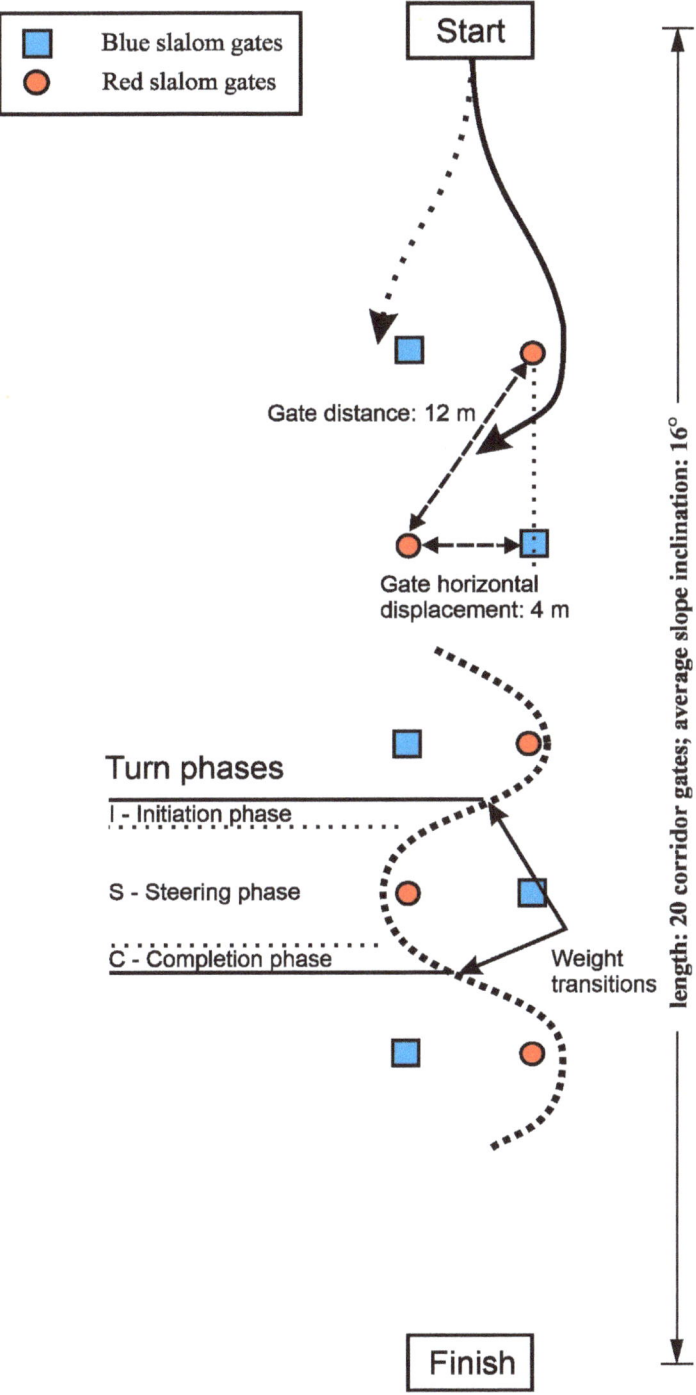

Figure 1. Schematic illustration of the corridor-shaped slalom course.

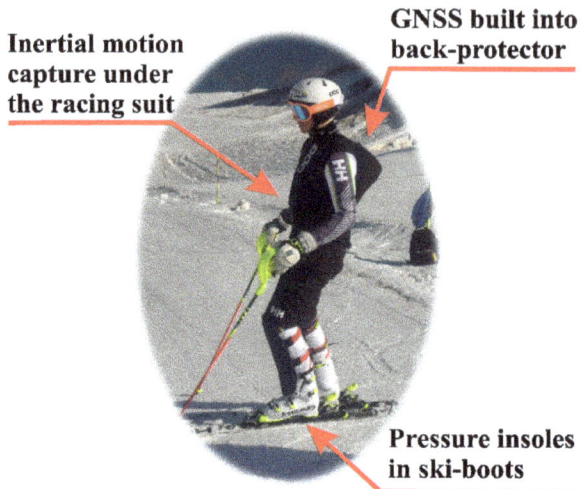

Figure 2. Equipment of the slalom skier with the global navigation satellite and inertial motion capture systems and pressure insoles.

In addition, the skier's boots were equipped with pressure insoles (Loadsol, Novel GmbH, Munich, Germany) that assessed the total ground reaction force acting perpendicular to the sole of the ski boot, the individual forces acting on the entire inside and outside foot and the distribution of force between the fore and rear foot. To assist analysis, all runs were also filmed at 50 Hz with a high-resolution camera (GC-PX100, The Japan Victor Company Ltd., Yokohama, Japan). To allow synchronization of all measurements, each skier performed three active squats and three hits with one of his skis on the ground before each start.

2.3. Computation

To match the frequency of the inertial system, the RTK GNSS system's captured trajectories at 20 Hz and the force measurements at 100 Hz were interpolated with cubic splines to 240 Hz. Following synchronization of the data collected by these three systems, these data were smoothed with the Rauch–Tung–Striebel algorithm [26], which utilizes a zero-lag two-way Kalman filter, in a manner similar to an earlier study [24]. The local coordinates provided by the inertial system were thereafter transformed into the global coordinates employed for RTK GNSS measurements by adding an extra node to the position of the RTK GNSS smart antenna. The data were subsequently transferred from Matlab R2016b (Mathworks, Natick, MA, USA) to the Visual 3D v6 software (C-Motion, Germantown, MD, USA), where the skier's center of mass (CoM) and the trajectory of the skis were calculated. The CoM was calculated utilizing Demster's regression equations [27], with inclusion of the mass of both the skiing and measuring equipment. The trajectory of the skis was defined as the arithmetic mean of the trajectories of the ankle joints [11].

The distance travelled and turn radius [7] were determined from the trajectory of the skis. From the trajectory of the CoM, the differential specific mechanical energy (i.e., the change in mechanical energy per unit change in altitude, normalized to the mass of the skier) [7] and mechanical energy for each specific section (normalized to the entrance speed) [5], which reflect instantaneous and sectional performance, respectively, were calculated. The definitions of both of these performance parameters mean that their values are negative when energy is dissipated. The flexion angles of the knee and hip joints on the left and right legs were provided directly by the inertial system. The angles of the inside and outside shanks, defined as the minimal tilt of the shank around the axis defined by the ski in relationship to the surface of the slope (Figure 3), were also calculated. Each turn was divided into initiation, steering and completion phases, as described previously [11] (Figure 1). To examine for temporal asymmetries, the left and right turning times were compared.

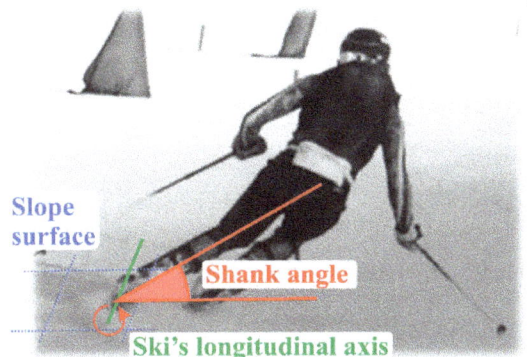

Figure 3. Photograph of a skier illustrating the angle of the shank.

Asymmetry between the left (L) and right (R) sides was expressed as the index SI = 1 − (|L − R|)/(L + R), where L and D represent the average values of parameters during the steering phase of the turn, with the exceptions of turn length, time, speed and sectional energy loss, which were determined for the entire turn. As an indicator of overall (as opposed to average) asymmetries throughout the entire turn, the Jaccard index (JI) [28] was also calculated. To obtain this index, the mean value and standard deviation of each parameter at each % of the turn were calculated. Then, the two curves obtained by adding or subtracting the standard deviation to the mean value were taken to represent the upper and lower boundaries, respectively, of the polygon delineating the turn. Thereafter, the overall JI was calculated as (A∩B)/(A∪B), where A and B represent the polygons associated with the left and right turns, respectively. In practice, when JI is equal to 1, the areas defined by the mean ± standard deviation boundaries for the left and right turns overlap entirely, whereas when JI is equal to zero, there is no overlap at all.

2.4. Statistical Analyses

All data are presented as mean values and standard deviations. The Shapiro–Wilk test was used to assess normality. Outliers detected employing standard Tukey's fences (1.5 interquartile range) were excluded from further analysis. A paired sample t-test was used for post hoc analysis of potential differences. In connection with the multivariable linear regression models, no more than two predictive (independent) variables were allowed. The dependent (predicted) variables were based on the objectives of the study related to performance (SI for turn time, turn length and average speed, and SI and JI for energy losses), while the independent (predictor) variables were related to skiing technique (SI and JI for the angles of flexion and inclination) and load (SI and JI for ground reaction forces). In connection with the multivariable linear regression models, no more than two predictive (independent) variables related to skiing technique (SI and JI for the angles of flexion and inclination) and load (SI and JI for ground reaction forces) were allowed, while the dependent (predicted) variables were related to performance (SI for turn time, turn length and average speed, and SI and JI for energy losses). All predictions in which G * Power (Faul et al., 2009, Heinrich University Heine Düsseldorf, Germany) was less than 0.8 were excluded. The level of statistical significance was set at $p < 0.05$. All statistical analyses were performed in the Matlab software.

3. Results

3.1. Descriptive Statistics, Symmetry and Jaccard Indices (SI and JI)

The descriptive statistics and symmetry indices for the independent variables (skiing technique and ground reaction forces) and dependent variables (skiing performance) during skiing are presented in Tables 1 and 2, respectively. In most cases, the differences in the independent variables during left and right turns were statistically insignificant (Table 1), the exception being GRF on the entire inside foot ($p < 0.05$). The mean symmetry indices (SI) for the independent variables related to skiing technique ranged from approximately 92 to 98%, with associated Jaccard indices (JI) during the steering phase ranging from approximately 29 to 53%. The corresponding values for the independent variables related to GRF ranged from approximately 85 to 98% and approximately 42 to 71%, respectively.

Table 1. The inclination, flexion of the joints and ground reaction forces (GRF) acting on various parts of the legs during the steering phase of left and right turns by elite slalom skiers, together with the corresponding symmetry (SI) and Jaccard (JI) indices (independent variables). All values presented are means ± standard deviations.

Variable	Left Turn	Right Turn	p-Value	SI [%]	JI [%]
Shank angle [°]					
Outside leg	30.8 ± 4.5	29.4 ± 4.6	0.49	93.8 ± 5.4	52.2 ± 19.5
Inside leg	33.2 ± 3.8	34.2 ± 2.4	0.84	92.8 ± 4.0	41.5 ± 16.2
Knee flexion [°]					
Outside leg	46.99 ± 8.9	52.20 ± 7.2	0.11	92.5 ± 4.4	28.7 ± 24.3
Inside leg	85.73 ± 9.3	81.25 ± 9.9	0.34	96.1 ± 2.2	39.1 ± 21.7
Hip flexion [°]					
Outside leg	37.4 ± 3.3	28.02 ± 3.0	0.70	95.71 ± 2.2	53.35 ± 14.9
Inside leg	71.8 ± 4.4	68.79 ± 5.5	0.22	97.52 ± 1.7	50.64 ± 15.5
GRF (pressure insoles) [% BW]					
On the entire foot					
Outside leg	126.2 ± 19.2	113.6 ± 21.6	0.21	92.9 ± 4.7	56.1 ± 18.9
Inside leg	66.8 ± 7.4	76.0 ± 10.0	0.04	91.4 ± 5.7	56.0 ± 19.6
On the fore foot [% BW]					
Outside leg	62.5 ± 20.6	58.7 ± 26.85	0.75	88.4 ± 8.4	47.2 ± 21.6
Inside leg	27.4 ± 9.2	37.8 ± 17.6	0.14	85.1 ± 10.1	42.7 ± 23.2
On the rear foot [% BW]					
Outside leg	63.8 ± 7.7	54.9 ± 16.6	0.17	87.8 ± 7.3	51.6 ± 14.4
Inside leg	39.4 ± 9.13	38.6 ± 15.8	0.85	85.8 ± 15.2	52.9 ± 23.2
GRF *					
Overall [% BW]	287.5 ± 26.3	283.7 ± 17.5	0.72	98.2 ± 1.1	71.3 ± 2.7

BW—body weight; SI—symmetry index; JI—Jaccard index; * approximated on the basis of the movement of the center of mass.

Moreover, none of the values for the dependent variables reflecting skiing performance differed significantly between the left and the right turns (Table 2). The mean SI for the dependent variables ranged from approximately 71% (in the case of instantaneous performance) to approximately 100% (average velocity). The nature of the parameters involved allowed the JI values to be calculated only for the turning radius and instantaneous performance during the steering phase as approximately 56% and 47%, respectively.

The patterns of the angle of the outside shank of all nine skiers during left and right turns, together with the corresponding JI during the steering phase (ranging from 14% for Skier I to 87% for Skier G), are shown in Figure 4. As depicted in the diagram, the mean angle of the outside shank during left and right turns differed during the entire steering phase for Skiers H and I, during the second half of the steering phase for Skiers B, D and E and during the first half of this phase in the case of Skier A. In contrast, the mean angle of the outside shank of Skier G was largely the same throughout the entire steering phase. With respect to the mean turning radius of left and right turns, most of the skiers demonstrated visible differences during the second half of the steering phase, with Skier G again being the exception (Figure 5). Moreover, the JI of 81% for the turning radius of Skier G was the largest observed, while the smallest JI of 56% in this regard was demonstrated by Skier C. Visually larger differences were observed between left and right turn instantaneous performance (Figure 6) with the JI ranging from 31% (Skier I) to 78% (Skier G).

Table 2. The time, trajectory, velocity and energy dissipation during left and right turns by elite slalom skiers, together with the corresponding symmetry (SI) and Jaccard indices (JI) (dependent variables). All values presented are means ± standard deviations.

Dependent Variable	Left Turn	Right Turn	p-Value	SI [%]	JI [%]
Time					
Turning time [s]	0.87 ± 0.03	0.87 ± 0.03	0.68	97.5 ± 1.7	n/a
Trajectory					
Turning length [m]	12.61 ± 0.30	12.51 ± 0.39	0.59	97.9 ± 1.5	n/a
Turning radius [m]	9.34 ± 0.44	9.32 ± 0.52	0.95	97.6 ± 1.5	56.1 ± 18.9
Velocity					
Average velocity [m/s]	14.5 ± 0.42	14.5 ± 0.37	0.97	99.6 ± 0.00	n/a
Energy associated with					
Instantaneous performance [J/kg/m]	−10.69 ± 4.67	−10.51 ± 2.98	0.92	70.6 ± 23.0	47.3 ± 14.1
Sectional performance [Js/kg/m]	−1.90 ± 0.39	−1.87 ± 0.50	0.91	84.2 ± 13.7	n/a

n/a—not applicable; SI—symmetry index; JI—Jaccard index.

3.2. Multivariable Regression Models

Altogether, our multivariable linear regression models, each involving no more than two predictor (independent) variables, included a total of 26 predictor and 8 predicted (dependent) variables. Models were discarded if the p-value was >0.05, R^2 < 0.7 or when the model's predictor coefficients did not differ significantly from 0 (t-statistic, $p < 0.05$). In addition, to restrict our analysis to results that could be meaningful, only the 13 models for which at least one of the predictor coefficient values was >0.1 are shown in Table 3. Of these, all included two independent variables, with the exception of Model #10, which only included one.

The largest predictor coefficients were associated with the SI values for instantaneous (differential specific mechanical energy) and sectional performance (mechanical energy for each specific section/turn normalized to the entrance speed) (Models #10–13, Table 3). The independent variables in Models #10 and 12 were related only to skiing technique, while those in Models #11 and 13 were related to skiing technique in combination with GRF. The remainder of the models had smaller predictive coefficients of 0.46 (Model #5) or lower, among which the coefficients for SI and JI for turning radius were largest (Models #4 and 5). Interestingly, the largest predictive coefficients obtained with Models #6–9, designed to predict the SI for average velocity, all corresponded to the SI for overall GRF.

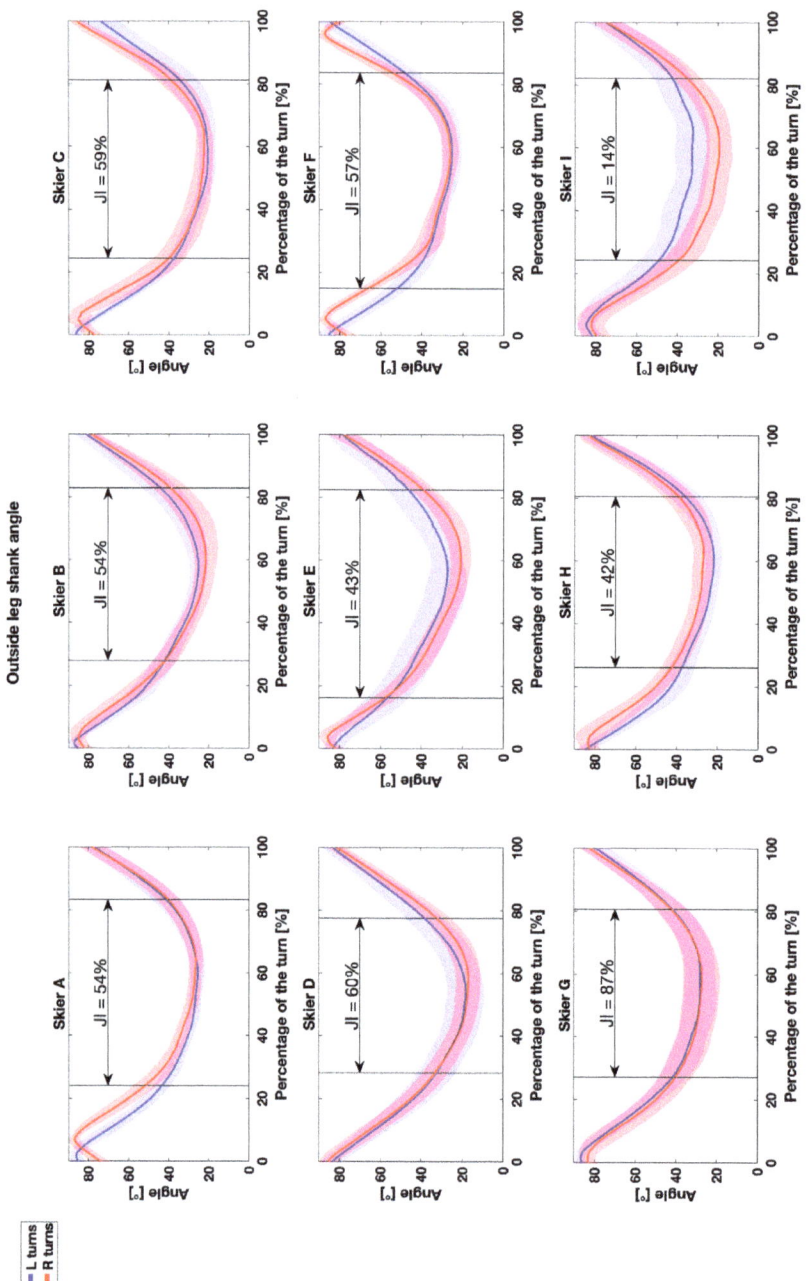

Figure 4. The angle of the outside shank of the 9 elite slalom skiers (A–I) during the steering phase of left and right turns, together with the corresponding Jaccard indices (JI). The two vertical lines indicate the beginning and end of the steering phase.

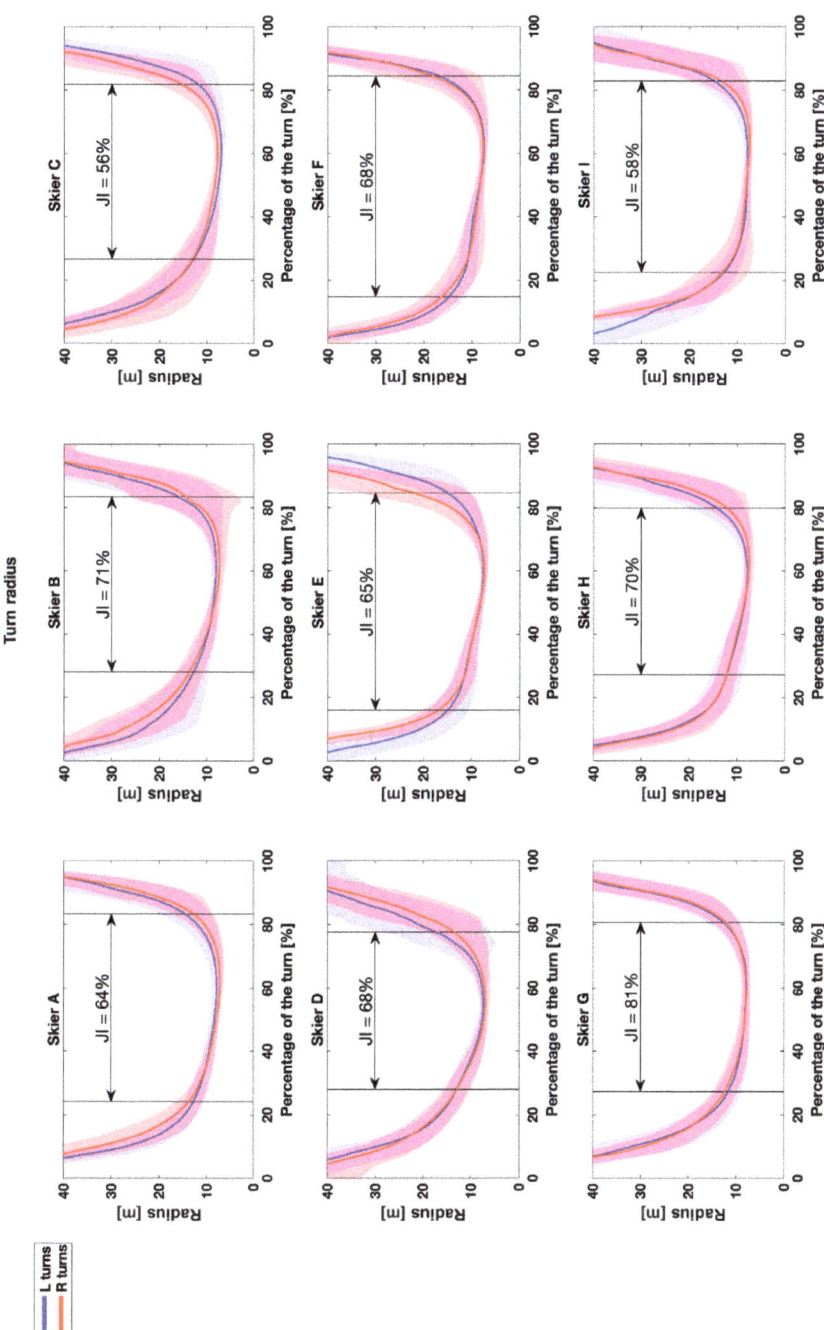

Figure 5. The turn radii during the steering phase of left and right turns by 9 elite slalom skiers (A–I) and corresponding Jaccard indices (JI). The two vertical lines indicate the beginning and end of the steering phase.

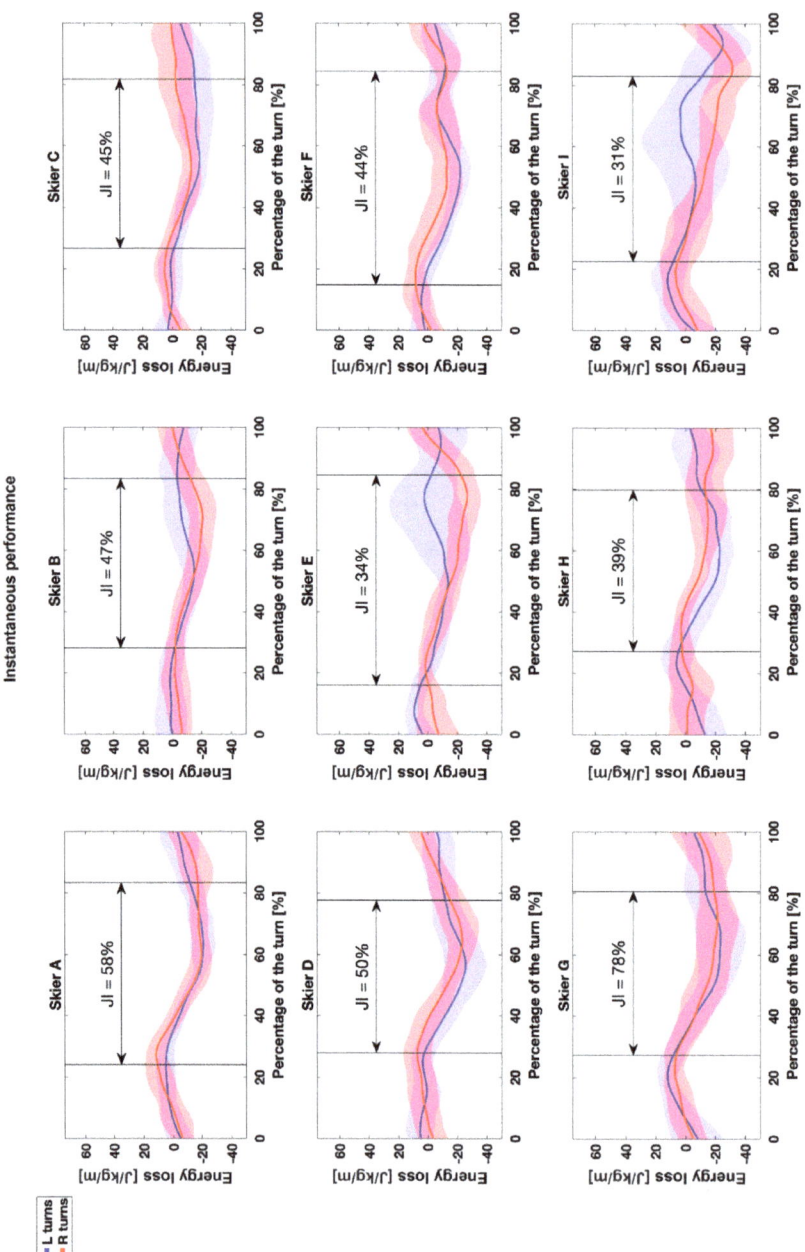

Figure 6. The instantaneous performance during the steering phase of left and right turns by 9 elite slalom skiers (**A–I**) and corresponding Jaccard indices (JI). The two vertical lines indicate the beginning and end of the steering phase. Instantaneous performance is defined as energy dissipation per change in altitude normalized relative to the mass of the skier and his equipment.

Table 3. Multivariable linear regression analysis of the relationships between the predicted (dependent, columns) and predictor (independent, rows) variables. The values in each column represent the coefficients of predictor variables.

Dependent Variables → Independent Variables ↓	SI for Turning Time	SI for Turning Length	JI for Turning Radius	SI for Turning Radius	SI for Average Velocity	SI for Instantaneous Performance	SI for Sectional Performance
Shank angle							
JI for outside leg	-	-	0.33 **,#4	-	-	-	-
SI for outside leg	0.08 *,#1	-	-	-	-	3.97 ***,#10	3.01 **,#13
JI for inside leg	-	0.07 **,#2	-	-	-	-	-
SI for inside leg	-	-	-	-	-	5.77 **,#11, 7.16 **,#12	-
Hip flexion							
JI for outside leg	-	-	-	−0.10 *,#5	0.01 *,#6	-	-
SI for outside leg	-	-	-	-	0.09 *,#7	8.33 *,#12	-
GRF on entire foot [a]							
JI for GRF outside leg	-	-	0.25 *,#4	0.46 **,#5	-	-	-
SI for GRF outside leg	-	-	-	-	-	-	-
SI for GRF inside leg	0.14 *,#1	0.13 **,#2, 0.11 *,#3	-	-	-	-	-
JI for GRF inside leg	-	-	-	-	−0.02 **,#8	-	-
GRF on rear foot [a]							
JI for outside leg	-	-	-	-	−0.03 **,#9	-	-
SI for GRF outside leg	-	-	-	-	-	-	-
Overall GRF [b]							
JI	-	-	-	-	0.10 **,#6, 0.12 **,#7, 0.15 ***,#8, 0.16 **,#9	-	-
SI	-	0.16 *,#3	-	-	-	−1.03 **,#11	0.56 *,#13
R^2	0.72 *,#1	0.80 **,#2, 0.75 *,#3	0.80 **,#4	0.74 *,#5	0.73 *,#6, 0.81 **,#7, 0.84 **,#8, 0.83 **,#9	0.86 ***,#10, 0.82 **,#11, 0.84 **,#12	0.76 **,#13

*—$p \leq 0.05$, **—$p \leq 0.01$, ***—$p \leq 0.001$; #—multivariable regression model number; GRF—ground reaction force; SI—symmetry index, JI—Jaccard index; [a] determined by pressure insoles; [b] approximated on the basis of the movements of the center of mass.

4. Discussion

The major novel finding here was confirmation of the hypothesis that asymmetries in technique and ground reaction forces are associated with asymmetries in the performance of elite, competitive slalom skiers. More specifically, (i) asymmetries in instantaneous and sectional performance were associated with the largest predictor coefficients for asymmetry in the angle of the shank and hip flexion on the outside leg; and (ii) asymmetry in turning radius demonstrated the largest predictor coefficients for asymmetry in the angle of the shank and GRF on the entire foot of the outside leg.

Our descriptive statistics showed that, on average, these elite alpine skiers performed left and right turns quite symmetrically (Tables 1 and 2), with the only statistically significant difference between these turns being the GRF on the entire foot of the inside leg. In particular, the average mean values for performance were almost identical for the left and right turns (Table 2). Furthermore, the symmetrical indices (SI) were all above 84% (sectional performance), except for instantaneous performance (70%).

This symmetry, which in light of the very small differences in performance of elite alpine skiers [9,29,30] was not unexpected, confirmed that our experimental setup was well suited for observing differences between left and right turns. Previously, the differences in the GRF and temporal parameters associated with left and right slalom turns by highly skilled ski instructors were also reported to be non-significant [23]. Similarly, the mean difference in strength between the dominant and non-dominant legs of elite Austrian alpine skiers was also small [31].

In the present case, the only SI that was markedly lower concerned instantaneous performance (70.6%). Overall, sectional and instantaneous performance demonstrated the most pronounced asymmetries, which was the initial rationale for employing these as measures of alpine skiing performance [5,7,30]. In giant slalom as well, utilization of energy-based performance over an entire section was found to be a valuable measure of performance [9].

However, the Jaccard indices (JI) revealed much more pronounced asymmetry between left and right turns, with the lowest value being only 28.6% (for flexion of the outside knee) and the highest 71.3% (for the overall GRF) (Table 1). The lowest individual JI value for the angle of the outside shank was only 14% (Skier I, Figure 4) and during the steering phase, a difference between left and right turns by this skier was clearly visible. This same skier exhibited the lowest JI for instantaneous performance (Figure 6) and the second lowest for turning radius (Figure 5). At the same time for Skier G, the largest JI for the angle of the outside shank (Figure 4) was associated with the largest JI values for both turning radius (Figure 5) and instantaneous performance (Figure 6). The dependence of sectional and instantaneous performance on the SI for the angles of both the inside and outside shank received further support from the multivariable regression analysis (Models #10–13, Table 3). Similarly, the JI for turning radius proved to be dependent on the corresponding value for the angle of the outside shank (Model #4, Table 3), an observation which in itself clearly demonstrates that asymmetry in technique is associated with asymmetry in performance. Such a relationship is not entirely unexpected, since according to the theory of carving skiing, the inclination of the ski is related to turning radius [32] and, moreover, in the case of slalom skiing, turning radius is related to instantaneous performance [5].

The SI for turning radius was not dependent on the SI for the angle of the outside shank. This independence demonstrates that the mean turn values taken into consideration when calculating SI did not take the profound turn cycle information into account as was the case with JI values in Model #4 (Table 3). The SI for turning radius was negatively correlated with the JI for flexion of the outside hip (predictor coefficient −0.10, Model #5, Table 3). This negative association means that less pronounced asymmetry in flexion of the outside hip should correspond to more asymmetry in the turning radius, an observation that we were unable to explain at present.

The predictor coefficients for JI and SI for the GRF acting on the entire foot of the outside leg were also relatively large in connection with the JI and SI for the turning radius (Models #4 and 5, Table 3). This finding can be explained by the action of radial forces, whose basic biomechanical modeling has shown to be dependent on the turning radius [32,33]. In this context, it is important to emphasize that only the GRF acting on the outside leg, not the overall GRF, was a predictor in the multivariable models. Indeed, in a previous study [5], this overall GRF did not differ between better and poorer slalom skiers. However, in the present investigation, the SI for average velocity was dependent on the corresponding value for the overall GRF in combination with several other "less important" variables with small predictor coefficients (Models #6–9, Table 3). This particularly interesting finding reveals that despite the virtually identical average velocity and overall GRF associated with left and right turns by our elite skiers, the asymmetries in these variables were actually large enough to demonstrate related dependency in the multivariable models (Tables 1 and 2).

The largest predictor coefficients observed in our multivariable models concerned the dependence of the SI for instantaneous performance on the combination of the SI values for the angle of the inside shank and flexion of the outside hip (Model #12, Table 3). The only apparent explanation for this dependency is the speculation that skiing technique influenced how smoothly the skis glide, (e.g., the attack angle defined as the angle between the longitudinal axis of the ski and the ski's center point's velocity vector projected onto a plane parallel to the surface of the snow) [14]) and/or the distribution of pressure under the ski and thereby the ski–snow interaction [34]. Either or both of these influences could exert an impact on energy dissipation.

Finally, some of the symmetry indices (SI) observed here, such as those for turning time, turn length and sectional performance, were dependent on various parameters related to the asymmetry of the inside leg (Models #1–3 and 13). This indicates that asymmetries in performance were also associated with the behavior of the inside leg, which has earlier been suggested to only play a role in maintaining stability while skiing [35]. Ski coaches already pay special attention to the inside leg in connection with training to optimize performance, but our findings provide the first experimental evidence that this is a valid concern.

Although the current investigation was extensive, assessing the full-body three-dimensional kinematics and GRF in connection with 720 slalom turns, like all studies, has certain limitations. Although some researchers question the reliability of inertial measurement systems and GNSS and/or pressure insoles, their reliability for in-field measurements on alpine skiers has already been demonstrated [23–25,35–39] and, moreover, we utilized state-of-the-art technology in this respect, i.e., one of the most up-to-date and accurate Leica Geosystems RTK GNSS systems and the latest version of the Xsens inertial motion capture hardware. However, since it was not possible to install an inertial sensor on a foot in a ski boot, we were unable to monitor flexion of the ankle joint. It would have been possible to measure bending of the ski boot, but this does not entirely reflect the more complicated three-dimensional behavior of the ankle joint (i.e., technique).

In addition, although GRF can certainly be measured most accurately with dynamometers/force-plates [40], the size and weight of these devices disturb the skiing equipment and, thereby, the performance of the skier. To avoid this, we used pressure insoles here, which do not always indicate the magnitude of GRF accurately [41]. On the other hand, direct measurement of the pressure on the soles, an important parameter when skiing [23,35], is especially useful for dealing with asymmetries in pressure on different parts of the foot. To assess a more precise magnitude of the GRF, we performed biomechanical modeling of this parameter based on the acceleration of the center of mass monitored by three-dimensional kinematics, as in our previous studies [11,42].

As is true of virtually all studies on alpine skiing, generalization of our present results, despite the relatively large size of our study population, is not straightforward. The snow, terrain and weather were nearly ideal during our testing and similar studies under varying conditions are now required.

5. Conclusions

In conclusion, the application of descriptive statistical analysis to left and right turns by elite slalom skiers revealed that with respect to technique, ground reaction forces and performance, these turns were quite symmetrical, with the only significant difference being related to the mean GRF on the entire inside foot. Furthermore, all symmetry indices for skiing technique and performance were >92%, with the exception of those for instantaneous (70.6%) and sectional performance (84.2%), demonstrating the relevance of these latter two parameters in connection with the analysis of skiing asymmetry. The Jaccard index, which takes into account behavior within the turn cycle, was found to be more sensitive to asymmetries than the symmetry index, which is based solely on the mean values of the parameters. Although the movements of elite slalom skiers were found to be quite symmetrical, this is the first demonstration that asymmetry in their skiing technique and ground reaction forces influences asymmetry in their performance. These findings constitute experimental support for the efforts of coaches to achieve symmetrical skiing technique, not only in order to decrease the risk of injury [31], but also to optimize overall performance.

Author Contributions: Conceptualization, M.S. and H.-C.H.; methodology, M.S. and J.O.; formal analysis, J.O. and M.S.; data collection and handling, M.S. and J.O.; writing—preparation of the first draft, M.S.; writing—review and editing, all authors; visualization, J.O. and M.S.; supervision, M.S.; project administration, M.S.; funding acquisition, H.-C.H. and N.Š. All authors have read and agreed to the published version of the manuscript.

Funding: This research was funded by the European Union's Horizon 2020 research and innovation programme (No 824984) and the Slovenian Research Agency (L5-1845 & P5-0147)

Acknowledgments: The authors would like to sincerely thank all the skiers and their coaches for their helpful cooperation. Many thanks also to Alessandro Galloppini and Mads Kjær Madsen Mads for their help with the data collection and to Uwe Kersting for performing inertial motion capture.

Conflicts of Interest: The authors have no conflict of interest to declare.

References

1. Supej, M.; Cernigoj, M. Relations between different technical and tactical approaches and overall time at men's world cup giant slalom races. *Kinesiol. Slov.* **2006**, *12*, 63–69.
2. Supej, M.; Holmberg, H.C. A new time measurement method using a high-end global navigation satellite system to analyze alpine skiing. *Res. Q. Exerc. Sport* **2011**, *82*, 400–411. [CrossRef] [PubMed]
3. Fasel, B.; Spörri, J.; Kröll, J.; Müller, E.; Aminian, K. A Magnet-Based Timing Tystem to Detect Gate Crossings in Alpine Ski Racing. *Sensors* **2019**, *19*, 940. [CrossRef]
4. Supej, M. Gate-to-Gate Synchronized Comparison of Velocity Retrieved from a High-End Global Navigation Satellite System in Alpine Skiing. In Proceedings of the 28th International Conference on Biomechanics in Sports, Melbourne, Australia, 2–6 July 2012.
5. Supej, M.; Kipp, R.; Holmberg, H.C. Mechanical parameters as predictors of performance in alpine World Cup slalom racing. *Scand. J. Med. Sci. Sports* **2011**, *21*, e72–e81. [CrossRef] [PubMed]
6. Hébert-Losier, K.; Supej, M.; Holmberg, H.C. Biomechanical factors influencing the performance of elite alpine ski racers. *Sports Med.* **2014**, *44*, 519–533. [CrossRef] [PubMed]
7. Supej, M. Differential specific mechanical energy as a quality parameter in racing alpine skiing. *J. Appl. Biomech.* **2008**, *24*, 121–129. [CrossRef]
8. Federolf, P.A. Quantifying instantaneous performance in alpine ski racing. *J. Sports Sci.* **2012**, *30*, 1063–1068. [CrossRef] [PubMed]
9. Spörri, J.; Kröll, J.; Schwameder, H.; Müller, E. The role of path length- and speed-related factors for the enhancement of section performance in alpine giant slalom. *Eur. J. Sport Sci.* **2018**, *18*, 911–919. [CrossRef]
10. Supej, M.; Nedergaard, N.J.; Nord, J.; Holmberg, H.C. The impact of start strategy on start performance in alpine skiing exists on flat, but not on steep inclines. *J. Sports Sci.* **2019**, *37*, 647–655. [CrossRef]
11. Supej, M.; Holmberg, H.C. How gate setup and turn radii influence energy dissipation in slalom ski racing. *J. Appl. Biomech.* **2010**, *26*, 454–464. [CrossRef]
12. Supej, M.; Kugovnik, O.; Nemec, B. New advances in racing slalom technique. *Kinesiol. Slov.* **2002**, *8*, 25–29.
13. Supej, M.; Kugovnik, O.; Nemec, B. Modelling and simulation of two competition slalom techniques. *Kinesiology* **2004**, *36*, 206–212.
14. Reid, R.C.; Haugen, P.; Gilgien, M.; Kipp, R.W.; Smith, G.A. Alpine Ski Motion Characteristics in Slalom. *Front. Sports Act. Living* **2020**, *2*. [CrossRef]
15. Meyer, F.; Le Pelley, D.; Borrani, F. Aerodynamic drag modeling of alpine skiers performing giant slalom turns. *Med. Sci. Sports Exerc.* **2012**, *44*, 1109–1115. [CrossRef]

16. Supej, M.; Sætran, L.; Oggiano, L.; Ettema, G.; Šarabon, N.; Nemec, B.; Holmberg, H.C. Aerodynamic drag is not the major determinant of performance during giant slalom skiing at the elite level. *Scand. J. Med. Sci. Sports* **2013**, *23*, e38–e47. [CrossRef]
17. Gilgien, M.; Kröll, J.; Spörri, J.; Crivelli, P.; Müller, E. Application of dGNSS in alpine ski racing: Basis for evaluating physical demands and safety. *Front. Physiol.* **2018**, *9*, 145. [CrossRef]
18. Federolf, P.; Scheiber, P.; Rauscher, E.; Schwameder, H.; Lüthi, A.; Rhyner, H.U.; Müller, E. Impact of skier actions on the gliding times in alpine skiing. *Scand. J. Med. Sci. Sports* **2008**, *18*, 790–797. [CrossRef] [PubMed]
19. Maloney, S.J. The Relationship Between Asymmetry and Athletic Performance: A Critical Review. *J. Strength Cond. Res.* **2019**, *33*, 2579–2593. [CrossRef]
20. Bell, D.R.; Sanfilippo, J.L.; Binkley, N.; Heiderscheit, B.C. Lean mass asymmetry influences force and power asymmetry during jumping in collegiate athletes. *J. Strength Cond. Res.* **2014**, *28*, 884–891. [CrossRef]
21. Hoffman, J.R.; Ratamess, N.A.; Klatt, M.; Faigenbaum, A.D.; Kang, J. Do bilateral power deficits influence direction-specific movement patterns? *Res. Sports Med.* **2007**, *15*, 125–132. [CrossRef]
22. Beck, O.N.; Azua, E.N.; Grabowski, A.M. Step time asymmetry increases metabolic energy expenditure during running. *Eur. J. Appl. Physiol.* **2018**, *118*, 2147–2154. [CrossRef]
23. Vaverka, F.; Vodickova, S. Laterality of the lower limbs and carving turn. *Biol.Sport* **2010**, *27*, 129–134. [CrossRef]
24. Supej, M. 3D measurements of alpine skiing with an inertial sensor motion capture suit and GNSS RTK system. *J. Sports Sci.* **2010**, *28*, 759–769. [CrossRef]
25. Krüger, A.; Edelmann-Nusser, J. Application of a full body inertial measurement system in alpine skiing: A comparison with an optical video based system. *J. Appl. Biomech.* **2010**, *26*, 516–521. [CrossRef]
26. Rauch, H.E.; Tung, F.; Striebel, C.T. Maximum likelihood estimates of linear dynamic systems. *AIAA J.* **1965**, *3*, 1445–1450. [CrossRef]
27. Dempster, W.T. *Space Requirements of the Seated Operator: Geometrical, Kinematic, and Mechanical Aspects of the Body with Special Reference to the Limbs*; Wright Air Development Center: Wright-Patterson Air Force Base, OH, USA, 1955.
28. Jaccard, P. Distribution florale dans une portio des Alpes du Jura. *Bull. Soc. Vaud. Sc. Nat.* **1901**, *37*, 547–579. [CrossRef]
29. Gilgien, M.; Reid, R.; Raschner, C.; Supej, M.; Holmberg, H.C. The Training of Olympic Alpine Ski Racers. *Front. Physiol.* **2018**, *9*, 1772. [CrossRef]
30. Supej, M.; Holmberg, H.C. Recent Kinematic and Kinetic Advances in Olympic Alpine Skiing: Pyeongchang and Beyond. *Front. Physiol.* **2019**, *10*, 111. [CrossRef]
31. Steidl-Muller, L.; Hildebrandt, C.; Muller, E.; Fink, C.; Raschner, C. Limb symmetry index in competitive alpine ski racers: Reference values and injury risk identification according to age-related performance levels. *J. Sport Health Sci.* **2018**, *7*, 405–415. [CrossRef] [PubMed]
32. Howe, J. *The New Skiing Mechanics: Including the Technology of Short Radius Carved Turn Skiing and the Claw Ski*; McIntire: Waterford, Ireland, 2001.
33. Lind, D.A.; Sanders, S.P. *The Physics of Skiing: Skiing at the Triple Point*; Springer: New York, NY, USA, 2013.
34. Federolf, P.; Roos, M.; Lüthi, A.; Dual, J. Finite element simulation of the ski–snow interaction of an alpine ski in a carved turn. *Sports Eng.* **2010**, *12*, 123–133. [CrossRef]
35. Falda-Buscaiot, T.; Hintzy, F.; Rougier, P.; Lacouture, P.; Coulmy, N. Influence of slope steepness, foot position and turn phase on plantar pressure distribution during giant slalom alpine ski racing. *PLoS ONE* **2017**, *12*, e0176975. [CrossRef]
36. Zorko, M.; Nemec, B.; Babic, J.; Lesnik, B.; Supej, M. The waist width of skis influences the kinematics of the knee joint in alpine skiing. *J. Sports Sci. Med.* **2015**, *14*, 606–619. [PubMed]
37. Spörri, J.; Kröll, J.; Fasel, B.; Aminian, K.; Müller, E. Course setting as a prevention measure for overuse injuries of the back in alpine ski racing: A kinematic and kinetic study of giant slalom and slalom. *Orthop. J. Sports Med.* **2016**, *4*, 2325967116630719. [CrossRef] [PubMed]
38. Spörri, J.; Kröll, J.; Fasel, B.; Aminian, K.; Müller, E. Standing Height as a Prevention Measure for Overuse Injuries of the Back in Alpine Ski Racing: A Kinematic and Kinetic Study of Giant Slalom. *Orthop. J. Sports Med.* **2018**, *6*, 2325967117747843. [CrossRef]
39. Spörri, J.; Kröll, J.; Haid, C.; Fasel, B.; Müller, E. Potential mechanisms leading to overuse injuries of the back in alpine ski racing: A descriptive biomechanical study. *Am. J. Sports Med.* **2015**, *43*, 2042–2048. [CrossRef]

40. Lüthi, A.; Federolf, M.; Fauve, M.; Oberhofer, K.; Rhyner, H.; Ammann, W.; Stricker, G.; Shiefermüller, C.; Eitzlmair, E.; Schwameder, H.; et al. Determination of forces in carving using three independent methods. In *Science and Skiing III*; Müller, E., Bacharach, D., Klika, R., Lindinger, S., Schwameder, H., Eds.; Meyer & Meyer Sport: Oxford, UK, 2005; pp. 96–106.
41. Stricker, G.; Scheiber, P.; Lindenhofer, E.; Müller, E. Determination of forces in alpine skiing and snowboarding: Validation of a mobile data acquisition system. *Eur. J. Sport Sci.* **2010**, *10*, 31–41. [CrossRef]
42. Supej, M.; Hébert-Losier, K.; Holmberg, H.C. Impact of the steepness of the slope on the biomechanics of World Cup slalom skiers. *Int. J. Sports Physiol. Perform.* **2015**, *10*, 361–368. [CrossRef]

Publisher's Note: MDPI stays neutral with regard to jurisdictional claims in published maps and institutional affiliations.

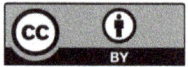

© 2020 by the authors. Licensee MDPI, Basel, Switzerland. This article is an open access article distributed under the terms and conditions of the Creative Commons Attribution (CC BY) license (http://creativecommons.org/licenses/by/4.0/).

Article

The Characteristics of Feet Center of Pressure Trajectory during Quiet Standing

Jacek Stodółka [1,*], Wieslaw Blach [2], Janez Vodicar [3] and Krzysztof Maćkała [1]

1 Department of Track and Field, University School of Physical Education, Wroclaw, Ul. Paderewskiego 35, 51-612 Wrocław, Poland; krzysztof.mackala@awf.wroc.pl
2 Department of Sport Didactics, University School of Physical Education in Wrocław, Wroclaw, Poland Ul. Paderewskiego 35, 51-612 Wrocław, Poland; wieslaw.blach@awf.wroc.pl
3 Faculty of Sport, University of Ljubljana, Gortanova ulica 22, 1000 Ljubljana, Slovenia; Janez.Vodicar@fsp.uni-lj.si
* Correspondence: jacek.stodolka@awf.wroc.pl; Tel.: +48-3473-147

Received: 1 April 2020; Accepted: 21 April 2020; Published: 23 April 2020

Abstract: To investigate the level of bilateral symmetry or asymmetry between right and left foot center of pressure (COP) trajectory in the mediolateral and anteroposterior directions, this study involved 102 participants (54 females and 48 males). Ground reaction forces were measured using two Kistler force plates during two 45-s quiet standing trials. Comparisons of COP trajectory were performed by correlation and scatter plot analysis. Strong and very strong positive correlations (from 0.6 to 1.0) were observed between right and left foot anteroposterior COP displacement trajectory in 91 participants; 11 individuals presented weak or negative correlations. In the mediolateral direction, moderate and strong negative correlations (from −0.5 to −1.0) were observed in 69 participants, weak negative or weak positive correlations in 30 individuals, and three showed strong positive correlations (0.6 to 1.0). Additional investigation is warranted to compare COP trajectories between asymptotic individuals as assessed herein (to determine normative data) and those with foot or leg symptoms to better understand the causes of COP asymmetry and aid clinicians with the diagnosis of posture-related pathologies.

Keywords: symmetry; asymmetry; foot; force; balance; postural stability; standing

---

1. Introduction

The force exerted by the body on the ground when standing is mirrored by a reaction force. The use of footwear during many activities of daily living not only provides a level of protection but also modifies the pressure distribution characteristics of the feet and, therefore, the forces that act on the foot. Depending on the type of footwear, these forces may be attenuated or "dampened". Additionally, the shape and construction of the sole, insole and heel may all modify the forces and load experienced by different foot regions [1–3].

From a mechanical perspective, balance preservation during upright standing is quite complex as the human body is never in a condition of perfect equilibrium and that balance must be maintained via two points of contact (both feet). The center of all external forces acting on the plantar surface of the foot is known as the center of pressure (COP). While providing a base of support, the feet can independently induce changes in COP trajectory in the coronal (anteroposterior direction) and sagittal (mediolateral direction) planes and, therefore, obfuscate right and left COP to create a condition of asymmetry. While COP displacement in the anteroposterior direction can be understood as bilaterally symmetrical when the trajectory (forward or backward) is concurrently equal between both feet, the level of bilateral symmetry in the mediolateral direction is far more problematic to measure. One possible method for assessing bilateral symmetry in mediolateral COP trajectory is by considering foot structure. Albeit an oversimplification, this paradigm allows us to treat COP displacement as symmetrical when left and right foot mediolateral COP both shift either to the inside or outside of the feet.

The literature is abound with studies investigating balance preservation during quiet standing primarily by analyzing COP-related variables. However, the vast majority is based on using a single force plate and thus measure the exerted force concurrently for both feet [4–10]. Few investigations have addressed the magnitude and distribution of force separately for the right and left foot with the use of more than one force platform. Although Soangra and Lockhart [11] and Brauer et al. [12] investigated the similarities and dissimilarities between right and left foot COP trajectories, no studies have yet addressed COP displacement in regards to the level of symmetry (or asymmetry) between the left and right foot. As COP has been identified as a measure of the neuromuscular response to maintain balance, differences in right and left foot COP trajectories can serve as a measure of sensorimotor control and function. In this way, the respective COP trajectories for either foot and the congruence between both points of application signify the ability of the central nervous system to integrate information from the sensory systems and then activate different postural muscles (exerting pressure at a specific foot region) so that upright stance is preserved.

While the foot can be assumed to hold two degrees of freedom relative to the lateral gastrocnemius (plantarflexion/dorsiflexion and inversion/eversion), COP displacement can independently shift not only in the anteroposterior and mediolateral directions but also combinations of the two, such as an anterior or posterior slant to either the medial or lateral side. If analyzed as a temporal series, this bivariate approach for each foot could help identify patterns in left and right foot COP trajectory. Knowledge of COP displacement between both feet across different population cohorts can help identify postural pathologies including foot deformities resulting from improper footwear or decreased neuromuscular control by some deficiency in central nervous system function.

Therefore, the purpose of the study was to define the incidence of right and left foot symmetry or asymmetry via displacement in COP trajectory by identifying what associations exist between left and right foot COP direction in an asymptomatic population. By knowing the value of the symmetry between left and right foot COP displacement, it could be possible to formulate criteria for evaluating postural balance during upright standing. We hypothesized that the temporal and spatial characteristics of right and left foot COP trajectories during upright stance would show little variability in a sample of healthy young adults.

2. Material and Methods

2.1. Subject

An age-homogeneous sample of 102 university students (54 females and 48 males) was recruited. Mean age was 21.08 ± 1.08 years, height 172.89 ± 9.56 cm and body mass 68.09 ± 13.12 kg. All individuals provided their written informed consent to participate in the study and ethical approval was obtained. All procedures were performed at a biomechanics research laboratory at the Opole University of Technology in Opole, Poland. The participants signed informed consent and were informed of the protocol and procedures for the experiment prior to the exercise. The study was approved by the Human Ethics Committee.

2.2. Ground Reaction Force (GRF) Measurement Procedure

The study protocol involved measuring ground reaction force during two 45-s trials of static standing. Ground reaction force (GRF) data were synchronously collected on two 600 × 400 mm piezoelectric force platforms (Kistler Type 9286B; Kistler Instruments AG, Winterthur, Switzerland) placed under each foot. Four tri-axial force sensors located in the corners of each platform quantified the ground reaction force signals at a sampling frequency of 50 Hz (measurement range was from 10 kN to 20 kN). The force platforms were calibrated before use and integrated with a base transceiver station (BTS) Smart optoelectronic system (BTS Bioengineering, USA) to register the force–time characteristics.

During signal acquisition, the participant was asked to assume a relaxed upright posture (minimizing head and trunk movements) with the upper extremities resting freely against the trunk and to fixate on a point placed at eye level 3 m from the subject. Only running shoes were allowed, and the participant stood with their feet completely parallel (no ankle rotation with a 30 cm stance width).

2.3. COP Measurement

GRF signals were recorded 10 s after trial commencement for 45 s. The two trials were executed one after the other with no change in foot position. The Bioware software automatically calculated x- and y-axis COP location (in mm) separately for right and left foot using the equations:

$$Ax = (Fx*az0 - My)/Fz = -My'/Fz \qquad (1)$$

where:
- Ax path of the lateral direction of the force component
- Fx magnitude of the component of the ground reaction force, caused by the pressure of the foot acting on the left to the right direction
- $az0$ constant value for a given measuring instrument (see Kistler platform) determining the distance of the piezoelectric sensor from the platform level
- My the moment of the component of the ground reaction force, caused by the pressure of the foot acting in the forward–backward direction
- Fz the magnitude of the component of the ground reaction force, caused by the pressure of the foot acting vertically

$$Ay = (Fy*az0 + Mx)/Fz = Mx'/Fz, \qquad (2)$$

where:
- Ay way of action of force component back and forth
- Fx the magnitude of the component of the ground reaction force, caused by the pressure of the feet acting on the left to the right direction
- $az0$ constant value for a given measuring instrument (see Kistler platform) determining the distance of the piezoelectric sensor from the platform level
- Mx the moment of the component of the ground reaction force, caused by the pressure of the foot acting in the direction to the left to the right
- Fz the magnitude of the component of the ground reaction force, caused by vertical pressure of the feet

In order to aid the quantification of COP trajectory as a function of time, the initial COP location was shifted to the mean COP location (calculated for each trial).

A mathematical coordinate system was used to present the test results. The x- and y-axes show the direction of action of ground reaction forces caused by foot pressure on the ground. This is called phase plane (ground). The x-axis represents the action of these forces in the left and right directions. The y-axis represents the action of these forces in the forward and reverse directions. In the context of these axes, anterior foot pressure means that the subject transfers weight to the toes and hind toes. There are people who transfer weight to the foot in opposite directions: outside, to the left foot to the left and to the right foot to the right; or inwards, to the left foot to the right and to the right foot to the left. Hence the term "mid-lateral".

The COP data (2250 measures per trial) were then plotted as a statokinesigram for COP spatial trajectory in the mediolateral and anteroposterior directions as well as a stabilogram showing the temporal domain of COP in both directions. An example of the COP trajectory as a stabilogram and statokinesigram is illustrated in Figures 1 and 2, respectively.

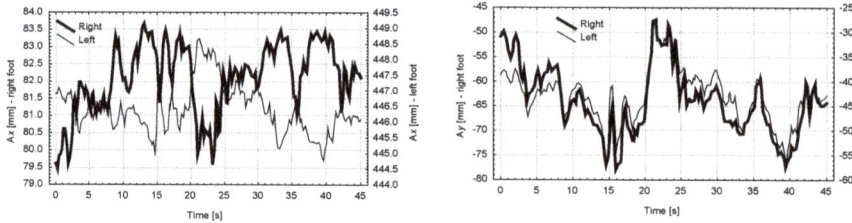

Figure 1. Exemplary stabilogram of center of pressure (COP) time series data in the mediolateral (Ax) and anteroposterior (Ay) directions.

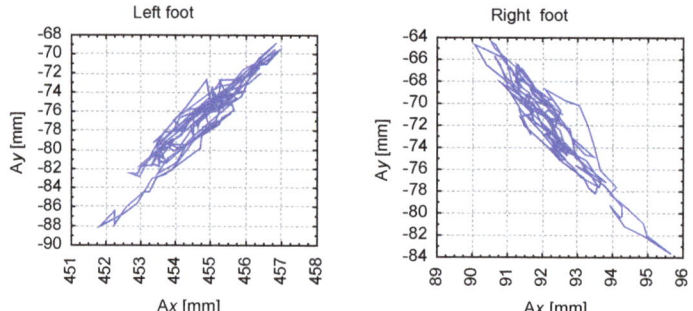

Figure 2. Exemplary statokinesigram of COP spatial data in the mediolateral (Ax) and anteroposterior (Ay) direction.

The selection of a right COP shift trajectory of the right and left foot may illustrate the motor abilities of the subject. The human may determine and choose a right COP displacement trajectory for the right or left foot. Namely, the human may decide on part of a foot which will put pressure on the surface.

2.4. Statistical Analysis

Basic descriptive statistics were calculated (means ± standard deviations). The Shapiro–Wilk test was used to determine if the data set was well-modeled by a normal distribution. Differences between the obtained values were assessed using Student's t-test. The level of symmetry or asymmetry in COP displacement trajectory between the right and left foot in both the mediolateral and anteroposterior directions was assessed with Pearson's correlation coefficients. Correlations between right and left foot COP trajectory were independently calculated in the mediolateral and anteroposterior directions for each participant. Additionally, the correlation coefficients of COP trajectory between the mediolateral and anteroposterior directions were also calculated independently for the right and left foot. The level of significance was set at $\alpha = 0.05$. All data processing was performed with the Statistica 10.0 software package.

3. Results

The assumption of normality was confirmed, indicating a normal distribution. As no significant between-sex differences for COP displacement trajectory were found, the data were analyzed for the entire sample ($n = 102$). Furthermore, t-tests revealed no significant differences between the first and second trial, hence analysis involved only data from the first trial.

The correlations between right and left foot COP trajectory in the mediolateral and anteroposterior directions are presented as a histogram (Figure 3). Strong and very strong positive correlations (0.6 to 1.0) for right and left foot COP displacement trajectory in the mediolateral direction were observed in

91 participants while 11 individuals presented weak or negative correlations. In the anteroposterior direction, moderate and strong negative correlations (−0.5 to −1.0) were observed in 69 participants while 30 were found with weak negative or positive correlations. Strong positive correlations (0.6 to 1.0) in the mediolateral direction were observed in only three individuals.

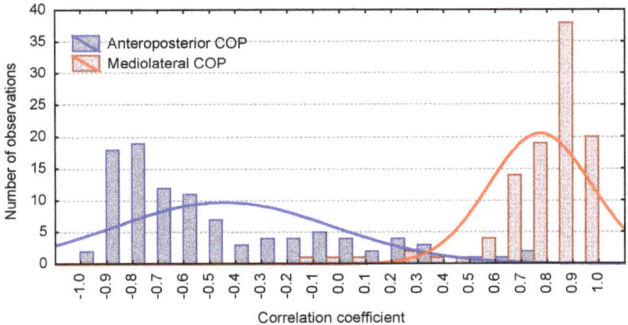

Figure 3. Histogram of correlation coefficients between right and left foot COP trajectory in the mediolateral and anteroposterior directions.

In order to better illustrate the correlations of COP trajectory between the mediolateral and anteroposterior directions, a scatter plot was generated in which the correlations were plotted for each participant (Figure 4). The x-axis was used to delineate the right foot correlations between COP trajectory directions whereas the y-axis represented the left foot. Based on this structure, four quadrants were defined.

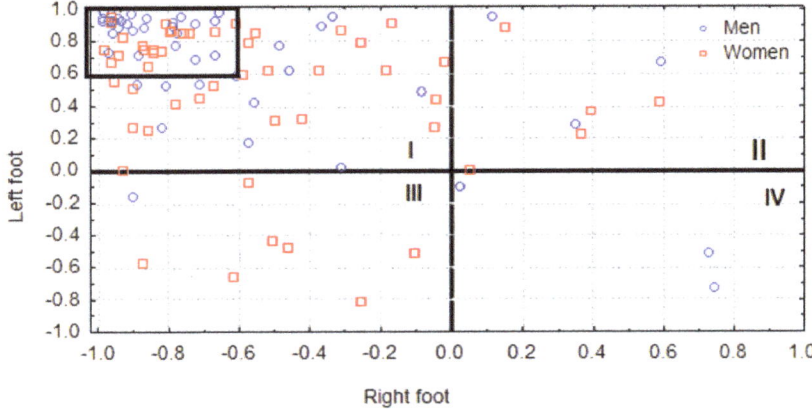

Figure 4. Scatter plot illustrating the correlations between right (x-axis) and left foot (y-axis) mediolateral and anteroposterior COP trajectories for each participant.

The first quadrant (Quadrant I) contains the participants (42 females and 41 males) presenting positive left foot and negative right foot correlations. The second quadrant (Quadrant II) represents those participants (five females and three males) with a positive correlation between the mediolateral and anteroposterior directions in both the right and left foot The third quadrant (Quadrant III), in turn, contains those participants (seven females and one male) with negative right and left foot correlations in both directions whereas the fourth quadrant (Quadrant IV) entails the small group of participants (three males) with positive right foot and negative left foot correlations.

The majority of the sample (n = 83) was grouped in the second quadrant (Quadrant II). A statokinesigram representative of this group was extracted from Participant 1 (Figure 5), who was found with a correlation coefficient of 0.94 for the left and −0.94 for the right foot. Furthermore, 57 participants (more than half the sample) in this quadrant presented strong correlations in both the left (r = 0.6 to 1.0) and right (r = −1.0 to −0.6) feet. A box was drawn in Figure 4 to highlight this congregation.

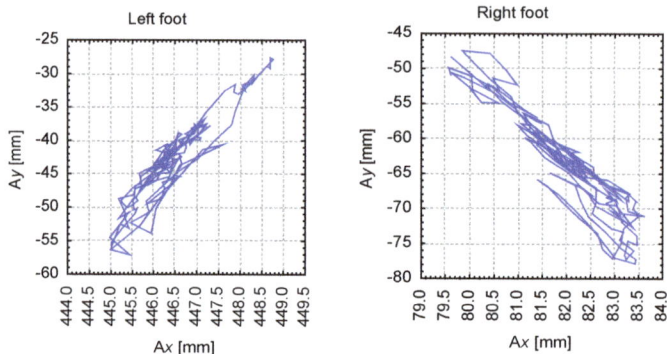

Figure 5. Stabilogram of right and left foot COP trajectories in the mediolateral (Ax) and anteroposterior (Ay) directions for Participant 1 (Quadrant II).

On the opposite spectrum, the three individuals composing the fourth quadrant (Quadrant IV) can be characterized by the statokinesigram of Participant 13 (Figure 6), who was found to present a correlation coefficient of −0.72 for the left and 0.74 for the right foot. The third quadrant (Quadrant III) can be represented by the statokinesigram of Participant 72 (Figure 7), with correlation coefficients of −0.65 for the left and 0.62 for the right foot. An exemplary statokinesigram of the participants located in the first quadrant (Quadrant I) is provided by Participant 93 (Figure 8), with correlation coefficients of 0.67 for the left and 0.59 for the right foot.

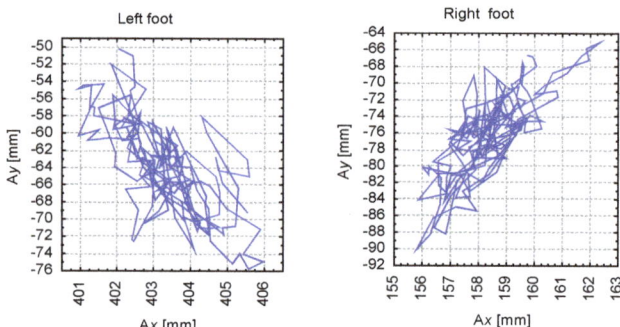

Figure 6. Stabilogram of right and left foot COP trajectories in the mediolateral (Ax) and anteroposterior (Ay) directions for Participant 13 (Quadrant IV).

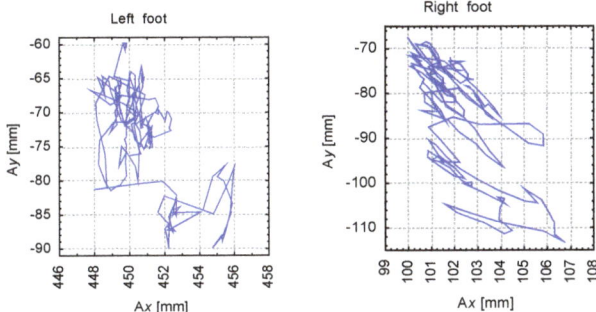

Figure 7. Stabilogram of right and left foot COP trajectories in the mediolateral (Ax) and anteroposterior (Ay) directions for Participant 72 (Quadrant III).

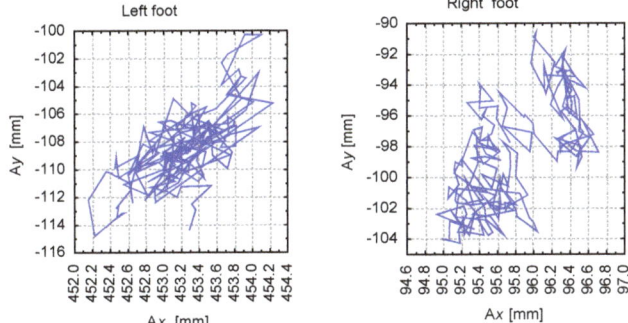

Figure 8. Stabilogram of right and left foot COP trajectories in the mediolateral (Ax) and anteroposterior (Ay) directions for Participant 93 (Quadrant I).

4. Discussion

This investigation considered how balance is maintained during an upright stance when COP is assessed over two points of application (both feet) with respect to the supporting surface. At first glance, it seems logical that the COP of each foot should be equal and, therefore, exhibit symmetry when balance is being maintained in a static position. The present study operated under the premise that a positive correlation between right and left foot COP trajectories (in the mediolateral and anteroposterior directions) indicates symmetry whereas a negative correlation indicates asymmetry. We hypothesized that the incidence of fluctuations or asymmetry between right and left foot COP can indicate foot pathology resulting from improper footwear or decreased neuromuscular control.

In our sample of healthy young adults, strong negative correlations between right and left foot COP in the mediolateral direction were found in approximately 67% of the participants. This indicates that during the quiet standing task the participants exerted pressure on the lateral boundary of the left foot while concurrently exerting pressure on the medial boundary of the right foot and, therefore, exhibit asymmetry. In turn, approximately 29% of the sample presented correlations coefficients between −0.4 and 0.3 between right and left foot mediolateral COP, which was considered to indicate more balanced symmetry albeit without any characteristic trend. More puzzling is the fact that the remaining 3% of the sample was found to show COP displacement simultaneously towards the medial and lateral sides of the right and left foot. From a biomechanical perspective, this type of balance control is difficult to understand. Interpretation of the correlation coefficients between right and left foot anteroposterior COP displacement found that approximately 88% of the sample presented considerable symmetry between both feet and that compared with mediolateral COP, anteroposterior

COP trajectory shows a greater level of symmetry between both feet. In effect, these results find that the majority of the sample presented asymmetry albeit defined as mediolateral COP trajectory traversing towards both the medial and lateral boundaries of the feet. Symmetry, in turn, was observed in the anteroposterior direction in which COP trajectory was along the toes or heel of the foot. This asymmetry and symmetry were presented by 86 participants ($n = 102$) and, therefore, suggests that this form of postural control defines healthy and active adults.

Research has suggested that the occurrence of asymmetry when maintaining balance to be the result of musculoskeletal dysfunction or lower extremity dominance. These conclusions were drawn by Ageberg [13], Lin [14] or Barone [15] who performed posturography on two force plates or by comparing COP variables between the dominant and non-dominant leg in static bilateral conditions. However, during single-leg testing, Hoffmann [16] and Greve [17] or Cuğ et al. [18] did not observe any differences in postural balance between the dominant and non-dominant leg in young adults. The aforementioned studies have mentioned that functional leg dominance may play an important role in bilateral postural stability, where, in most individuals, the left leg is the functionally dominant extremity and the right leg the functionally non-dominant extremity. Interestingly, Micarelli et al. [19] found greater COP displacement in the right rather than left leg during quiet standing in a group of children 4–13 and 4–7 years old. Research on the development of postural control by Assaiante [20] found that the trunk serves as an important reference frame in the emergence of structured postural strategies. It has been suggested that shifting the center of mass over the left increases weight-bearing load of the left leg over time.

Of consideration is the use of a scatter plot as presented herein as it can provide facile comparisons with other cohorts or normative data or illustrate more clearly the relationships of COP trajectories between the right and left foot. For example, when considering left foot COP trajectory in both directions, over half of the sample was found to present a pattern in which COP displacement traversed in the anteroposterior direction with a rightwards slant (medial direction) whereas right foot COP followed an anteroposterior displacement with a leftwards shift (medial direction). This medial shift of right and left foot COP trajectory with an anteroposterior displacement in the majority of the sample is contrasted by the marginal number of participants (three individuals) who presented an inverse pattern. In this small group, anteroposterior COP trajectory was associated with a lateral COP displacement (towards the outside of both feet) in the forward direction whereas in the backward direction COP transversed in the medial direction (towards the outside of the feet). In addition, the visualization of COP data by mapping its trajectory in the spatial domain can show patterns in COP trajectory over the base of the support, i.e., the feet. The trends that we observed in the majority of the sample (Quadrant II, Figure 5) confirm the findings of Oba et al. [21], Rival et al. [22] and Cumberworth et al. [23], who concluded that postural stability (COP displacement) is limited to an area between the heel and toe alongside the lateral edge in adults.

Our sample, as previously mentioned, was composed of young and asymptotic individuals free of lower extremity injury or disability. Although not assessed in the present study, it can be presumed that the incidence of foot or leg pathologies can modify the maximum displacement of COP trajectory and, therefore, stability. The literature contains numerous reports that utilize data on COP area and its relation to the base of support as a measure of postural stability [24–26]. Riach and Starkes [20] sound that children show a larger area of stability than adults and that the limit of stability decreases with age. Young adults aged 18–27 years appropriate on average 73% of the anteroposterior and 75% of the mediolateral base of support during upright standing. By ages 40–70, individuals use only 54% and 59%, respectively [22]. Clifford and Holder-Powell [23] indicated that the elderly show an even further reduced base of support for postural stability. Bottaroa [24] reported that this observation is associated with the fact that young asymptotic adults use up to 80% while older adults only up to 50% of foot length to maintain balance.

The present findings raise a number of questions concerning the etiology of disturbed COP displacement trajectory between the right and left foot and indicate the need for additional investigation in this area. Further research on COP symmetry in various populations (athletes, physically impaired, sedentary individuals) can provide further insight on the causes of asymmetry (e.g., decreased neuromuscular control) and aid clinicians with the diagnosis of various posture-related pathologies.

5. Conclusions

Approximately 88% of the participants exhibited left and right foot symmetry for anteroposterior COP trajectory magnitude and direction. Asymmetry was noted in 67% of participants for mediolateral COP trajectory, in which COP displacement was observed along the lateral boundary of one foot and along the medial boundary of the other. In 82% of the samples, COP displacement followed an anteroposterior trajectory with a medial slant for left foot and lateral slant for right foot COP, whereas the remaining 12% showed other variations. These findings raise a number of questions concerning the etiology of asymmetric COP displacement trajectory between the right and left foot. Additional investigation is warranted to compare COP trajectories between asymptotic individuals and various populations (e.g., sedentary individuals, patients with foot or leg pathologies or athletes engaged in sports with strong lateralization) to better understand the causes of asymmetry and aid clinicians with the diagnosis of various posture-related pathologies.

Author Contributions: Conceptualization, J.S., J.V. and K.M.; methodology, K.M., W.B. and J.S.; software, W.B. and J.V.; validation, W.S., M.K. and J.S.; formal analysis, K.M. and J.S.; investigation, W.B., K.M. and J.S.; resources, J.S. and W.B.; data curation, W.B. and K.M.; writing—original draft preparation, J.S., J.V., K.M. and M.C.; writing—review and editing, J.S., J.V. and K.M.; visualization, J.S. and K.M.; supervision, J.S. and K.M. All authors have read and agreed to the published version of the manuscript.

Funding: This research received no external funding.

Acknowledgments: The authors would like to acknowledge the involvement of the participants for their contribution to this study.

Conflicts of Interest: The authors have no conflict of interest to declare. The results do not constitute endorsement of any product or device. The authors would like to thank the sprinters who participated in this study.

References

1. Fuller, J.T.; Bellenger, C.R.; Thewlis, D.; Tsiros, M.D.; Buckley, J.D. The effect of footwear on running performance and running economy in distance runners: A systematic review. *Sports Med.* **2015**, *45*, 411–422. [CrossRef] [PubMed]
2. Mohr, M.; Meyer, C.; Nigg, N.; Nigg, B. The relationship between footwear comfort and variability of running kinematics. *J. Footwear Sci.* **2017**, *9*, 45–47. [CrossRef]
3. Squadrone, R.; Rodano, R.; Preatoni, E.; Andreoni, G.; Pedotti, A. The EUROSHOE approach to ergonomics of foot and shoe. *Ergon. IJE HF* **2005**, *27*, 43–51.
4. Winter, D.A. Human balance and posture control during standing and walking. *Gait Posture* **1995**, *3*, 193–214. [CrossRef]
5. Winter, D.A. *Biomechanics and Motor Control of Human Movement*; John Wiley and Sons, Inc.: Hoboken, NJ, USA, 2009.
6. Prieto, T.E.; Myklebust, J.B.; Hoffmann, R.G.; Lovett, E.G.; Myklebust, B.M. Measures of postural steadiness: Differences between healthy young and elderly adults. *IEEE Trans. Biomed. Eng.* **1996**, *43*, 956–966. [CrossRef] [PubMed]
7. Winter, D.A.; Patla, A.E.; Prince, F.; Ishac, M.; Gielo-Perczak, K. Stiffness control of balance in quiet standing. *J. Neurophysiol.* **1998**, *80*, 1211–1221.
8. Karlsson, A.; Frykberg, G. Correlations between force plate measures for assessment of balance. *Clin. Biomech.* **2000**, *15*, 365–369. [CrossRef]
9. Gage, W.H.; Winter, D.A.; Frank, J.S.; Adkin, A.L. Kinematic and kinetic validity of the inverted pendulum model in quiet standing. *Gait Posture* **2004**, *19*, 124–132. [CrossRef]
10. Kleipool, R.P.; Blankevoort, L. The relation between geometry and function of the ankle joint complex: A biomechanical review. *Knee Surg. Sports Traumatol. Arthrosc.* **2010**, *18*, 618–627. [CrossRef]

11. Soangra, R.; Lockhart, T.E. Determination of stabilogram diffusion analysis coefficients and invariant density analysis parameters to understand postural stability associated with standing on anti-fatigue mats. *Biomed. Sci. Instrum.* **2012**, *48*, 415–422.
12. Brauer, S.G.; Burns, Y.R.; Galley, P.A. prospective study of laboratory and clinical measures of postural stability to predict community-dwelling fallers. *J. Gerontol. A Biol. Sci. Med. Sci.* **2000**, *55*, 469–476. [CrossRef] [PubMed]
13. Ageberg, E.; Roberts, D.; Holmström, E.; Fridén, T. Balance in single-limb stance in healthy subjects—Reliability of testing procedure and the effect of short-duration sub-maximal cycling. *BMC Musculoskelet Disord.* **2003**, *27*, 4–14. [CrossRef] [PubMed]
14. Lin, W.H.; Liu, Y.F.; Hsieh, C.C.; Lee, A.J. Ankle eversion to inversion strength ratio and static balance control in the dominant and non-dominant limbs of young adults. *J. Sci. Med. Sport* **2009**, *12*, 42–49. [CrossRef] [PubMed]
15. Rosario, B.F.; Macaluso, M.T.; Leonardi, V.; Farina, F.V. Soccer players have a better standing balance in nondominant one-legged stance. *J. Sports Med.* **2011**, *2*, 1–6.
16. Hoffman, M.; Schrader, J.; Applegate, T.; Koceja, D. Unilateral postural control of the functionally dominant and nondominant extremities of healthy subjects. *J. Athl. Train.* **1998**, *33*, 319–322.
17. Greve, J.; Alonso, A.; Bordini, A.C.; Camanho, G.L. Correlation between body mass index and postural balance. *Clinics (Sao Paulo)* **2007**, *62*, 717–720. [CrossRef]
18. Cuğ, M.; Özdemir, A.R.; AK, E. Influence of leg dominance on single-leg stance performance during dynamic conditions: An investigation into the validity of symmetry hypothesis for dynamic postural control in healthy individuals. *Turk. J. Phys. Med. Rehabil.* **2014**, *60*, 22–26.
19. Micarelli, A.; Viziano, A.; Augimeri, I.; Micarelli, B.; Alessandrini, M. Age-related assessment of postural control development: A cross-sectional study in children and adolescents. *J. Mot. Behav.* **2019**. [CrossRef]
20. Assaiante, C.; Mallau, S.; Viel, S.; Jover, M.; Schmitz, C. Development of postural control in healthy children: A functional approach. *Neural Plast.* **2005**, *12*, 109–118. [CrossRef]
21. Oba, N.; Sasagawa, S.; Yamamoto, A.; Nakazawa, K.; Glasauer, S. Difference in postural control during quiet standing between young children and adults: Assessment with center of mass acceleration. *PLoS ONE* **2015**, *10*, e0140235. [CrossRef]
22. Rival, C.; Ceyte, H.; Olivier, I. Developmental changes of static standing balance in children. *Neurosci. Lett.* **2005**, *376*, 133–136. [CrossRef]
23. Cumberworth, V.L.; Patel, N.N.; Rogers, W.; Kenyon, G.S. The maturation of balance in children. *J. Laryngol. Otol.* **2007**, *121*, 449–454. [CrossRef] [PubMed]
24. Lacour, M.; Bernard-Demanze, L.; Dumitrescu, M. Posture control, aging, and attention resources: Models and posture-analysis methods. *Neurophysiol. Clin.* **2008**, *38*, 411–421. [CrossRef] [PubMed]
25. Clifford, A.M.; Holder-Powell, H. Postural control in healthy individuals. *Clin. Biomech.* **2010**, *25*, 546–551. [CrossRef] [PubMed]
26. Bottaroa, A.; Yasutakeb, Y.; Nomurab, T.; Casaidioma, M.; Morassoa, P. Bounded stability of the quiet standing posture: An intermittent control model. *Hum. Mov. Sci.* **2008**, *27*, 473–495. [CrossRef] [PubMed]

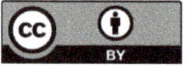

© 2020 by the authors. Licensee MDPI, Basel, Switzerland. This article is an open access article distributed under the terms and conditions of the Creative Commons Attribution (CC BY) license (http://creativecommons.org/licenses/by/4.0/).

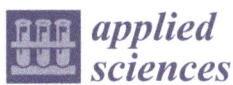 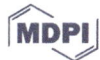

Article

Elbow Extensors and Volar Flexors Strength Capacity and Its Relation to Shooting Performance in Basketball Players—A Pilot Study

Darjan Smajla [1,2], Žiga Kozinc [1,3] and Nejc Šarabon [1,2,3,4,*]

1. Faculty of Health Sciences, University of Primorska, 6310 Izola, Slovenia; darjan.smajla@fvz.upr.si (D.S.); ziga.kozinc@fvz.upr.si (Ž.K.)
2. Innorenew CoE, Livade 6, 6310 Izola, Slovenia
3. Andrej Marušič Institute, University of Primorska, 6000 Koper, Slovenia
4. Laboratory for Motor Control and Motor Behaviour, S2P, Science to Practice, Ltd., 1000 Ljubljana, Slovenia
* Correspondence: nejc.sarabon@fvz.upr.si; Tel.: +38-6040-429-505

Received: 23 September 2020; Accepted: 17 November 2020; Published: 19 November 2020

Abstract: Rate of force/torque development scaling factor (RFD-SF/RTD-SF) has been used as a tool for assessing neuromuscular quickness. The aim was to investigate strength capacities of two major shooting muscle groups and their relationship to basketball shooting performance, and to compare the RFD-SF as well as shooting performance between junior and senior basketball players, and finally to examine the differences in RTD-SF between elbow extensors and volar flexors. In 23 male basketball players (13 juniors and 10 seniors) we assessed maximal isometric torque (T_{MVC}), maximal rate of torque development and RTD-SF slope (k_{RTD-SF}) for elbow extensors and volar flexors. The subjects performed 10 throws at 2.3 m (short) and 8.9 m (long) from the basket. Our results showed similar k_{RTD-SF} and T_{MVC} in both groups. Better shooting performance from short distance was observed in senior players. Significant associations between k_{RTD-SF}, T_{MVC} and shooting performance were found only in juniors. Elbow extensors T_{MVC} was found to have a significant positive large association with shooting performance from long distance. It seems that muscle capacity has an important role in shooting performance in junior compared to players. Sufficient strength capacity of major shooting muscles is important for juniors' shooting performance from a long distance.

Keywords: wrist; elbow; shot; accuracy; RFD-SF

1. Introduction

Rate of force development scaling factor (RFD-SF) has been used to quantify the ability to generate force rapidly, which is described as neuromuscular quickness [1]. A large number of studies have reported the RFD-SF as a reliable method for a number of muscle groups such as index finger abductors [1,2], elbow extensors [1,3], knee extensors [1,4] and various hip muscles [5]. However, the relationship between RFD-SF and performance in functional or sports-related tasks has not been yet investigated. It is known that muscle quickness decreases with age [2] or disease [6], while the influence of the specific training history on this ability is still, to a great extent, unknown.

Explosive and quick release during basketball shot is important to avoid the defender reaction. One of the studies showed positive effects of explosive strength training on the shot percentage level. However, explosive strength training was performed for upper and lower limb; therefore, it is unknown if upper limb strength capacities play important role in basketball shooting performance [7]. We speculate that upper limb strength capacities may be important for accurate shooting performance because it has been reported that an increase in maximum strength of elbow extensors positively affected the shoot accurately in the three-point shot [8].

Basketball shot is among the sports-specific movements in which rapid production of submaximal force by muscles that act across multiple arm joints is considered important. During a basketball throw, the players manipulate their shoulder, elbow, and wrist to generate the optimal ball speed and angular velocity of the joint at the time of the release [9], depending on the distance and the position from the basket. The angular velocity of the upper arm joints and the speed of ball release increase with the shooting distance [10], which suggests that higher submaximal involvement of the major muscle groups is required as the distance increases. The elbow extensors have been suggested as major contributors to release speed in basketball shooting [11,12] as they extend the elbow joint before release, while the activation of the volar flexors is an important component of shooting that optimises impulse applied to the ball at release [13]. Previous studies have reported that the angular velocity of the elbow joint of the shooting arm at release increases with distance from the basket, while the opposite is observed for the wrist [11], suggesting that the roles of the two joints vary with the shooting distance. Some earlier studies reported that players with more training experience had better shooting performance [12,14] and lower average duration of arm muscle activation [15,16]. Based on this, we assumed that junior and senior players might also differ in the neuromuscular quickness of the major shooting muscles (i.e., elbow extensors and volar flexors). Furthermore, the relationship between neuromuscular quickness and performance of sport-specific tasks has not yet been investigated. Filling these missing gaps could contribute to better understanding of RFD-SF and its use during routine testing of the athletes and possibly, based on these assessments, to individualized guidance of training programmes (e.g., more emphasis on speed-power training for individuals with lower RTD or RTD-SF).

To contribute our part in clarification of the functional role of the RTD-SF in sport-specific performance, we conducted a study to investigate strength capacities of elbow extensors and volar flexors in two groups of basketball players (juniors and seniors) and their relationship to shooting performance, put into the sport-specific training history. Specifically, the first aim of our study was to investigate the differences in the strength capacities (RTD-SF slope (k_{RTD-SF}), maximum torque (T_{MVC}), and peak rate of torque development (RTD_{PEAK}) of elbow extensors (EE) and volar flexors (VF) and the shooting performance between junior and senior basketball players. We hypothesised that senior players, based on their longer training history and complete physical development, have significantly higher strength capacities of elbow extensors and volar flexors and better shooting performance compared to junior players. The second aim of the study was to investigate the relationship between the strength capacities (k_{RTD-SF}, T_{MVC}, and RTD_{PEAK}) and shooting performance. We hypothesised that in both groups, shooting performance would be significantly positively associated with k_{RTD-SF}, T_{MVC}, and RTD_{PEAK} of elbow extensors and volar flexors, at least from the long shooting distance. The third aim of the study was to investigate associations of elbow extensors and volar flexors as previous studies showed positive associations of k_{RTD-SF} ability for different muscle groups, while this association between elbow extensors and volar flexors has not yet been confirmed. We hypothesised that there will be a large and statistically significant association in k_{RTD-SF} between elbow extensors and volar flexors in both groups of players, which might support the idea of a central regulation and upper extremity (not a single joint, i.e., muscle group) related characteristics of RTD-SF ability.

2. Materials and Methods

2.1. Subjects

A total of 23 male basketball players from the top-ranked Slovenian basketball club were included in the study (Table 1). All subjects reported their right arm as the preferred shooting arm. Subjects with previous upper limb injuries (past 6 months), neurological disorders, low back pain, or recent general illness were excluded from the study. The inclusion criteria were regular basketball training in past 3 years at least 4 times per week. The subjects and their parents/guardians were informed about the testing procedures and provided written informed consent prior to commencing the study.

The experiment was approved by the Slovenian Medical Ethics Committee (approval no. 0120-99/2018/5) according to the Declaration of Helsinki.

Table 1. Characteristics of Subjects.

Group	N	Age (years)	Body Height (cm)	Body Mass (kg)	BMI	Training History (Years)
Junior	13	16.5 ± 0.9	192.7 ± 7.8	81.5 ± 9.1	21.9 ± 2.0	5.5 ± 1.8
Senior	10	24.0 ± 4.2	198 ± 7.9	95.5 ± 10.9	24.2 ± 1.6	14.1 ± 3.8
Total	23	19.7 ± 4.8	195.2 ± 8.2	87.6 ± 11.9	22.9 ± 2.1	9.3 ± 5.2

N—the number of participants; BMI—Body mass index.

2.2. Study Design and Testing Procedures

For each subject, we captured measurements of (i) k_{RTD-SF}, T_{MVC}, and RTD_{PEAK} for EE and VF of the self-reported preferred arm and (ii) shooting performance at two different distances from the basket in two separate visits. On the first measurement day, the subjects performed isometric strength tests for EE and VF (random order) preceded by a 10 min warm-up consisting of 5 min of light running, 4 min of dynamic stretching, and 1 min of activation exercises (10 repetitions of squats, push-ups, and V-ups). The isometric strength tests were performed before their regular training in the laboratory setting. The next day, on the second measurement day, the subjects performed 10 throws at two different distances (random order) from the basket after the standardized warm-up protocol described before. The shooting performance was assessed in the gym basketball gym before their regular training. The flowchart of the study is outlined on the Figure 1.

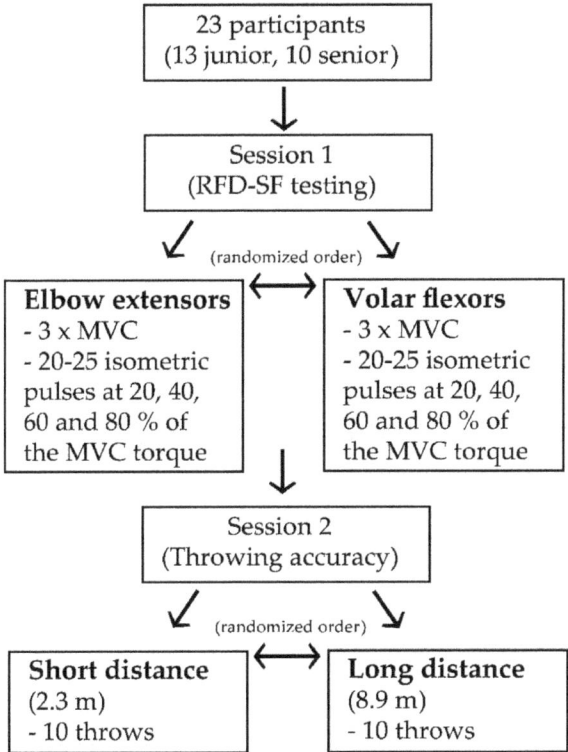

Figure 1. The flowchart of the measurement protocols. MVC—maximal voluntary isometric contraction.

Following the warm-up, the subject was positioned in a custom-made dynamometer (S2P, Science to Practice, ltd., Ljubljana, Slovenia) which was used for T_{MVC} and RTD_{PEAK} and k_{RTD-SF} assessment. Participants position during elbow extension or volar flexion T_{MVC}, RTD_{PEAK}, and k_{RTD-SF} assessment is presented and described in Figure 2. In all cases, the lever arm (i.e., the linear distance from the axis of the joint and the centre of the distal force-detecting support) was measured and considered in the torque calculation. The signals from force transducers during elbow extension (Bending beam load cell 1-Z6FC3/200kg, HBM, Darmstadt, Germany) and volar flexion (Tension compression load cell FL25-50 kg, Forsentek, Shenzhen, China) were amplified (Isotel, Logatec, Slovenia) and converted from analogue to digital signal (NI USB-6211, National Instruments, Austin, TX, USA). Signals were sampled at 1000 Hz by a custom-made LabView 2015 software (National Instruments Corp., Augustin, TX, USA). In case of T_{MVC} and RTD_{PEAK}, the raw signals were smoothed (moving average filter, 5 ms time-window). In RTD-SF analyses the signals were filtered using a lowpass Butterworth filter with cut-off frequency at 5 Hz, while corresponding RTD of each contraction was calculated as a peak value of derivate of the torque curve [4]. All measurements were processed by a single investigator.

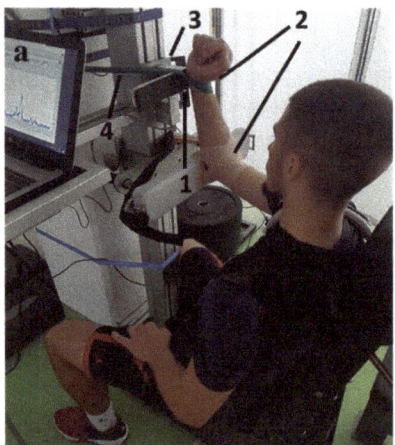
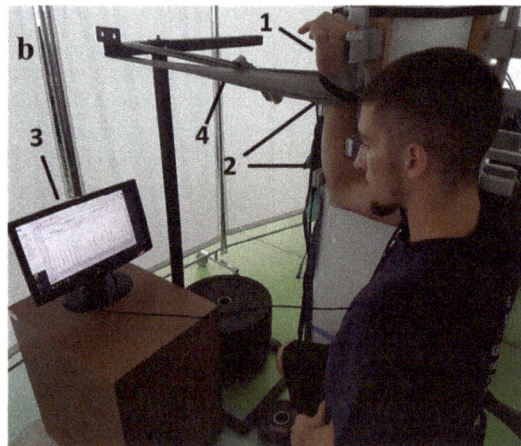

Figure 2. Measurement set-up: (**a**) Subject in the custom-built elbow extensor dynamometer. Subjects were seated (knee and hip in 90° position, trunk in upright position) on a bench with back support, while their shoulder and elbow were flexed at 90° in sagittal plane (forearm was in neutral position). The trunk and the shoulder of the performing arm were fixed to the back support, while the elbow was fixated to the lower support of the dynamometer. The force sensor was at the upper support, where the subject placed the wrist, which was fixated using elastic bands (to provide tension and proper contact between wrist and dynamometer support). (**b**) Subject in the custom-built volar flexor dynamometer. Subjects were seated on a chair. The subject's shoulder and elbow were both flexed at 90°, while their forearm (pronated position) was placed in a custom-made dynamometer which allows full forearm fixation. Wrist was in neutral position. 1—force sensor, 2—joint fixations, 3—monitor for visual feedback, 4—elastic band

2.3. Testing T_{MVC} and RTD_{PEAK}

In T_{MVC} testing subjects were instructed to gradually increase the force and push as hard as possible against the elbow (Figure 2a) and wrist dynamometer's support (Figure 2b). Contractions were sustained for at least 3 s; meanwhile, verbal encouragement was given to the subject. T_{MVC} for each muscle group was calculated (Nm/kg) as the maximal mean value on a 1 s time interval. Each participant performed three repetitions for each muscle group. The greatest T_{MVC} was used for statistical analysis.

Three isometric MVCs for each muscle group (EE and VF) with a 60 s rest between trials were repeated, while in this case subjects were instructed to push as hard and explosive as possible to calculate their RTD_{PEAK} (maximum of the toque-time derivative). Greatest RTD_{PEAK} (Nm/kg s) was used for statistical analysis.

2.4. Testing RTD-SF

The RTD-SF relationship for each muscle group was computed from sets of 20–25 explosive isometric contractions at four different submaximal intensities (20%, 40%, 60%, and 80% of T_{MVC}) (Figure 3a,c) in a random order, as previously described [1]. Subjects rested for 60 s between different contraction intensities and 3 min between each task, i.e., muscle group. The target torque was displayed as a horizontal line on a graph on a computer screen placed at the subject's eye level (Figure 2). The subjects were instructed to contract and relax as fast as possible.

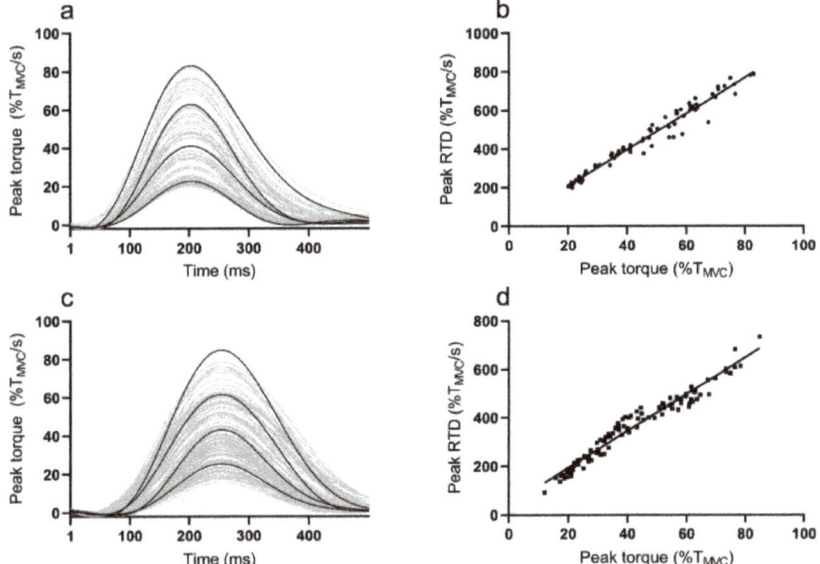

Figure 3. Sample recording of rapid torque pulses of (**a**) elbow extensors and (**c**) volar flexors to a variety of amplitudes. Rate of torque development scaling factor (RTD-SF) plot of (**b**) elbow extensors (**b**) and (**d**) volar flexors with data points taken from the peaks of the preferred arm.

The regression parameters k_{RTD-SF} (/s) and r^2_{RTD-SF} were obtained from the relationship between the peak torque and the corresponding peak RTD.

2.5. Testing Shooting Performance

During the second visit, the subjects performed 10 throws at two different distances, orientated frontally towards the basket. Shooting distances were selected in random order for each subject. Shooting performance from short distance was performed from half the distance between the basket and free throw line (2.3 m), while shooting form the longer distance was performed from 8.9 m (three-point line + distance between free throw and three-point line). From each subject shooting performance from each distance was assessed (n/10).

2.6. Statistical Analysis

Descriptive data of the dependent variables are presented as means and standard deviations. The Shapiro–Wilk test was used to assess data normality. Fisher's z-transformation was used to transform $r^2_{RTD\text{-}SF}$ in case of RTD-SF to obtain normal distribution. The differences in $k_{RTD\text{-}SF}$, T_{MVC}, and RTD_{PEAK} between groups were evaluated with a two-tailed independent sample t-test and Cohen's d effect size (ES). The ES was interpreted as negligible (<0.2), small (0.2–0.5), moderate (0.5–0.8), and large (≥0.8) [17]. Pearson correlation coefficients were used to determine the relationship between $k_{RTD\text{-}SF}$, T_{MVC}, and RTD_{PEAK} of EE and VF and shooting performance from short and long distance. The correlation coefficient was interpreted in as (0.00–0.19 trivial; 0.10–0.29 small; 0.30–0.49 moderate; 0.50–0.69 large; 0.70–0.89 very large; 0.90–0.99 nearly perfect; and 1.00 perfect) [18]. Moreover, we assessed the reliability of $k_{RTD\text{-}SF}$, T_{MVC}, and RTD_{PEAK} by calculating two-way random model intra-class correlation coefficients (ICC) for single measures and standard error of measurement, expressed as the coefficient of variation (CV). For T_{MVC} and RTD_{PEAK}, we conducted inter-repetition reliability, while for the RFD-SF, we split the data from each intensity into two halves, and compared $k_{RTD\text{-}SF}$ $r^2_{RTD\text{-}SF}$ obtained from both subsets of the data. The level of statistical significance was set at $p < 0.05$. Statistical analyses were performed using the SPSS (IBM SPSS version 26.0, Chicago, IL, USA) software package.

3. Results

The reliability of the outcome variables is shown in Table 2. For both muscle groups RTD-SF and T_{MVC} showed very good reliability (all ICC ≥ 0.85; all CV ≤ 5.66%); however, the reliability was somewhat lower for RTD_{PEAK}, especially for the VF muscles (ICC = 0.54; CV = 15.21%).

Table 2. Reliability of the outcome variables.

Muscle Group/Variable		ICC	CV
Elbow extensors	T_{MVC}	0.91 (0.85–0.96)	2.34 (1.02–3.49)
	RTD_{PEAK}	0.78 (0.55–0.92)	7.89 (3.44–12.75)
	$k_{RFD\text{-}SF}$	0.99 (0.97–1.00)	1.23 (0.97–2.03)
	$r^2_{RFD\text{-}SF}$	0.88 (0.76–0.96)	1.05 (0.54–1.61)
Volar flexors	T_{MVC}	0.85 (0.72–0.94)	5.66 (2.81–8.44)
	RTD_{PEAK}	0.54 (0.23–0.84)	15.211 (8.76–21.12)
	$k_{RFD\text{-}SF}$	0.99 (0.96–1.00)	1.71 (1.11–2.58)
	$r^2_{RFD\text{-}SF}$	0.87 (0.67–0.96)	5.45 (2.36–9.21)

$k_{RTD\text{-}SF}$—slope of regression line, $r^2_{RTD\text{-}SF}$—linearity of regression line, T_{MVC}—maximal torque normalized on body weight, RTD_{PEAK}—maximal rate of torque development normalized on body weight.

Junior players had a significantly lower average number of training years (5.5 ± 1.8 years) compared to senior players (14.1 ± 3.8 years) ($t_{(21)} = -7.2, p < 0.013$). There was no statistically significant difference in height between groups ($t_{(21)} = -1.6, p = 0.11$), while senior players had statistically significantly higher body mass ($t_{(21)} = -3.4, p = 0.003$) and body mass index (BMI)($t_{(21)} = -3.0, p = 0.007$). Average $k_{RTD\text{-}SF}$, T_{MVC}, and RTD_{PEAK} values of elbow extensors and volar flexors in junior and senior group are presented in Table 3. Junior and senior players had similar values of T_{MVC} in both muscle groups, while junior players had significantly greater RTD_{PEAK} of EE and VF ($p = 0.003$–0.005, ES = 0.35–0.36). For both groups, a strong linear relationship ($r^2_{RTD\text{-}SF} = 0.93$–0.95) between the peak force and the RFD across submaximal contractions was calculated for both muscle groups (sample recordings are presented in Figure 3). There was no statistically significant difference in $k_{RTD\text{-}SF}$ between junior and senior players for elbow extensors or volar flexors. There was no difference in shooting performance from long distance, whereas senior players were more successful from short distance.

Table 3. Descriptive statistics and differences in measured parameters between junior and senior basketball players.

Muscle Group/Variable		Junior	Senior	t	p	ES
Elbow extensors	k_{RTD-SF} (/s)	8.9 ± 0.9	8.5 ± 1.2	0.46	0.65	0.009
	r^2_{RTD-SF}	0.95 ± 0.04	0.93 ± 0.07	0.98	0.34	0.04
	T_{MVC} (Nm/kg)	0.70 ± 0.13	0.74 ± 0.16	−0.65	0.6	0.01
	RTD_{PEAK} (Nm/kg s)	9.9 ± 0.9	8.3 ± 1.3	3.45	0.005	0.36
Volar flexors	k_{RTD-SF} (/s)	7.5 ± 1.0	7.3 ± 1.8	0.87	0.39	0.04
	r^2_{RTD-SF}	0.93 ± 0.04	0.94 ± 0.05	−0.35	0.73	0.006
	T_{MVC} (Nm)	0.21 ± 0.07	0.23 ± 0.03	−0.5	0.63	0.02
	RTD_{PEAK} (Nm/kg s)	9.2 ± 1.5	7.2 ± 1.3	3.3	0.003	0.35
Shooting performance	Short distance (%)	8.6 ± 1.2	10.0 ± 0.0	−3.9	0.02	0.56
	Long distance (%)	4.8 ± 2.2	6.3 ± 2.1	−1.7	0.1	0.12

k_{RTD-SF}—slope of regression line, r^2_{RTD-SF}—linearity of regression line, T_{MVC}—maximal torque normalized on body weight, RTD_{PEAK}—maximal rate of torque development normalized on body weight, Short distance—shooting distance at 2.3 m from the basket, Long distance—shooting distance at 8.9 m from the basket.

Significant associations between k_{RTD-SF}, T_{MVC}, RTD_{PEAK} (EE and VF) with shooting performance for junior players are presented in Figure 4. We calculated a large positive association between k_{RTD-SF} of EE and VF and shooting performance from short distance (Figure 4a,b), while significant negative large associations were seen between k_{RTD-SF} of both muscle groups and shooting performance from long distance (Figure 4c,d). Moreover, a significant positive large association was calculated between T_{MVC} of EE and shooting performance from long distance (Figure 4e), while the association between T_{MVC} of VF and shooting performance was not statistically significant (Figure 4f). No statistically significant associations were calculated in junior players between RTD_{PEAK} of both muscle groups and shooting performance (r = 0.246–0.315, p = 0.48–0.49). There were no significant associations between T_{MVC}, RTD_{PEAK}, or k_{RTD-SF} (EE and VF) and any shooting performance in senior basketball players (r = −0.481–0.481, p = 0.15–0.55) or in both groups combined (r = −0.366–0.271, p = 0.16–0.87).

Significant positive large associations between k_{RTD-SF} of elbow extensors and volar flexors were calculated for senior group (r = 0.677, p < 0.05) and when both groups were evaluated together (r = 0.615, p < 0.001), while associations between k_{RTD-SF} of elbow extensors and volar flexors in junior group were not statistically significant (r = 0.514, p = 0.72).

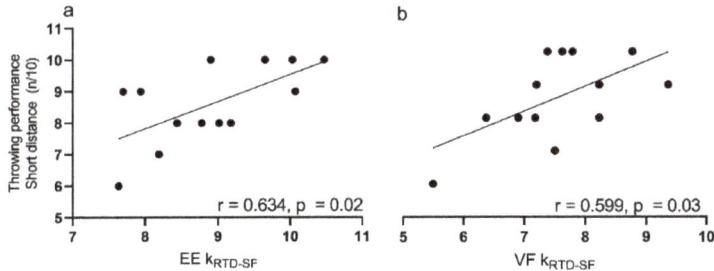

Figure 4. Cont.

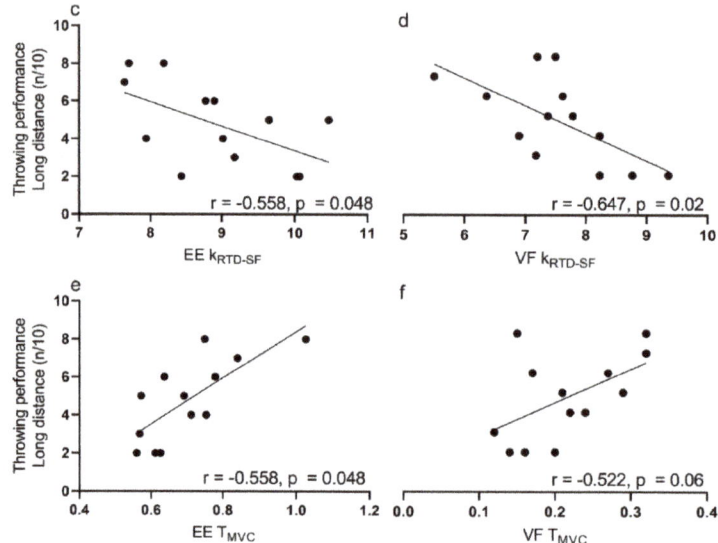

Figure 4. Associations between k_{RTD-SF} (**a–d**), T_{MVC} (**e,f**) of elbow extensors (EE) or volar flexors (VF) and shooting performance from short and long distance.

4. Discussion

The first aim of our study was to investigate differences in strength capacities of elbow extensors and volar flexors and shooting performance between junior and senior basketball players. Our results showed similar k_{RTD-SF} of both muscle groups between juniors and seniors regardless of significant differences between the two groups regarding training history, body mass and BMI. Similar values were also observed for T_{MVC} of both groups, while juniors had significantly greater RTD_{PEAK} (normalized to body weight). Seniors showed better shooting performance only at short distance compared to junior players. The second aim was to investigate associations between strength capacities and shooting performance. Significant associations between k_{RTD-SF} of both muscle groups and shooting performance were found only in juniors. Our results revealed significant positive association between k_{RTD-SF} of elbow extensors, volar flexors and shooting performance from short distance. On the contrary, a significant negative large association was found between k_{RTD-SF} of both muscle groups and shooting performance from long distance. T_{MVC} of elbow extensors was found to have a significant positive large association with shooting performance from long distance. Our third aim was to investigate associations in k_{RTD-SF} of elbow extensors and volar flexors. Our results showed significant positive large associations between k_{RTD-SF} of elbow extensors and volar flexors.

In this study, we investigated the k_{RTD-SF}, T_{MVC}, and RTD_{PEAK} of two major groups of arm muscles that generate force that is necessary for the execution of the basketball shot. RTD-SF has already been shown to be sensitive to changes in neuromuscular function associated with age [2] and disease [6]. As it was shown that explosive strength training positively influences shooting accuracy in basketball players [7], and moreover, there are some indices that maximum strength of elbow extensors is positively associated with shooting accuracy in the three-point shot, our goal was to further investigate the relationship between upper limb strength capacity and shooting performance. We hypothesized that a sport-specific movement that is constantly repeated (such as basketball shooting) might have an influence on strength capacities (k_{RTD-SF}, T_{MVC}, and RTD_{PEAK}) of the responsible muscle groups, and in addition, it might be dependent on the training history and physical development. On this basis, we evaluated differences between junior and senior basketball players in terms of k_{RTD-SF}, T_{MVC}, and RTD$_{PEAK}$ of EE and VF. The senior basketball players had significantly longer participation in basketball training and consequently greater experience and completed maturation.

Previous studies have shown that players with more training experience had better free-throw performance compared to less-experienced players [12,14]. Moreover, it was shown that explosive strength training of upper and lower limb improves basketball shooting accuracy [7]. In our study, we investigated shooting performance from shorter and longer, as different shooting distances may require different involvement of muscle strength capacities. Although it is known that muscle growth is occurring in boys until 17.5 years of age [19], our results showed that juniors and seniors had similar strength capacities of elbow extensors and volar flexors, with the exception of RTD$_{PEAK}$. Significantly larger normalized RTD$_{PEAK}$ in junior players can be explained with their lower body mass index (Table 1), since it is known that lean body mass is associated with greater RFD/RTD [20]. On the other hand, differences in abilities such as k$_{RTD-SF}$, which is independent of the body mass and muscle size, have not yet been investigated in relation to age. T$_{MVC}$ of elbow extensors, volar flexors as well as k$_{RTD-SF}$ values of both muscle groups showed similar values in junior and senior basketball players (Table 3). There is a paucity of literature analysing the differences in muscle capacity between junior and senior elite basketball players, especially regarding the upper body. A previous study reported that senior basketball players produce significantly higher absolute power with lower extremities [21]. Our data suggest that there is no difference in neuromuscular quickness (as tested by k$_{RTD-SF}$), between juniors and seniors. On the other hand, some studies that assessed shooting and passing actions showed that more experienced basketball players exhibit a shorter duration of muscle activation of the arm muscles [15,16]. This could be due to the changes in motor pattern activity associated with increasing skill [22] and not due to the changes in neuromuscular quickness. In accordance with previous studies [12,14], we have also confirmed that the players with more training experience have better shooting performance, but only from short distance. It is known that the shooting movement pattern changes with greater shooting distance, while its accuracy significantly decreases [23]. Overall, our results suggest that senior players do not have higher strength capacities compared to junior players, while they are equalized in shooting performance at long shooting distance. Thus, we can reject our first hypothesis.

Shooting performance was related with k$_{RTD-SF}$ and T$_{MVC}$ only in junior players. This result suggests that muscle abilities such as neuromuscular quickness and T$_{MVC}$ play an important role in shooting performance only in junior players, whereas in seniors their shooting muscles exceed the level of strength capacities required for successful shooting performance. In more experienced players, the shooting performance is influenced by the pattern of muscle activity (i.e., shorter or longer duration from the beginning of muscle activity, lower average activation time) [15,16] and likely not by the capacity of the shooting muscles. A very strong positive association between elbow extensor T$_{MVC}$ and shooting performance from long distance shows that muscle strength is more important for shooting performance from longer distance in juniors compared to seniors. On the contrary there was no associations between T$_{MVC}$ and shooting performance from short distance. Junior players with higher elbow extensors T$_{MVC}$ were more successful at shooting performance from a long distance (Figure 4e), which highlights the importance of muscle strength in the accuracy task from such distance. We can speculate that junior players with a smaller T$_{MVC}$ were closer to their maximum strength capacity when they performed shots from a greater distance. This can be supported with findings from one study, which showed that the accuracy decreases when the shot is performed closer to the maximal strength capacity [24]. Such associations have been only approaching statistical significance for volar flexors. Likely, it seems that the elbow extensors play a more important role than wrist muscles in providing the force required for the ball to reach the basket at greater distances [11]. On the other hand, RTD$_{PEAK}$ was not associated with shooting performance which could be explained by the fact that basketball shots are not performed under conditions that acquire maximal rate of force development.

Significant large positive associations were calculated between k$_{RTD-SF}$ of both muscle groups and the shooting performance from short distance in juniors, while k$_{RTD-SF}$ of both groups was in large negative association with long distance. It seems that the execution of the shot from short distance was better suited to junior players with greater k_{RTD-SF}, while the opposite holds true for the long-distance shots. A negative association between k_{RTD-SF} and shooting performance from long distance indicates that players with greater k_{RTD-SF} have worse shooting performance from long distance. It is already known that basketball shots are performed at higher velocities as the distance from the basket is increased [13], while lower velocities are related to greater movement accuracy [25]. It has been shown that weaker players who are unable to generate sufficient force must use a strategy of generating greater segmental velocities in order to execute a shot [26]. Shot execution at higher velocities (due to the greater distance) increases body segments movement variability and decreased movement consistency [27], while shooting performance at lower velocities provides additional time and thus allows players to perform movement corrections with visual and proprioceptive feedback [28]. This could be supported by the results of another study in which novice handball players reduced their shooting accuracy when the shooting speed was increased, while this had no effect on the shooting accuracy of expert players [29]. However, we did not measure the kinematic characteristics of shot execution, which would be valuable information for further explanations of measured associations.

In addition, similar investigation on a larger sample size would be needed for further conclusions together with the kinematic analysis of the shot from few shooting distances, while contribution from lower limb should be also considered. Finally, although the sensors used to acquire force data were high-quality load cell models, the reliability of the exact set-up, as used in this study, has not been checked before. The inter-repetition reliability of the outcome variables was, however, mostly very good. Notably, RFD_{PEAK} had k_{RTD-SF}, which supports that the latter could be an important addition or alternative to commonly performed assessments (T_{MVC} and RTD_{PEAK}).

5. Limitations of the Study

An important limitation of our study is the lack of data about the kinematics of the shot execution (especially movement velocity), which could further explain the relationship between shooting performance and strength capacity. There are potentially other additional variables that influenced the shooting performance and were not controlled (e.g., release angle, release height, physical characteristics of the players, additional basketball skills and movements that occur before shot, the power generated by the leg muscles, etc.). Moreover, only male gender was evaluated so our conclusion refers only to young male basketball players.

6. Conclusions

This was the first study to investigate differences in k_{RTD-SF} and other strength capacities between juniors and seniors with significantly different training histories. It appears that the specific training history (performing basketball shot) has no influence on neuromuscular quickness of elbow extensors and volar flexors. Our results suggest that strength capacities, specifically T_{MVC} is a limiting factor for successful shooting performance only in juniors, while in seniors there was no associations with strength capacities and shooting accuracy. This should be taken into account in training programmes of young male basketball players. Appropriate strength capacities, specifically maximum strength of elbow extensors should be developed for successful shooting performance for longer distance in young male basketball players. Detailed kinematic assessment of shooting performance should be measured in the future to confirm our assumptions that players with higher k_{RTD-SF} use higher movement velocities at longer shooting distance, resulting in poorer shooting performance.

Author Contributions: Conceptualization, N.Š.; methodology, D.S., N.Š., and Ž.K.; software, N.Š.; formal analysis, D.S., N.Š., and Ž.K.; investigation, D.S.; resources, N.Š.; data curation, D.S. and Ž.K.; writing—original draft preparation, D.S.; writing—review and editing, N.Š. and Ž.K.; visualization, N.Š.; supervision, N.Š.; project administration, N.Š.; funding acquisition, N.Š. All authors have read and agreed to the published version of the manuscript.

Funding: This research was funded by Slovenian research agency, grant number L5-1845: Body asymmetries as a risk factor in musculoskeletal injury development: studying etiological mechanisms and designing corrective interventions for primary and tertiary preventive care, (2) bilateral project between Slovenia and Serbia ARRS-BI-RS/18-19-010 and by the research program fund P5-0147 Kinesiology of monostructural, polystructural, and conventional sports.

Acknowledgments: Authors thank a student at the University of Primorska, Jure Muršec, for his help at subject's recruitment and data acquisition.

Conflicts of Interest: The authors declare no conflict of interest.

References

1. Bellumori, M.; Jaric, S.; Knight, C.A. The rate of force development scaling factor (RFD-SF): Protocol, reliability, and muscle comparisons. *Exp. Brain Res.* **2011**, *212*, 359–369. [CrossRef] [PubMed]
2. Bellumori, M.; Jaric, S.; Knight, C.A. Age-related decline in the rate of force development scaling factor. *Motor Control* **2013**, *17*, 370–381. [CrossRef] [PubMed]
3. Mathern, R.M.; Anhorn, M.; Uygur, M. A novel method to assess rate of force relaxation: Reliability and comparisons with rate of force development across various muscles. *Eur. J. Appl. Physiol.* **2019**, *119*, 291–300. [CrossRef] [PubMed]
4. Djordjevic, D.; Uygur, M. Methodological considerations in the calculation of the rate of force development scaling factor. *Physiol Meas* **2017**, *39*, 015001. [CrossRef] [PubMed]
5. Casartelli, N.C.; Lepers, R.; Maffiuletti, N.A. Assessment of the rate of force development scaling factor for the hip muscles. *Muscle Nerve* **2014**, *50*, 932–938. [CrossRef]
6. Uygur, M.; de Freitas, P.B.; Barone, D.A. Rate of force development and relaxation scaling factors are highly sensitive to detect upper extremity motor impairments in multiple sclerosis. *J. Neurol. Sci.* **2020**, *408*, 116500. [CrossRef]
7. Savaş, S.; Yüksel, M.F.; Uzun, A. The effects of rapid strength and shooting training applied to professional basketball players on the shot percentage level. *Univers. J. Educ. Res.* **2018**, *6*, 1569–1574. [CrossRef]
8. Justin, I.; Strojnik, V.; Sarabon, N. The effect of increased maximum strength of elbow extensors on the ability to shoot accurately in darts and the three-point shot in basketball. *Rev. Šport Rev. za Teor. Prakt. Vprašanja Športa* **2006**, *2*, 51–55.
9. Okubo, H.; Hubbard, M. Kinematics of arm joint motions in basketball shooting. *Procedia Eng.* **2015**, *112*, 443–448. [CrossRef]
10. Miller, S.; Federation, I.T. The relationship between basketball shooting kinematics, distance and playing position. *J. Sports Sci.* **1996**, *14*, 243–253. [CrossRef]
11. Miller, S.; Bartlett, R.M. The effects of increased shooting distance in the basketball jump shot. *J. Sports Sci.* **1993**, *11*, 285–293. [CrossRef] [PubMed]
12. Button, C.; Macleod, M.; Sanders, R.; Coleman, S. Examining movement variability in the basketball free-throw action at different skill levels. *Res. Q. Exerc. Sport* **2003**, *74*, 257–269. [CrossRef] [PubMed]
13. Okazaki, V.H.A.; Rodacki, A.L.F.; Satern, M.N. A review on the basketball jump shot. *Sports Biomech.* **2015**, *14*, 190–205. [CrossRef] [PubMed]
14. Zuzik, P. Free Throw Shooting Effectiveness in Basketball Matches of Men and Women. *Sport Sci. Rev.* **2012**, *20*, 149–160. [CrossRef]
15. Pakosz, P.; Konieczny, M. Time Analysis of Muscle Activation during Basketball Free Throws. *Cent. Eur. J. Sport Sci. Med.* **2016**, *15*, 73–79. [CrossRef]
16. Pakosz Paweł Emg Signal Analysis of Selected Muscles During Shots and Passes in Basketball. *J. Heal. Promot. Recreat. Rzesz.* **2011**, *2*, 8–14.
17. Cohen, J. *Statistical Power Analysis for the Behavioral Sciences*, 2nd ed.; Routlege Academic: New York, NY, USA, 1988.
18. Hopkins, W.G. Measures of Reliability in Sports Medicine and Science. *Sport. Med.* **2000**, *30*, 1–15. [CrossRef]
19. Malina, R.; Bouchard, C.; Bar-Or, O. *Growth, Maturation, and Physical Activity*, 2nd ed.; Human Kinetics: Champaign, IL, USA, 2004.
20. Kavvoura, A.; Zaras, N.; Stasinaki, A.N.; Arnaoutis, G.; Methenitis, S.; Terzis, G. The importance of lean body mass for the rate of force development in taekwondo athletes and track and field throwers. *J. Funct. Morphol. Kinesiol.* **2018**, *3*, 1–20. [CrossRef]

21. Balsalobre-Fernández, C.; Tejero-González, C.M.; Del Campo-Vecino, J.; Bachero-Mena, B.; Sánchez-Martínez, J. Differences of muscular performance between professional and young basketball players. *Cult. Cienc. y Deport.* **2016**, *11*, 61–65. [CrossRef]
22. Wissel, H. *Basketball: Steps to Success*; Human Kinetics: Champaign, IL, USA, 1994.
23. Liu, S.; Burton, A.W. Changes in basketball shooting patterns as a function of distance. *Percept. Mot. Skills* **1999**, *89*, 831–845. [CrossRef]
24. Etnyre, B.R. Accuracy characteristics of throwing as a result of maximum force effort. *Percept. Mot. Skills* **1998**, *86*, 1211–1217. [CrossRef] [PubMed]
25. Knudson, D. Biomechanics of the Basketball Jump Shot—Six Key Teaching Points. *J. Phys. Educ. Recreat. Dance* **1993**, *64*, 67–73. [CrossRef]
26. Hudson, J. Shooting techniques for small players. *Athl. J.* **1985**, *11*, 22–24.
27. Darling, W.; Cooke, J. Changes in the variability of movement trajectories with practice. *J. Mot. Behav.* **1987**, *19*, 291–309. [CrossRef] [PubMed]
28. Schmidt, R.; Zelaznik, H.; Hawkings, B.; Frank, J.; Quinn, J., Jr. Motor-output variability: A theory for the accuracy of rapid motor acts. *Psychol. Rev.* **1979**, *47*, 415–451. [CrossRef]
29. García, J.A.; Sabido, R.; Barbado, D.; Moreno, F.J. Analysis of the relation between throwing speed and throwing accuracy in team-handball according to instruction. *Eur. J. Sport Sci.* **2013**, *13*, 149–154. [CrossRef]

Publisher's Note: MDPI stays neutral with regard to jurisdictional claims in published maps and institutional affiliations.

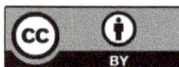

© 2020 by the authors. Licensee MDPI, Basel, Switzerland. This article is an open access article distributed under the terms and conditions of the Creative Commons Attribution (CC BY) license (http://creativecommons.org/licenses/by/4.0/).

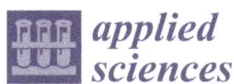 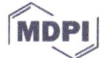

Article

Anthropometric Characteristics, Maximal Isokinetic Strength and Selected Handball Power Indicators Are Specific to Playing Positions in Elite Kosovan Handball Players

Jeton Havolli [1,2], Abedin Bahtiri [1], Tim Kambič [3,4], Kemal Idrizović [2], Duško Bjelica [2] and Primož Pori [4,*]

1. Department of Physical Culture, Sport and Recreation, Kolegji Universi (Universi College) Prishtina, 10000 Prishtina, Kosovo; jeton.havolli@kolegjiuniversi-edu.net (J.H.); abedinbahtiri@gmail.com (A.B.)
2. Faculty of Sport and Physical Education, 81400 Nikšić, Montenegro; kemali@ucg.ac.me (K.I.); dbjelica@ucg.ac.me (D.B.)
3. Department of Research and Education, General Hospital Murska Sobota, 9000 Murska Sobota, Slovenia; tim.kambic@gmail.com
4. Department of Sports Medicine, Faculty of Sport, University of Ljubljana, 1000 Ljubljana, Slovenia
* Correspondence: primoz.pori@fsp.uni-lj.si; Tel.: +386-(0)-520-77-64

Received: 30 July 2020; Accepted: 24 September 2020; Published: 27 September 2020

Abstract: Anthropometric characteristics and physical performance are closely related to the game demands of each playing position. This study aimed to first examine the differences between playing positions in anthropometric characteristics and physical performance with special emphasis on the isokinetic strength of elite male handball players, and secondly to examine the correlations of the latter variables with ball velocity. Anthropometric characteristics, maximal isokinetic strength, sprinting and vertical jumping performance, and ball velocity in the set shot and jump shot were obtained from 93 elite handball players (age 22 ± 5 years, height 184 ± 8 cm, and weight 84 ± 14 kg) pre-season. Wing players were shorter compared to other players, and pivots were the heaviest. Wings had the fastest 20 m sprints, and, along with backcourt players, jumped higher, had better maximal knee isometric strength, and achieved the highest ball velocity compared to pivots and goalkeepers, respectively. There were no significant differences between playing positions in unilateral and bilateral maximal leg strength imbalances. Ball velocity was significantly correlated with height, weight, squat jump and maximal torque of extensors and flexors. Our study suggest that shooting success is largely determined by the player's height, weight, muscle strength and power, while it seems that anthropometric characteristics and physical performance are closely related to the game demands of each playing position.

Keywords: morphology; isokinetic; sprints; vertical jump performance; handball shooting

1. Introduction

Handball is an Olympic team sport [1,2], split into two periods (each 30 min long) and consisting of a high degree of body contact and predominantly aerobic activities separated by anaerobic bouts of sprints, jumps, throws, changes of directions in the offense (counterattack and attack buildup) and defense [2,3]. Therefore, competition success in elite handball is not only closely related to the technical and tactical skills of each individual or team, but also to the players' anthropometric characteristics, physical performance (e.g., maximal strength and power as measured using strength, sprinting, and jumping tests), and handball shooting performance [3–5].

To date, only a few studies evaluating the physical and physiological demands in handball matches have shown significant differences between playing positions [6–8]. Results obtained during gameplay have shown that backcourt players cover larger distances and spend less time standing and walking, and, together with pivots, have higher in-game heart rates and spend longer durations at higher intensities (>80% maximal heart rate) [7]. In contrast, wing players are faster than other playing positions, and pivots endure more body impact than other players [6]. Furthermore, similar differences between playing positions were also obtained in anthropometric characteristics [9,10] and physical performance [11–16]. Wings are the shortest, have significantly lower body mass and body mass index (BMI) than other players; pivots are the heaviest, whereas other playing positions do not differ in height [9–16]. Research comparing playing positions in sprinting (e.g., sprints on 20–30 m) and jumping performance (squat jump (SJ) and/or countermovement jumps (CMJs)) is relatively scarce, and there are some discrepancies in sprinting times and jump heights among studies [11,14–16]. Nevertheless, backcourt players and wings demonstrated the fastest sprinting times [14,15], while CMJ height was the highest in wings [14], compared to pivots and goalkeepers [15].

Isokinetic dynamometry has long been the gold standard for assessing changes to an athlete's maximal muscle strength/torque during the season [17,18] and risk of injury (measured as imbalances between agonist and antagonist muscles or bilateral differences) in different types of a team sport [19]. In the past, only a few studies have evaluated isokinetic maximal knee strength and strength imbalances in male handball players [19–21], with the majority of studies having been performed on female handball players, focusing on shoulder muscle strength, and several on knee muscle strength in relation to shoulder and knee injuries [18,22–25]. Evidence from two studies evaluating isokinetic maximal strength in male handball players has suggested no differences between dominant and nondominant lower limb knee extensor and flexor strength, as well as normal hamstring-to-quadriceps ratio on both limbs at 60°/s and 180°/s [19,20]. However, no studies in handball have investigated isokinetic maximal strength of the knee joint according to playing position. Furthermore, it also remains to be elucidated the potential role of playing position on development of muscle strength imbalances between and within legs as a product of specific game demands. Such findings would serve as excellent feedback to practitioners to focus on preventing potential injuries and to improve player performance.

Ball velocity has been recognized as one of the most important determinants of game performance [14]. Maximal ball velocity is achieved through a proximal-to-distal manner; this movement allows momentum of force to transfer from the lower limb and/or pelvis through the trunk to the throwing arm, thereby enabling higher velocities of the shot [26]. During the game, the majority of shots are performed using two shooting techniques: a three-step jump shot and a standing set shot from the ground. Both techniques use two different kinetic strategies (braking the body with lead leg in the standing set shot vs. opposed leg movement during the flight phase of the three-step jump shot) [27,28], while ball velocity in both is influenced by an optimal proximal–distal principle, trunk movement, and maximal arm rotation [26,28]. It is well established that elite players are able to maintain an optimal proximal-to-distal principle and arm movement while performing different shooting techniques [27]. Lower ball velocity has been associated with lower strength in the lower and upper limbs, leading to inefficient transfer of power from the proximal (pelvis, trunk) to distal (shooting arm) parts of the body [29]. Backcourt players and wings shoot the ball faster compared to pivots or goalkeepers [14,15,30]. For overhead throws, only inconsistent correlations have been reported between ball velocity and anthropometric characteristics or physical performance, and this is likely due to the complex nature of this movement [10,11,13,31,32]. Body height and weight were the only anthropometric characteristics significantly correlated with ball velocity of the standing shot [11] and/or three-step running shot [10,13,31], whereas two additional studies reported significant correlations with lower limb strength (1-RM half back squat) [31], standing long jump, 30 m sprint, and maximal oxygen uptake (estimated from 20 m shuttle run) [31]. Other studies have failed to detect such correlations [11,13]; therefore, additional studies are warranted to transfer these findings into training settings.

Based on the identified gaps in the knowledge of the anthropometric characteristics, maximal strength and power performance, and handball shooting performance of elite handball players, our study consisted of three aims. The first aim of the study was to provide further evidence on the isokinetic maximal strength and potential limb imbalances between playing positions in elite male handball players. The second aim was to examine the differences in anthropometric characteristics, sprinting and vertical jump performance between playing positions, and the last aim was to investigate the correlations between handball-specific performance (e.g., ball velocity) and selected anthropometric characteristics and physical performance indicators.

2. Materials and Methods

2.1. Study Design

The study was designed as a cross-sectional study of a sample of elite Kosovo handball players. Measurements were conducted two weeks before the start of a competitive season, at the end of August 2019. Testing procedures were split into three days. On the first day anthropometric characteristics (height, weight, wingspan, and thigh circumference) and body composition (skeletal muscle mass and fat mass) were measured, and familiarization with all testing procedures was conducted. On the second day, following a standardized warm-up procedure, sprinting performance (20 m sprints), vertical jump performance (CMJ and SJ), and shooting performance (shooting velocity of three-step set shot and jump shot) were assessed. Finally, during the last day measurements of unilateral isokinetic knee flexor and extensor torque at 60°/s and 180°/s were conducted after the standardized warm-up. Forty-eight hours of rest were given between the second and third testing day to minimize any potential effects of fatigue. Testing procedures were performed by experienced strength and conditioning specialists.

2.2. Subjects

A total of 93 elite male handball players from Kosovo's first handball league were enrolled into the study, age (mean (SD)) 22 (1) years, height 184.0 (7.83) cm, weight 84.10 (13.74) kg, and with 8 (4) years of professional playing experience. The sample consisted of 35 (37.63%) backcourt players, 26 (27.96%) wing players, 15 (16.13%) pivots, and 17 (18.28%) goalkeepers. Playing positions were determined according to registration data obtained from the Handball Federation of Kosovo. Players' adherence was consistent throughout the study, and no injuries or other health issues were reported.

Prior to enrolment into the study, we informed all participants about the aims of our study, methods and procedures, and potential testing risks. Measurements were performed at the end of the last week of the specific preparation phase for the upcoming season, with at least 48 h of rest after the last training session, and 10–14 days prior to beginning of the season. The exclusion criteria were: fewer than two years of professional playing experience, age younger than 18 years, and any recent musculoskeletal injuries (<6 months). All participants signed a written consent prior to inclusion in the study. The study design was approved by the Ethics Committee of Universi College Prishtina (document number: 488/18), while the study was conducted according to the Declaration of Helsinki guidelines for the use of human participants.

2.3. Procedures

2.3.1. Anthropometric and Body Composition Measurement

Prior to physical performance measurements on the first testing day, anthropometric and bioimpedance measurements were obtained according to the international guidelines [33]. Body height and weight were measured while standing barefoot using a SECA 763 stadiometer with electronic scale (Seca Instruments Ltd., Hamburg, Germany) to the nearest cm and kg, respectively. The wingspan was measured using a horizontal wall-mounted scale to the nearest cm, with arms abducted at 90° from a neutral position and back facing towards the wall, and thigh circumference was measured using a tape measure while standing at 2/3 of the distance between the lateral epicondyle of the knee and the greater trochanter on the dominant leg. Skeletal muscle mass and fat mass measurements were obtained using a Biospace Inbody 720 bioimpedance device (Inbody Co., Leicester, United Kingdom). Participants were asked to place toes and heels on the anterior and posterior electrodes of the weighting platform, and to firmly grasp the hand grip with both hands. Measurements were taken early in the morning, and participants were advised to avoid any moderate to vigorous physical activity a day before the measurement [34].

2.3.2. Sprint Performance Measurement

After the general 15-min warm-up (10 min running, and 5 min of whole-body dynamic mobility exercises) and an additional three repetitions of progressive acceleration from faster to sprint running, participants performed two 20 m sprints, with 3 min of rest between each exertion. Prior to testing, four photocell gates (Polifemo Radio Light, Microgate, Bolzano, Italy) were placed at the start, at 5 m, at 10 m, and at 20 m. The dominant foot (lead-off foot) [35] was placed one meter behind the first photocell. The time recording was automatically initialized when a participant crossed the first photocell gate and stopped when the participant crossed the last photocell gate at 20 m distance. Participants were instructed to sprint at least 25 m in order to reach the highest maximum sprinting speed. The fastest of the two split times on 5 m, 10 m, and 20 m distances was used in the final analysis [4]. All measurements were performed indoors.

2.3.3. Vertical Jump Performance Measurement

Vertical jump performance, measured as jump height (cm), was evaluated from the CMJ and SJ using an OptoJump infrared timing system (Microgate, Bolzano, Italy). The participants first performed three trials of CMJs followed by three trials of SJs [15]. One minute of rest was given between two trials. Prior to performing both jumps, participants were instructed about the jumping technique and later performed at least two submaximal familiarization repetitions of CMJs and SJs to learn proper jumping techniques [4]. The CMJ was performed by flexing the knee to a squat position (approximately 90° of knee flexion) from an upright position and then immediately extending the hips and the knee into a vertical jump, whereas the SJ was performed by jumping to vertical from squat position (90° of knee flexion) [20]. When approaching the landing position, participants were advised to land with extended knees to avoid any measurement error resulting from prolonged flight time. Both jumps were performed with hands placed on hips and with legs straightened during the flight. The jump height was calculated from the recorded flight time (height = [gravitational acceleration (9.81 m/s^2) × flight time2] × 8 − 1) [4], and the highest jump was used in the final analysis.

2.3.4. Handball Shooting Performance Measurement

Handball shooting performance was evaluated by measuring the ball velocity of a three-step set shot from the ground and the ball velocity of a three-step jump shot from the 9-m line, using the Bushnell Radar (Bushnell, Overland Park, KS, USA) with a measurement error of ±1.60 km/h (www.bushnellspeedster.com). The investigator measured ball velocity while standing at the 9-m line within 1 m of the participant performing the throw. After the warm-up, each participant performed one familiarization shot and two test shots of each shot type, with one minute of rest between shots [14,15].

2.3.5. Maximal Isokinetic Strength Measurement

Isokinetic concentric torque of knee extensors and flexors was measured using an isokinetic dynamometer Biodex Pro 4 (Biodex Medical Systems, Shirley, New York, NY, USA) at 60°/s and 180°/s according to previous guidelines and studies [18,36]. Prior to testing day, the machine was calibrated according to manufacturer guidelines, using a long shoulder attached to the axis of the apparatus, generating a standard torque of 67.8 Nm.

Prior to testing, each participant completed a standardized warm-up protocol consisting of 10 min of light jogging, followed by short dynamic stretching exercises for lower limbs, and ending with a single 8-repetition set of squat and hip thrust exercises. After the general warm-up, the participants were seated upright in the dynamometer chair with restraining belts fastened across the chest, pelvis, and leg thigh to minimize body movement or any potential compensation of synergist muscles. Later, we aligned the dynamometer axis of rotation to the participant's knee joint axis of rotation using the lateral epicondyle as the anatomic mark. Additionally, gravitation torque error was measured prior to each trial, and the starting leg was randomly selected for each participant. The range of motion was set at 80°, from 90° to 10° of knee flexion.

Prior to measuring maximal effort, each participant first performed a specific warm-up on the dynamometer consisting of 10 submaximal concentric contractions of knee flexion and extension at 60°/s. The maximal test was conducted after 2 min of rest, with participants performing five maximal concentric knee extensions and flexions. Verbal encouragement was given by the investigator during the test to ensure participants performed at their maximal effort. The maximal value out of five measurements was normalized to body weight (N/kg) and used in the final statistical analysis. In addition, bilateral differences between left and right maximal isometric torque (left leg/right leg maximal isometric torque × 100%) and unilateral hamstring-to-quadriceps maximal isometric torque (hamstring/quadriceps maximal isometric torque × 100%) [37] was calculated prior to further statistical analysis.

2.4. Statistical Analysis

Categorical variables are presented as frequencies and percentages, and numeric variables are presented as means and standard deviations, unless otherwise stated. All numeric variables were firstly screened for assumptions of normality of distribution and homogeneity of variances using the Shapiro–Wilk test and the Levene's test, respectively. This was screened for the whole sample and according to each playing position. The difference between playing positions was calculated using one-way analysis of variance (ANOVA) for normally distributed variables and homogeneous variances, otherwise, the Kruskal–Wallis test was applied. When one-way ANOVA detected significant differences between playing positions, an additional post hoc analysis was performed using the Tukey's honest significance test or pairwise comparisons, depending on the dispersion of variances between playing positions. Correlations between anthropometric, physical, and handball performance were assessed using Spearman's rank correlation coefficient. All statistical analyses were performed using IBM SPSS version 21 (SPSS Inc., Armonk, New York, NY, USA), and the level of significance was set at p-value < 0.05.

3. Results

There were statistically significant differences for playing positions in all measured anthropometric characteristics and skeletal muscle mass and fat mass (all p-values < 0.01; Table 1). The wings were significantly shorter compared to backcourt players ($p < 0.001$), pivots ($p = 0.035$), and goalkeepers ($p = 0.018$). Similar significant differences were obtained in weight (pivots vs. wing, $p < 0.001$; wings vs. backcourt players, $p < 0.001$), wingspan (wings vs. pivots, $p < 0.001$; wings vs. backcourt players, $p < 0.001$; wings vs. goalkeepers, $p = 0.038$), and thigh circumference (wings vs. pivots, $p < 0.001$; wings vs. backcourt players, $p = 0.041$). Additionally, pivots were heavier than goalkeepers ($p < 0.001$) and backcourt players ($p = 0.003$) and had larger thigh circumference compared to goalkeepers ($p < 0.001$) and backcourt players ($p < 0.001$), whereas backcourt players were heavier than goalkeepers ($p = 0.015$).

Table 1. Differences between playing positions in anthropometric characteristics and body composition.

	Backcourt Player (N = 34)	Wing (N = 26)	Pivot (N = 15)	Goalkeeper (N = 17)	p
Height (cm)	187 (8)[1]	179 (7)	185 (7)[1]	185 (6)[1]	<0.001
Weight (kg)	87 (11)[1,2]	75 (9)	102 (11)[1,2]	78 (10)	<0.001
Wingspan (cm)	190 (9)[1]	180 (8)	191 (9)[1]	186 (8)[1]	<0.001
Thigh circ. (cm)	60 (5)[1]	57 (5)	68 (5)[1,2,3]	58 (5)	<0.001
Skeletal muscle mass (kg)	44 (5)[1,2]	38 (4)	47 (5)[1,2]	37 (4)	<0.001
Body fat mass (kg)	12 (5)	10 (4)	23 (8)[1,2,3]	15 (7)[1]	<0.001

Cir.–circumference, [1]—significantly different from the wing, [2]—significantly different from the goalkeeper, [3]—significantly different from backcourt players.

Body composition measurements revealed that goalkeepers had significantly less skeletal muscle mass than backcourt players ($p < 0.001$) and pivots ($p < 0.001$), while wings had less skeletal muscle mass than backcourt players ($p < 0.001$) and pivots ($p < 0.001$). Pivots, on the other hand, had significantly more fat mass than wings ($p < 0.001$), backcourt players ($p < 0.001$) and goalkeepers ($p = 0.005$). Lastly, goalkeepers also had significantly more muscle mass than wings ($p = 0.010$).

Similar to the anthropometric characteristics, the playing positions differed in maximal isokinetic concentric extensor strength at 60°/s and 180°/s ($p < 0.001$), concentric knee flexion of the left knee at 60°/s ($p = 0.007$), and borderline significance of the right knee ($p = 0.070$) (Table 2). Pivot players displayed lower isokinetic concentric torque of knee extensors and flexors compared with wings and backcourt players at 60°/s and 180°/s, respectively, whereas backcourt players were superior compared to goalkeepers at 60°/s and 180°/s of knee flexion and extension. Additionally, wings performed better than goalkeepers at 60°/s and 180°/s of knee extension and flexion. Otherwise, no differences between playing positions were obtained in hamstring-to-quadriceps ratio (HQR) and in bilateral differences in maximal concentric torque of extensors and flexors at 60°/s and 180°/s.

Table 2. Differences among playing positions in isokinetic concentric torque.

	Backcourt Player (N = 34)	Wing (N = 26)	Pivot (N = 15)	Goalkeeper (N = 17)	p
Extension left knee at 60°/s (Nm/kg)	2.80 (0.58)	2.88 (0.55)	2.23 (0.45)[1,2]	2.53 (0.32)[1,2]	<0.001
Extension right knee at 60°/s (Nm/kg)	2.86 (0.45)	2.83 (0.56)	2.30 (0.43)[1,2]	2.50 (0.35)[2]	<0.001
Extension left knee at 180°/s (Nm/kg)	1.80 (0.32)	1.85 (0.28)	1.42 (0.28)[1,2]	1.49 (0.29)[1,2]	<0.001
Extension right knee at 180°/s (Nm/kg)	1.79 (0.27)	1.73 (0.36)	1.45 (0.27)[1,2]	1.51 (0.24)[2]	<0.001
Flexion left knee at 60°/s (Nm/kg)	1.74 (0.38)	1.74 (0.38)	1,50 (0.63)[1,2]	1.52 (0.24)[1,2]	0.007
Flexion right knee at 60°/s (Nm/kg)	1.78 (0.25)	1.70 (0.39)	1.57 (0.59)	1.53 (0.39)	0.070
Flexion left knee at 180°/s (Nm/kg)	1.33 (0.29)	1.33 (0.30)	1.07 (0.34)[1,2]	1.11 (0.26)[1,2]	0.002
Flexion right knee at 180°/s (Nm/kg)	1.32 (0.25)	1.21 (0.28)	1.08 (0.34)[2]	1.12 (0.22)[2]	0.012
Bilateral ratio left–right knee extension at 60°/s (%)	98.23 (15.08)	102.36 (9.97)	95.95 (7.04)	96.95 (7.04)	0.251
Bilateral ratio left–right knee flexion at 60°/s (%)	98.50 (21.14)	103.16 (11.35)	95.17 (10.47)	102.86 (20.42)	0.059
Bilateral ratio left–right knee extension at 180°/s (%)	101.89 (19.47)	110.65 (16.02)	100.71 (13.56)	98.58 (11.86)	0.112
Bilateral ratio left–right knee flexion at 180°/s (%)	101.43 (17.55)	109.70 (19.37)	97.76 (9.74)	98.59 (13.11)	0.068
HQR left knee at 60°/s (%)	63.23 (17.97)	60.84 (11.78)	70.29 (36.66)	59.93 (6.39)	0.725
HQR right knee at 60°/s (%)	63.56 (12.52)	60.54 (11.69)	69.40 (28.23)	61.06 (12.21)	0.958
HQR left knee at 180°/s (%)	74.18 (15.22)	71.55 (11.83)	77.35 (27.68)	74.67 (13.42)	0.596
HQR right knee at 180°/s (%)	74.32 (14.73)	70.90 (12.91)	74.58 (21.80)	74.17 (10.87)	0.704

HQR–hamstring-to-quadriceps torque ratio, [1]—significantly different from the wing, [2]—significantly different from backcourt players.

Measurements of sprinting and vertical jump performance showed significant differences between playing positions (all p-values < 0.01; Table 3). Wing players were significantly faster than backcourt players (5 m, $p = 0.042$; 10 m, $p = 0.001$; and 20 m, $p = 0.027$), goalkeepers (5 m, $p = 0.013$; 10 m, $p = 0.001$; and 20 m, $p = 0.001$), and pivots (5 m, $p = 0.001$ and 20 m, $p < 0.001$). At the 10-m time gate, backcourt players were significantly faster than goalkeepers ($p < 0.001$). Moreover, backcourt players and wings jumped significantly higher compared to pivots (backcourt players vs. pivots: CMJ, $p = 0.007$, SJ, $p = 0.027$; wings vs. pivots: CMJ, $p < 0.001$, SJ, $p < 0.001$) and goalkeepers (backcourt players vs. pivots: CMJ, $p = 0.006$; wings vs. goalkeepers: CMJ, $p < 0.001$, SJ, $p = 0.004$), respectively.

Table 3. Differences between playing positions in sprinting, vertical jump performance, and handball shooting performance.

	Backcourt Player (N = 34)	Wing (N = 26)	Pivot (N = 15)	Goalkeeper (N = 17)	p
Sprint 5 m (s)	1.05 (0.08) [1]	1.01 (0.08)	1.11 (0.09) [1]	1.10 (0.12) [1]	0.006
Sprint 10 m (s)	1.83 (0.20) [1]	1.75 (0.24)	1.93 (0.30)	1.97 (0.13) [1,3]	0.003
Sprint 20 m (s)	3.31 (0.24) [1]	3.15 (0.19)	3.44 (0.22) [1]	3.42 (0.17) [1]	<0.001
SJ (cm)	30 (5)	32 (6)	25 (6) [1,3]	26 (4) [1,3]	<0.001
CMJ (cm)	34 (4)	37 (6)	29 (6) [1,3]	31 (5) [1]	<0.001
Set shot (km/h)	89 (7) [1,2]	84 (9) [2]	89 (5) [2]	79 (6)	<0.001
Jump shot (km/h)	88 (7) [1,2]	83 (9) [2]	87 (9) [2]	77 (6)	<0.001

SJ—squat jump, CMJ—countermovement jump, [1]—significantly different from the wing, [2]—significantly different from the goalkeeper, [3]—significantly different from backcourt players.

There were also significant differences in ball velocity among playing positions (both p-values <0.001). Post hoc analysis showed that goalkeepers shoot the ball at significantly lower velocity while shooting from ground position (all p-values < 0.01) or while performing a three-step jump shot (all p-values < 0.01).

Correlations between handball shooting performance and sprinting, jumping, and maximal strength performance are shown in Table 4. With the exception of body fat mass and thigh circumference, all other anthropometric characteristics were significantly correlated with the ball velocity of a three-step set shot and jump shot. A higher SJ was significantly correlated with the ball velocity of the set shot, and borderline significant with the ball velocity of the jump shot. Maximal isokinetic torque of knee flexors and extensors was significantly correlated with ball velocity of both shot types. Lastly, HQR at 60°/s was significantly correlated with the ball velocity of the set shot.

Table 4. Correlations between playing positions in sprinting, vertical jump performance, and handball shooting performance.

	Set Shot (m/s)		Jump Shot (m/s)	
	Spearman Rho	p	Spearman Rho	p
Height (cm)	0.330	0.001	0.263	0.011
Weight (kg)	0.303	0.003	0.282	0.006
Skeletal muscle mass (kg)	0.522	<0.001	0.473	<0.001
Body fat mass (kg)	−0.116	0.267	−0.083	0.428
Wingspan (cm)	0.387	<0.001	0.349	0.001
Thigh circumference (cm)	0.183	0.080	0.166	0.112
Sprint 20 (s)	0.061	0.566	−0.018	0.862
SJ (cm)	0.210	0.043	0.185	0.076
CMJ (cm)	0.128	0.221	0.057	0.585
Knee extension torque at 60°/s (Nm)	0.219	0.035	0.340	0.001
Knee extension torque at 180°/s (Nm)	0.352	0.001	0.419	<0.001
Knee flexion torque at 60°/s (Nm)	0.493	<0.001	0.465	<0.001
Knee flexion torque at 180°/s (Nm)	0.477	<0.001	0.460	<0.001
HQR at 60°/s (%)	0.317	0.002	0.171	0.101
HQR at 180°/s (%)	0.139	0.185	0.061	0.564

SJ—squat jump, CMJ—countermovement jump, HQR—hamstring-to-quadriceps torque ratio.

4. Discussion

In the present study, we identified differences between playing positions in anthropometric characteristics, isometric maximal leg strength, sprinting and vertical jumping performance, and established new evidence on the relationship between anthropometry, physical performance, and ball velocity as an indicator of game performance. The most novel findings of this study were related to isokinetic performance, adding to the few reports of the isokinetic maximal strength and strength imbalances in elite male handball players that have been published to our knowledge [19–21]. Our results suggest that maximal knee flexor and extensor strength is related to playing position, whereas no differences between playing positions were observed in bilateral muscle imbalances or the ratios between knee joint agonists and antagonists.

In the previous studies of sports performance in elite handball, the investigators applied different methods to assess maximal leg strength. Most of those studies on elite male handball players used different variations of maximal squat tests to determine maximal leg strength [4,11,15,32], while (only) a small body of evidence used isokinetic testing [19,20], despite it being considered the gold standard for assessing quadriceps and hamstring maximal strength and muscle imbalances [17,18]. Most studies measuring maximal isokinetic knee strength were performed with females [18,24,38,39], likely due to higher rates of anterior cruciate ligament injuries, compared with males [40], while only two isokinetic studies included male handball players [19,20]. In the latter studies, male handball players were recognized as functionally balanced athletes, where maximal unilateral (50–69%) and bilateral (10–15%) muscle strength differences were in the normal range [19,20]. This was similarly demonstrated in our study, although there were no bilateral differences in maximal strength of flexors and extensors, or muscle imbalances between hamstrings and quadriceps on each leg at 60°/s and 180°/s. Our relative values of maximal flexion and extension torque at 60°/s and 180°/s (N/kg) were also similar to a report by Gonzalez-Rave et al. [20]. Additionally, our study also evaluated the difference between playing positions in relative maximal strength and muscle imbalances. Backcourt and wing players were the strongest in extension and flexion, independent of muscle mass at both angular velocities. These results may potentially be associated with game demands, as wings and backcourt players perform the most jumps and throws [7]. In contrast, all playing positions showed symmetrical strength (unilateral and bilateral ratios in the normal range) between legs and within each leg analysis.

Studies have suggested that anthropometric characteristics are related to playing position. In our study, wing players were the shortest, had the lowest body weight, shortest wingspan and smallest thigh circumference, while pivots had the highest body weight, skeletal muscle mass, and body fat mass content. These results were in line with previous studies [7,10,13–16] from elite and sub-elite male handball players. Despite the similar ages of players and the differences between playing positions in body weight and height, our subsample of backcourt players, pivots, and goalkeepers was generally shorter and lighter than players competing on elite German [10,14], Norwegian [15], and national teams playing in the World Championship [9]. Thus, these differences can be explained by the level of play and age. Players competing in lower leagues were generally shorter [10], independent of playing position, whereas pivots in higher leagues were heavier and had the highest body mass index [14]. Also, younger elite handball players were shorter, lighter, had lower free fat mass and body mass index values compared to elite adult players [16].

The fastest sprint times were recorded in wing players compared to other playing positions on each of three time gates (5 m, 10 m, and 20 m). Similar variations in sprinting performance at 20 m were observed in the other two studies consisting of handball players performing in elite European leagues [14,15]. In addition to the fastest times recorded by wings, backcourt players were also faster than goalkeepers on 10-m sprints, similar to data obtained by Haugen et al. [15] (wings, 2.78 (0.08) s; backcourt players, 2.83 (0.11) s; goalkeepers, 2.94 (0.10) s). Partly contrary to our findings, one study reported significant differences between playing positions only on longer sprint distances (30 m), postulating equal starting acceleration of all playing positions, which likely contributed to the longer competitive career and a higher level of competition [14]. Moreover, sprinting performance is closely related to the in-game demands of each playing position. Data derived from game movement analysis has shown that wing players have a higher frequency of performed sprints, with the longest duration, time, and fraction of distance covered compared to pivots and backcourt players [7].

Vertical jumping is an important movement performed during the course of the game [7]. In previous studies, the best vertical jumps were performed by the wings (39–50 cm) and backcourt players (38–47 cm), compared to pivots (35–43 cm) and goalkeepers (35–47 cm) [14,15]. Similar differences between playing positions were also obtained in our study. Nevertheless, jump performance was lower compared to data from two samples of elite European Championship players [14,15], but comparable to a similar level of play [16], thus, our results were likely influenced by the level of play and quality of the training regime.

Handball scoring efficiency is largely dependent on ball velocity. In our study, ball velocity was highest in backcourt players and lowest in wings and goalkeepers. A similar superiority was also obtained in other samples of elite players [13–15], although the maximal shooting velocities of our participants (88.94 km/h) were only comparable to one study (90.72 km/h) [14], while others performed better (94.32–96.84 km/h) [13,15]. The best shooting performance from three-step shots was reported in a sample of Tunisian national team players (99.67 km/h), although it showed no significant difference between playing positions, likely due to its small sample size (N = 21) [11].

The kinematics of overhead shoots is a highly complex whole-body movement [26], with many studies undertaken to identify the possible determinants of shooting success [10,11,13,31,32]. Our results supported previous findings that suggest body height and mass may influence shooting velocities from a standing [11] and/or jumping position [10,13,31]. In contrast, several studies investigating the correlations between physical performance and ball velocity have been inconclusive [11,13,31,32]. Others, including our study, reported significant correlations between ball velocity and sprinting time, lower limb maximal strength, and endurance [31,32], while others failed to reach such conclusions [11,13]. Furthermore, our results also highlighted the importance of lower limb muscle mass and strength as an initiator of proximal-to-distal principal during the shot [41]. When an optimal sequence of force translation from proximal muscles of legs, pelvis, and trunk to throwing arm is achieved, the highest force production in the leg muscles can substantially contribute to higher ball velocities [27,29,32], as confirmed in our study. Similarly, recent study has suggested that jump height in the CMJ is significantly correlated with jump height while performing a jump shot in a game-based performance test [42]. During the handball game, this may present an advantage over the opponent, as the three-step jump jump shot is the most frequently executed shot [26]. In addition to faster ball-shooting velocity, the importance of jump height may also explain the higher frequency of jumps and shots performed during the game by backcourt players compared to pivots and goalkeepers [7]. However, as a handball shot is a complex, multi-joint movement, more research is needed to determine new potential physical performance determinants of shooting success (e.g., ball velocity).

In summary, the results of this study may further clarify several important aspects of the anthropometric and physical aspects of handball performance with special reference to playing position. Firstly, we confirmed previously reported variations between playing positions in anthropometric characteristics, sprinting, jumping, and handball shooting performance. Secondly, and most importantly, our study was one of the first to establish new evidence on the isokinetic maximal strength of lower limbs. We provided novel data for maximal torque of extensors and flexors in elite handball as well as demonstrated that male handball players are symmetrical with no significant maximal strength deficits between, and within, knee extensors and flexors. Lastly, our study also established further evidence on the potential role of various physical performance aspects in handball success as measured by ball velocity. Despite presenting novel findings on one of the largest samples in male handball performance research, some limitations must be acknowledged. Most of our sample were members of Kosovo's national handball team, but none of them played abroad in higher-ranking leagues or the European Championship league. As Kosovo is a young country with very few professional handball opportunities, our results may be affected by the playing level, training process, and relative lack of experience of the players. Nevertheless, our data showed results comparable to other elite playing countries, e.g., Germany and Norway, therefore, we believe that strong professional handball foundations have been built in Kosovo.

5. Conclusions

In conclusion, our study clearly demonstrated the importance of anthropometry, jumping performance, and maximal isometric strength to handball performance. In future sports practice, more emphasis should be given to handball-specific resistance training for players to gain more muscle mass of lower (legs and pelvis) and upper limbs (shoulders and arms), which will afterwards manifest in better jumping, sprinting, and shooting performance. Special consideration must be given to resistance training of pivots and goalkeepers to improve their muscle strength and shooting performance [2], as they were outperformed by wings and backcourt players. Furthermore, we also propose the routine inclusion of isometric measurement of shoulder and knee joint maximal torques to monitor changes of maximal muscle strength during the course of the handball season and to detect potential muscle imbalances, which may contribute to higher injury incidence. In line with this, more studies on elite and sub-elite handball players should be conducted to provide new practical evidence of the importance of isokinetic testing and to further determine several important aspects of physical performance in relation to handball shooting performance.

Author Contributions: Conceptualization, J.H., T.K., K.I., D.B. and P.P.; methodology, J.H., T.K., K.I., D.B. and P.P.; software, J.H., A.B.; validation, J.H., A.B. and P.P.; formal analysis, J.H., T.K. and P.P.; investigation, J.H., A.B. and P.P; resources, J.H. and A.B.; data curation, T.K.; writing—original draft preparation, J.H., T.K. and P.P.; writing—review and editing, J.H., A.B.,T.K., K.I., D.B. and P.P.; visualization, J.H., T.K. and P.P.; supervision, K.I., D.B.,P.P.; project administration, J.H., A.B. and P.P. All authors have read and approved the final version of the manuscript.

Funding: This research received no external funding.

Acknowledgments: The authors would like to thank all participants for their efforts during the study, and Jožef Šimenko, for his valuable feedback during the preparation of the manuscript. No external funds were used in the present study.

Conflicts of Interest: The authors declare no conflict of interest.

References

1. Saavedra, J.M. Handball Research: State of the Art. *J. Hum. Kinet.* **2018**, *63*, 5–8. [CrossRef] [PubMed]
2. Ziv, G.A.L.; Lidor, R. Physical characteristics, physiological attributes, and on-court performances of handball players: A review. *Eur. J. Sport Sci.* **2009**, *9*, 375–386. [CrossRef]
3. Karcher, C.; Buchheit, M. On-court demands of elite handball, with special reference to playing positions. *Sport Med.* **2014**, *44*, 797–814. [CrossRef] [PubMed]
4. Ortega-Becerra, M.; Pareja-Blanco, F.; Jiménez-Reyes, P.; Cuadrado-Peñafiel, V.; González-Badillo, J.J. Determinant Factors of Physical Performance and Specific Throwing in Handball Players of Different Ages. *J. Strength Cond. Res.* **2018**, *32*, 1778–1786. [CrossRef]
5. Gorostiaga, E.M.; Granados, C.; Ibanez, J.; Izquierdo, M. Differences in physical fitness and throwing velocity among elite and amateur male handball players. *Int. J. Sports Med.* **2005**, *26*, 225–232. [CrossRef]
6. Barbero, J.C.; Granda-Vera, J.; Calleja-González, J.; Del Coso, J. Physical and physiological demands of elite team handball players. *Int. J. Perform. Anal. Sport* **2014**, *14*, 921–933. [CrossRef]
7. Póvoas, S.C.A.; Ascensão, A.A.M.R.; Magalhães, J.; Seabra, A.F.; Krustrup, P.; Soares, J.M.C.; Rebelo, A.N. Physiological demands of elite team handball with special reference to playing position. *J. Strength Cond. Res.* **2014**, *28*, 430–442. [CrossRef]
8. Michalsik, L.; Aagaard, P. Physical demands in elite team handball: Comparisons between male and female players. *J. Sport Med. Phys. Fit.* **2015**, *55*, 878–891.
9. Ghobadi, H.; Rajabi, H.; Farzad, B.; Bayati, M.; Jeffreys, I. Anthropometry of world-class elite handball players according to the playing position: Reports from men's handball world championship 2013. *J. Hum. Kinet.* **2013**, *39*, 213–220. [CrossRef]

10. Fieseler, G.; Hermassi, S.; Hoffmeyer, B.; Schulze, S.; Irlenbusch, L.; Bartels, T.; Delank, K.S.; Laudner, K.G.; Schwesig, R. Differences in anthropometric characteristics in relation to throwing velocity and competitive level in professional male team handball: A tool for talent profiling. *J. Sports Med. Phys. Fit.* **2017**, *57*, 985–992.
11. Chaouachi, A.; Brughelli, M.; Levin, G.; Boudhina, N.B.B.; Cronin, J.; Chamari, K. Anthropometric, physiological and performance characteristics of elite team-handball players. *J. Sports Sci.* **2009**, *27*, 151–157. [CrossRef] [PubMed]
12. Hermassi, S.; Laudner, K.G.; Schwesig, R. Playing level and position differences in body characteristics and physical fitness performance among male team handball players. *Front. Bioeng. Biotechnol.* **2019**, *7*, 149. [CrossRef] [PubMed]
13. Schwesig, R.; Hermassi, S.; Fieseler, G.; Irlenbusch, L.; Noack, F.; Delank, K.-S.; Shephard, R.J.; Chelly, M.S. Anthropometric and physical performance characteristics of professional handball players: Influence of playing position. *J. Sports Med. Phys. Fit.* **2017**, *57*, 1471–1478.
14. Krüger, K.; Pilat, C.; Üçkert, K.; Frech, T.; Mooren, F.C. Physical Performance Profile of Handball Players Is Related to Playing Position and Playing Class. *J. Strength Cond. Res.* **2014**, *28*, 117–125. [CrossRef] [PubMed]
15. Haugen, T.A.; Tønnessen, E.; Seiler, S. Physical and physiological characteristics of male handball players: Influence of playing position and competitive level. *J. Sports Med. Phys. Fit.* **2016**, *56*, 19–26.
16. Nikolaidis, P.T.; Ingebrigtsen, J.; Póvoas, S.C.; Moss, S.; Torres-Luque, G.; Pantelis, N. Physical and physiological characteristics in male team handball players by playing position-Does age matter. *J. Sports Med. Phys. Fit.* **2015**, *55*, 297–304.
17. Maurelli, O.; Bernard, P.L.; Dubois, R.; Ahmaidi, S.; Prioux, J. Effects of the Competitive Season on the Isokinetic Muscle Parameters Changes in World-Class Handball Players. *J. Strength Cond. Res.* **2019**, *33*, 2778–2787. [CrossRef]
18. Xaverova, Z.; Dirnberger, J.; Lehnert, M.; Belka, J.; Wagner, H.; Orechovska, K. Isokinetic strength profile of elite female handball players. *J. Hum. Kinet.* **2015**, *49*, 257–266. [CrossRef]
19. Teixeira, J.; Carvalho, P.; Moreira, C.; Santos, R. Isokinetic assessment of muscle imbalances and bilateral differences between knee extensores and flexores' strength in basketball, footbal, handball and volleyball athletes. *Int. J. Sport Sci.* **2014**, *4*, 1–6.
20. Gonzalez-Rave, J.M.; Juarez, D.; Rubio-Arias, J.A.; Suarez, V.J.; Martinez-Valencia, M.A.; Abian-Vicen, J. Isokinetic leg strength and power in elite handball players. *J. Hum. Kinet.* **2014**, *41*, 227–233. [CrossRef]
21. Carvalho, A.; Mourão, P.; Abade, E. Effects of Strength Training Combined with Specific Plyometric exercises on body composition, vertical jump height and lower limb strength development in elite male handball players: A case study. *J. Hum. Kinet.* **2014**, *41*, 125–132. [CrossRef] [PubMed]
22. Andrade, M.D.S.; Fleury, A.M.; de Lira, C.A.B.; Dubas, J.P.; da Silva, A.C. Profile of isokinetic eccentric-to-concentric strength ratios of shoulder rotator muscles in elite female team handball players. *J. Sports Sci.* **2010**, *28*, 743–749. [CrossRef] [PubMed]
23. Dos Santos Andrade, M.; de Lira, C.A.B.; Vancini, R.L.; de Almeida, A.A.; Benedito-Silva, A.A.; da Silva, A.C. Profiling the isokinetic shoulder rotator muscle strength in 13-to 36-year-old male and female handball players. *Phys. Ther. Sport* **2013**, *14*, 246–252. [CrossRef] [PubMed]
24. Risberg, M.A.; Steffen, K.; Nilstad, A.; Myklebust, G.; Kristianslund, E.; Moltubakk, M.M.; Krosshaug, T. Normative quadriceps and hamstring muscle strength values for female, healthy, elite handball and football players. *J. Strength Cond. Res.* **2018**, *32*, 2314. [CrossRef]
25. Steffen, K.; Nilstad, A.; Kristianslund, E.K.; Myklebust, G.; Bahr, R.; Krosshaug, T. Association between lower extremity muscle strength and noncontact ACL injuries. *Med. Sci. Sport Exerc.* **2016**, *48*, 2082–2089. [CrossRef]
26. Bencke, J.; van den Tillaar, R.; Møller, M.; Wagner, H. Throwing Biomechanics: Aspects of Throwing Performance and Shoulder Injury Risk. In *Handball Sports Medicine*; Laver, L., Landreau, P., Seil, R., Popović, N., Eds.; Springer: Berlin/Heidelberg, Germany, 2018; pp. 69–79.
27. Wagner, H.; Pfusterschmied, J.; Klous, M.; von Duvillard, S.P.; Müller, E. Movement variability and skill level of various throwing techniques. *Hum. Mov. Sci.* **2012**, *31*, 78–90. [CrossRef]
28. Wagner, H.; Pfusterschmied, J.; von Duvillard, S.P.; Müller, E. Performance and kinematics of various throwing techniques in team-handball. *J. Sports Sci. Med.* **2011**, *10*, 73.
29. Wagner, H.; Buchecker, M.; Von Duvillard, S.P.; Müller, E. Kinematic description of elite vs. low level players in team-handball jump throw. *J. Sports Sci. Med.* **2010**, *9*, 15.

30. Michalsik, L.; Madsen, K.; Aagaard, P. Physiological capacity and physical testing in male elite team handball. *J. Sport Med. Phys. Fit.* **2015**, *55*, 415–429.
31. Zapartidis, I.; Kororos, P.; Christodoulidis, T.; Skoufas, D.; Bayios, I. Profile of young handball players by playing position and determinants of ball throwing velocity. *J. Hum. Kinet.* **2011**, *27*, 17–30. [CrossRef]
32. Hermassi, S.; Chelly, M.S.; Wagner, H.; Fieseler, G.; Schulze, S.; Delank, K.-S.; Shephard, R.J.; Schwesig, R. Relationships between maximal strength of lower limb, anthropometric characteristics and fundamental explosive performance in handball players. *Sport. Sport.* **2019**, *33*, 96–103. [CrossRef] [PubMed]
33. Stewart, A.D.; Marfell-Jones, M.; Olds, T.; De Ridder, J.H. *International Standards for Anthropometric Assessment*; International Society for the Advancement of Kinanthropometry: Wellington, New Zealand, 2012.
34. Lee, L.-W.; Liao, Y.-S.; Lu, H.-K.; Hsiao, P.-L.; Chen, Y.-Y.; Chi, C.-C.; Hsieh, K.C. Validation of two portable bioelectrical impedance analyses for the assessment of body composition in school age children. *PLoS ONE* **2017**, *12*, e0171568. [CrossRef] [PubMed]
35. Van Melick, N.; Meddeler, B.M.; Hoogeboom, T.J.; Nijhuis-van der Sanden, M.W.G.; van Cingel, R.E.H. How to determine leg dominance: The agreement between self-reported and observed performance in healthy adults. *PLoS ONE* **2017**, *12*, e0189876. [CrossRef] [PubMed]
36. Kovaleski, J.E.; Heitman, R.J. Testing and training the lower extremity. In *Isokinetics in Human Performance*; Brown, L.E., Ed.; Human Kinetics: Champagne, IL, USA, 2000; pp. 171–195.
37. Croisier, J.-L.; Ganteaume, S.; Binet, J.; Genty, M.; Ferret, J.-M. Strength Imbalances and Prevention of Hamstring Injury in Professional Soccer Players: A Prospective Study. *Am. J. Sports Med.* **2008**, *36*, 1469–1475. [CrossRef] [PubMed]
38. Andrade, M.D.S.; De Lira, C.A.B.; Koffes, F.D.C.; Mascarin, N.C.; Benedito-Silva, A.A.; Da Silva, A.C. Isokinetic hamstrings-to-quadriceps peak torque ratio: The influence of sport modality, gender, and angular velocity. *J. Sports Sci.* **2012**, *30*, 547–553. [CrossRef] [PubMed]
39. Lund-Hanssen, H.; Gannon, J.; Engebretsen, L.; Holen, K.; Hammer, S. Isokinetic muscle performance in healthy female handball players and players with a unilateral anterior cruciate ligament reconstruction. *Scand. J. Med. Sci. Sports* **1996**, *6*, 172–175. [CrossRef] [PubMed]
40. Myklebust, G.; Maehlum, S.; Holm, I.; Bahr, R. A prospective cohort study of anterior cruciate ligament injuries in elite Norwegian team handball. *Scand. J. Med. Sci. Sports* **1998**, *8*, 149–153. [CrossRef]
41. Herring, R.M.; Chapman, A.E. Effects of changes in segmental values and timing of both torque and torque reversal in simulated throws. *J. Biomech.* **1992**, *25*, 1173–1184. [CrossRef]
42. Wagner, H.; Sperl, B.; Bell, J.W.; Von Duvillard, S.P. Testing specific physical performance in male team handball players and the relationship to general tests in team sports. *J. Strength Cond. Res.* **2019**, *33*, 1056–1064. [CrossRef]

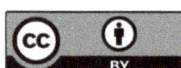

© 2020 by the authors. Licensee MDPI, Basel, Switzerland. This article is an open access article distributed under the terms and conditions of the Creative Commons Attribution (CC BY) license (http://creativecommons.org/licenses/by/4.0/).

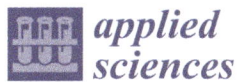 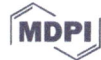

Commentary

Supramaximal Eccentric Training for Alpine Ski Racing—Strength Training with the Lifter

Carson Patterson * and Christian Raschner

Olympiazentrum, Department of Sport Science, University of Innsbruck, 6020 Innsbruck, Austria; christian.raschner@uibk.ac.at
* Correspondence: carson.patterson@uibk.ac.at

Received: 27 October 2020; Accepted: 7 December 2020; Published: 10 December 2020

Featured Application: The Intelligent Motion Lifter is a new mechatronic strength training device that allows safe and effective strength training with supramaximal loads.

Abstract: Eccentric muscular work plays a large role in alpine ski racing. Training with supramaximal eccentric loads (SME) is highly effective to improve eccentric strength but potentially dangerous. Most SME training devices do not allow the athlete to move a barbell freely as they would when performing conventional barbell training. The Intelligent Motion Lifter (IML) allows for safe SME training with a free barbell and no spotters. The IML can be used for free barbell training: a spotter for normal training, eccentric only, concentric only, and squat jumps. It is also a training and testing device for isokinetic and isometric exercise. This commentary addresses the necessity of eccentric training for elite alpine ski racers, the development of the IML and its use in training.

Keywords: eccentric; alpine ski racing; strength training; supramaximal loads; athlete safety

1. Eccentric Exercise in Alpine Ski Racing

Scientific analysis of world class Swedish alpine ski racers in the 1990s [1,2] showed that eccentric muscular work predominated over concentric work in the disciplines of slalom, giant slalom and super G. More current work with elite Swiss racers corroborated this [3–5], with Vogt and Hoppeler stating that alpine skiing is "the only sport activity dominated by eccentric muscle activity" [5].

The introduction of carving (greater side-cut) skis in World Cup ski racing in 1999 changed ski turns [6]. Ferguson [7] concluded that ski racing is characterized by isometric and eccentric muscular actions. New studies with Austrian [8] and French [9] elite ski racers have indicated that a "quasi-isometric" phase exists in ski racing and that this phase of the ski turn has been overlooked but must be considered.

There is still an incomplete understanding of what is happening during a high-speed ski turn. More research is needed for a full understanding of the metabolic and muscular functional demands of ski racing [10], and there is "a lack of functional and biomechanical understanding of the performance relevant parameters" in ski racing [11].

The dominance of eccentric muscular actions in ski racing can be debated, but eccentric muscular control is important in the sport. Gravity propels the ski racer down the hill [12,13] and the racer must efficiently use potential energy to maintain speed on a racecourse. A kinematic analysis of a World Cup slalom race [13] found that faster racers better controlled the dissipation of potential energy and could more effectively reduce ground reaction forces compared to slower performers. Reid et al. [14] also demonstrated that more energy is dissipated in skidded turns than in carved turns with Norwegian national team ski racers.

We believe that high levels of eccentric strength are necessary to control the dissipation of energy during a skiing turn. Higher strength levels allow the ski racer to work with less relative strength, which may lead to more control in turns (less energy dissipation) and less fatigue during races.

Swiss sport scientists working with the Swiss ski team [3] have built an "Eccentric-Trainer". This special cycle ergometer forces the athlete to eccentrically "brake" the machine to achieve the selected power output and cadence. They found that the ability of the racer to precisely control the eccentric work correlated with International Ski Federation points, which is the system of grading ski racers' racing success. The better control of the eccentric work, the better the ski racer.

The effectiveness of eccentric training in improving maximal strength has been known for some time [15]. The most effective uses of eccentric training seem to be high speed eccentric work and heavy eccentric loading [16]. Many athletes employ supramaximal eccentric training (SME) to improve maximal strength, which may improve performance. World class powerlifters can use 105–110% of their one repetition maximum and lower-level athletes can use 120–130% for SME training [17].

The Norwegian alpine ski team trained with SME squats regularly in the 1990s [17]. A minimum requirement for the squat (hip joint at least same level or lower than knee joint) was 2.5 times bodyweight for the men's Europe and World Cup teams. They also tested for maximal eccentric force with a negative (from top to bottom with control) squat.

Elite sport training centers have developed their own SME squat machines in Austria [18], Norway [17] and Sweden [19], and as mentioned above, the Swiss have designed an eccentric cycle ergometer for ski racers [3]. There are anecdotal references of athletes using supramaximal squats to prepare for ski racing. Bode Miller, a very successful American ski racer, built his own training device in order to perform eccentric squats. We have had personal communications with Canadian and American coaches and know that supramaximal eccentric squats are used in the training of alpine ski racers in other nations. In reviews of the training of alpine ski racers, eccentric training is recommended [20,21].

In a recent review of nine different eccentric training devices [22], the Intelligent Motion Lifter© (IML), from Intelligent Motion GmbH (Wartberg an der Krems, Austria) is the only device which allowed the athlete to move the barbell freely in all planes as they would when performing conventional barbell training.

Free weights, when compared to machines, allow movement in multiple planes, require balance, and mimic natural acceleration and velocity patterns, resulting in a greater transfer of training effect [23]. Electromyographic (EMG) activity is greater when training with free weights, perhaps due to the action of stabilizing muscle groups [24]. A free barbell bench press elicited more muscle activity than a machine bench press [24], and free weight squats showed 43% higher EMG activity than Smith machine squats [25].

Weight releasers are a cost-effective method for barbell SME training, and their use has been documented in scientific studies [26–28]. However, this system is strenuous for coaches or helpers and the athlete must have very good lifting technique to ensure that the two releasers hit the floor simultaneously.

Patterson and Raschner [29] reported a case study with an Austrian world champion ski racer utilizing the Intelligent Motion Lifter© (IML), from Intelligent Motion GmbH (Wartberg an der Krems, Austria) for SME training.

Coaches and athletes must be aware that SME barbell squat training is extremely strenuous and potentially dangerous. Spotters must be properly trained to safely spot the squatter, and SME training requires multiple spotters. The IML makes safe SME barbell training possible without spotters.

2. Development of the IML

The initial goal was to develop a device to allow safe SME training. A high priority was that the barbell would have 100% freedom to move in all three planes during SME loading, so that the normal demands of free weight training would be met (see Figure 1).

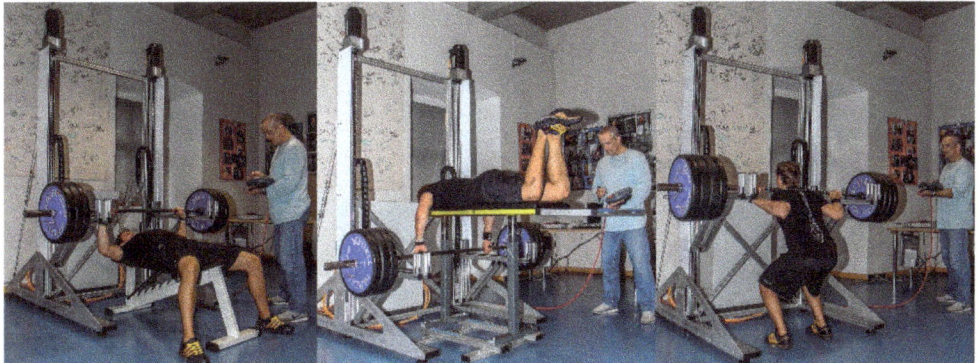

Figure 1. The Intelligent Motion Lifter© (IML) prototype in 2010. From left to right: bench press, bench pull and squat.

A needs analysis concluded that the following conditions must be met:

- The device will safely and quickly stop the bar if the athlete "fails" during a lift.
- The barbell will move freely (in all planes) during the eccentric portion of lift.
- There will be no external adjustments to the barbell load during a multiple repetition set.
- Automated assistance will be provided to safely return the barbell to the starting position of the eccentric phase (no concentric phase for the athlete).
- The range of motion (top and bottom of lift) can be adjusted for each athlete.
- The range of motion for all lifts performed by an athlete will be saved by the device.
- The device will provide training data which can be exported for training documentation.
- The machine can be used as a spotting device during normal lifts.
- The machine will have dimensions similar to a normal power rack.
- The machine cannot be used without a coach or training partner to operate the device.

The Lifter was originally conceived for SME training, but further developments allow the device to be used for concentric-only training, isometric training, and testing, and as a spotter for normal barbell lifts and jumping. The additional functions that were added to later versions of the Lifter included:

- Automated assistance will be provided to safely return the barbell to the starting position of the concentric phase (no eccentric phase for the athlete).
- The arms will move fast enough that an athlete can perform a loaded squat jump or countermovement jump and the arms will catch the barbell at the top of the jump.
- Isokinetic movements can be performed with a bar attached to the arms in both concentric and eccentric movements. The force applied by the athlete on the arms will be measured and recorded.
- Isometric testing and training can be performed with a bar coupled to the arms. The force applied to the bar by the athlete will be measured and recorded.
- The velocities of the concentric and eccentric phases of the isokinetic movements can be independent of each other; one phase can be faster than the other.

These conditions were taken into consideration when developing and constructing the IML. The IML is a safe automated mechatronic SME device which requires one operator and no external load adjustments during training. A prototype of this training device was introduced at the International Conference on Strength Training 2010 [30].

3. Description of the IML

The IML is essentially two lifting systems utilizing mechatronic technology. Each system has a lifting arm and consists of a column with a drive spindle, guide rails and a synchronized servomotor. The two drives can be virtually coupled via the software and the arms can operate independently of each other. The system is controlled by a real-time capable central processing unit (CPU).

The arms move with the barbell as it is lowered or raised without contacting the barbell. The displacement and speed of the barbell is tracked by two draw-wire encoders attached to the barbell with lightweight plastic plates, which slide onto the barbell similar to weight plates (see Figure 2).

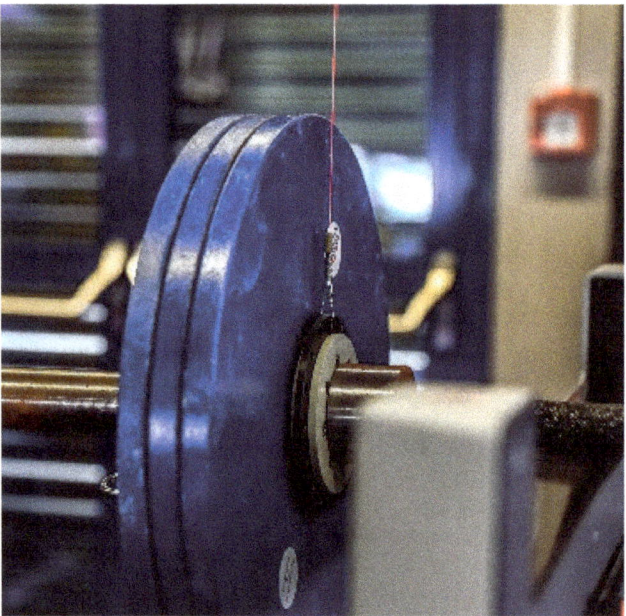

Figure 2. The draw-wire and plate of the draw-wire encoder.

The height difference between the two arms is automatically limited to 100 mm. If the difference exceeds 100 mm, the machine will automatically move one of the arms to stay within 100 mm. The arms can work independently so that the athlete must balance the bar as in a normal free barbell squat. The arms can also be programmed to work together, so that the barbell still moves freely, but the athlete does not have to concentrate on keeping the barbell level. The arms can be programmed to follow the barbell at a distance of 12.5 to 100 mm, allowing a tolerance limit for keeping the barbell level.

A free barbell can be raised and lowered to heights of 1850 mm and 550 mm, respectively, and the simulation bar can be raised and lowered to heights of 1750 mm and 450 mm, respectively. The maximum barbell load is 400 kg and the maximum simulated load is 250 kg.

The maximum velocity of the arms is 2000 mm/s and the minimum velocity is 10 mm/s. The maximum acceleration of the arms (full load or empty) is 4000 mm/s^2.

The entire machine is controlled by a mobile handheld control unit, which has a touchscreen display, an emergency stop switch, and an override switch. This unit is attached by cable to the IML. There is also a screen on the IML for athlete instructions.

4. Safety Standards of the IML

Various safety functions ensure maximum safety during training with the IML. The IML has two CPUs which monitor the programed safety elements. These are:

- All emergency stop switches,
- The speed of the barbell,
- The displacement of the barbell, and
- The bottom movement limits of the exercise.

There are four emergency switches. Two are on the sides of the IML, one is on the handheld control unit and one is mounted on the front wall facing the athlete at foot height (see Figure 3). If an emergency switch is activated, the arms will stop. The programmed movement range and speed of the barbell is monitored by the safety CPUs. In order to actively move to the lowest positions in training, the override switch on the handheld unit must be pressed during the entire exercise. If the override switched is not pressed, the arms will automatically stop.

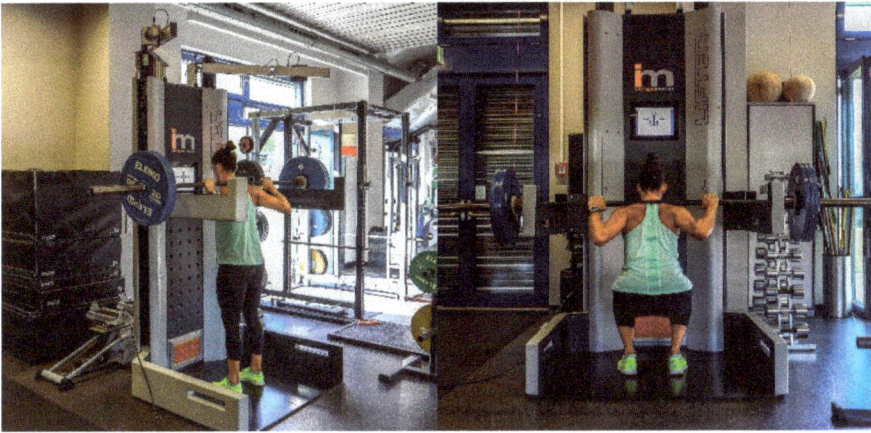

Figure 3. The present IML model: squat top position and squat bottom position.

All safety elements, including the safety CPUs, have the highest safety level in control technology and automation available at the time of manufacture: safety integrity level (SIL) 3. A discussion of how safety standards and risk assessment systems for manufacturers and approval agencies are developed has been presented by Stavrianidis and Bhimavarapu [31].

An additional safety feature has been developed. In the bench press, the barbell or the coupled bar is lowered to the chest and the athlete may fear that the bar will crush them. A mechanical safety pin system can be placed onto the floor supports and this will brake the arms so that the coupled bar or barbell will not crush the athlete. The safety CPUs prevent this, but the safety pin system assures the athlete that he or she is safe (see Figure 4).

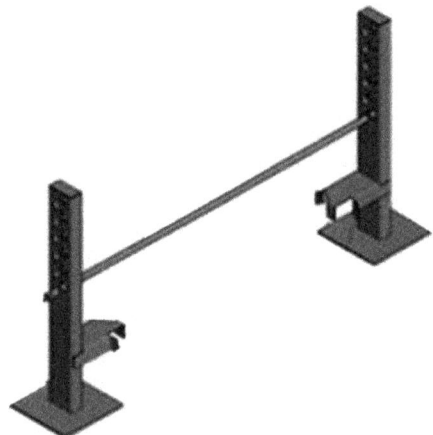

Figure 4. The mechanical safety pin system.

5. Training and Testing with the IML

5.1. Training Mode

5.1.1. Training with a Free Barbell

First, the upper and lower limits and lift off position of the lift are set for the athlete. The number of sets and repetitions can be prescribed. The coach can operate the machine manually, or program the number of sets, repetitions, and rest periods between repetitions and sets. The velocity and the acceleration of the arms can be programmed, dictating the speed of movement and the "hardness" or "softness" of the change of direction between the raising and lowering of the arms. There is also an "aggressiveness" setting, which controls how quickly the arms follow the movement of the barbell.

5.1.2. Spotter Mode

The arms are positioned under the barbell (but without contact) and follow the path of the bar at a predetermined distance (12.5–100 mm). The athlete is able to train normally with no help from the machine. When the set is done, the athlete can rack the bar onto the arms (see Figure 3).

5.1.3. Eccentric Only Mode

The athlete loads the barbell onto the back from the lift off position and lowers the barbell under control to the lower limit. The arms lift the barbell back to the lift-off or upper limit. The rest at the top can be programmed or determined manually by the coach.

5.1.4. Concentric Only Mode

The athlete starts with the barbell at the lower limit and lifts the barbell to the upper limit. The arms lower the barbell back to the lower limit. The rest at the bottom can be programmed or determined manually by the coach.

5.1.5. Throw or Jump Mode

The barbell is caught by the device in loaded jumps or bench press throws (or other dynamic exercises). For a jump, after lift-off, the athlete lowers into a controlled countermovement and when the lower limit is reached, a beep signals the athletes that he/she can jump. The arms are then "triggered"

The increased central nervous system load during SME leads to greater strength gains, but coaches and athletes must be wary of overtraining. In the present case study, SME twice a week elicited satisfactory strength gains without adverse effects. Norwegian sport scientists have recommended that athletes train with SME only once per week [17].

The 1080 Quantum Synchro by 1080 Motion is a new device that also allows SME with a barbell, but in a Smith machine, so the athlete does not have to control the path of the barbell. This is an unnatural way to perform barbell exercises and the athlete does not have to balance the barbell. The 1080 Quantum Synchro can be used with the following forms of resistance: isokinetic, normal mass, isotonic and ballistic. It appears that the eccentric barbell movements are isokinetic, but isokinetic movements do not exist in sport. It has a maximum eccentric resistance load of 325 kg; the IML can be loaded up to 400 kg. The 1080 Quantum Synchro can also be used with a cable system to allow sport-specific movements. This device looks very promising, and has been used in research [40].

The IML allows an athlete to train heavy with EOL squats with just one coach or partner to control the IML. Eccentric training is becoming more popular in GPP strength programs for alpine ski racers, and the authors believe that this trend will continue.

8. Conclusions

Properly planned strength training programs incorporating SME, which the IML supports, can improve maximal strength. The use of the IML as a SME training device for athletes who do not have an advanced level of strength is not advised. Athletes need to have the technical abilities and adequate strength to manage supramaximal loading. Athletes without high strength levels can utilize the device for other methods of training.

Author Contributions: Conceptualization, C.P. and C.R.; Methodology, C.P.; Investigation, C.P.; Data collection and curation, C.P.; Writing—original draft preparation, C.P.; Writing—review and editing, C.P. and C.R.; Supervision, C.R.; Photography, C.P. and C.R. All authors have read and agreed to the published version of the manuscript.

Funding: This research received no external funding.

Conflicts of Interest: The authors declare no conflict of interest.

References

1. Berg, H.E.; Eiken, O.; Tesch, P.A. Involvement of eccentric muscle actions in giant slalom racing. *Med. Sci. Sports Exerc.* **1995**, *27*, 1666–1670. [CrossRef] [PubMed]
2. Berg, H.E.; Eiken, O. Muscle control in elite alpine skiing. *Med. Sci. Sports Exerc.* **1999**, *31*, 1065–1067. [CrossRef] [PubMed]
3. Vogt, M.; Dapp, C.; Blatter, J.; Weisskopf, R.; Suter, G.; Hoppeler, H. Training for optimization of the dosage of eccentric muscle action. *Schweiz. Z. Sportmed. Sporttraumol.* **2003**, *51*, 188–191.
4. Hoppeler, H.; Vogt, M. Eccentric exercise in alpine skiing. In *Science and Skiing IV*; Mueller, E., Lindinger, S., Stoeggl, T., Eds.; Meyer & Meyer: Maidenhead, UK, 2009; pp. 33–42.
5. Vogt, M.; Hoppeler, H. The role of eccentric exercise training in alpine ski racers. In *Eccentric Exercise, Physiology and Application in Sport and Rehabilitation*, 1st ed.; Hoppeler, H., Ed.; Routledge: London, UK, 2016; pp. 132–147.
6. Supej, M.; Holmberg, H.-C. Recent kinematic and kinetic advances in Olympic alpine skiing: Pyeongchang and beyond. *Front. Physiol.* **2019**, *10*, 111. [CrossRef] [PubMed]
7. Ferguson, R.A. Limitations to performance during alpine skiing. *Exp. Physiol.* **2010**, *95*, 404–410. [CrossRef]
8. Kröll, J.; Spörri, J.; Fasel, B.; Müller, E.; Schwameder, H. Type of muscle control in elite alpine skiing—Is it still the same than in 1995? In *Skiing and Science VI*; Müller, E., Kröll, J., Lindinger, S., Eds.; Meyer and Meyer Sport Ltd.: Oxford, UK, 2014; pp. 56–64.
9. Alhammoud, M.; Hansen, C.; Meyer, F.; Hautier, C.; Morel, B. On-field ski kinematic according to leg and discipline in elite alpine skiers. *Front. Sports Act. Living* **2020**, *2*, 56. [CrossRef]
10. Turnbull, J.R.; Kilding, A.E.; Keogh, J.W.L. Physiology of alpine skiing. *Scand. J. Med. Sci. Sports* **2009**, *19*, 146–155. [CrossRef]

11. Spörri, J.; Kröll, J.; Schwameder, H.; Müller, E. Turn characteristics of a top world class athlete in giant slalom: A case study assessing current performance prediction concepts. *Int. J. Sports Sci. Coach.* **2012**, *7*, 647–659. [CrossRef]
12. Stöggl, T.; Schwarzl, C.; Müller, E.; Nagasaki, M.; Stöggl, J.; Scheiber, P.; Niebauer, J. A comparison between alpine skiing, cross-country skiing and indoor cycling on cardiorespiratory and metabolic response. *J. Sports Sci. Med.* **2016**, *15*, 184–195.
13. Matej, M.; Kipp, R.; Holmberg, H.-C. Mechanical parameters as predictors of performance in alpine World Cup slalom racing: 1247. *Scand. J. Med. Sci. Sports* **2011**, *21*, e72–e81.
14. Reid, R.; Gilgien, M.; Moger, T.; Tjorhom, H.; Haugen, P.; Kipp, R.; Smith, G. Mechanical energy dissipation and performance in alpine ski racing. *Med. Sci. Sports Exerc.* **2008**, *40*, S165. [CrossRef]
15. Schmidtbleicher, D.; Bührle, M. Vergleich von konzentrischem und exzentrischem Maximalkrafttraining. *Ber. Inst. Sport Sportwiss. Univ. Freibg.* **1980**, *1*, 1–59.
16. Suchomel, T.J.; Wagle, J.P.; Douglas, J.; Taber, C.B.; Harden, M.; Haff, G.G.; Stone, M.H. Implementing Eccentric Resistance Training—Part 1: A Brief Review of Existing Methods. *J. Funct. Morphol. Kinesiol.* **2019**, *4*, 38. [CrossRef]
17. Refsnes, P.E. Testing and training for top Norwegian athletes. In *Science in Elite Sport*; Mueller, E., Ludescher, F., Zallinger, G., Eds.; E & FN Spon: London, UK, 1999; pp. 91–114.
18. Raschner, C.; Kroell, J.; Zallinger, G.; Koesters, A.; Mueller, E. Trainingswissenschaftliche Aspekte eines exzentrischen Krafttrainings bei unterschiedlichen Bewegungsgeschwindigkeiten für alpine Skirennläufer. In *Skilauf und Wissenschaft*; Mueller, E., Lindinger, S., Raschner, C., Schwameder, H., Eds.; Österreichischer Skiverband: Innsbruck, Austria, 2001; Volume 15, pp. 92–101.
19. Frohm, A.; Halvorsen, K.; Thorstensson, A. A new device for controlled eccentric overloading in training and rehabilitation. *Eur. J. Appl. Physiol.* **2005**, *94*, 168–174. [CrossRef] [PubMed]
20. Gilgien, M.; Reid, R.; Raschner, C.; Supej, M.; Holmberg, H.-C. The training of olympic alpine ski racers. *Front. Physiol.* **2018**, *9*, 1772. [CrossRef] [PubMed]
21. Hydren, J.R.; Volek, J.S.; Maresh, C.M.; Comstock, B.A.; Kraemer, W.J. Review of strength and conditioning for alpine ski racing. *Strength Cond. J.* **2013**, *27*, 927–934. [CrossRef]
22. Tinwala, F.; Cronin, J.; Haemmerle, E.; Ross, A. Eccentric strength training: A review of the available technology. *Strength Cond. J.* **2017**, *39*, 32–47. [CrossRef]
23. Stone, M.; Plisk, S.; Collins, D. Training principles: Evaluation of modes and methods of resistance training—A coaching perspective. *Sports Biomech.* **2002**, *1*, 79–103. [CrossRef]
24. McCaw, S.T.; Friday, J.J. A comparison of muscle activity between a free weight and machine bench press. *J. Strength Cond. Res.* **1994**, *8*, 259–264.
25. Schwanbeck, S.; Chilibeck, P.D.; Binsted, G. A comparison of free weight squat to Smith machine squat using electromyography. *J. Strength Cond. Res.* **2009**, *23*, 2588–2591. [CrossRef]
26. Doan, B.K.; Newton, R.U.; Marsit, J.L.; Triplett-McBride, N.T.; Koziris, L.P.; Fry, A.C.; Kraemer, W.J. Effects of increased eccentric loading on bench press 1RM. *J. Strength Cond. Res.* **2002**, *16*, 9–13. [PubMed]
27. Ojasto, T.; Hakkinen, K. Effects of different accentuated eccentric loads on acute neuromuscular, growth hormone, and blood lactate responses during a hypertrophic protocol. *J. Strength Cond. Res.* **2009**, *23*, 946–953. [CrossRef] [PubMed]
28. Walker, S.; Blazevich, A.J.; Haff, G.G.; Tufano, J.J.; Newton, R.U.; Häkkinen, K. Greater strength gains after training with accentuated eccentric than traditional isoinertial loads in already strength-trained men. *Front. Physiol.* **2016**, *7*, 149. [CrossRef] [PubMed]
29. Patterson, C.; Raschner, C. Eccentric overload squats with the intelligent motion lifter strength training for alpine ski racing. In *Skiing and Science VI*; Müller, E., Kröll, J., Lindinger, S., Eds.; Meyer and Meyer Sport Ltd.: Oxford, UK, 2014; pp. 260–267.
30. Patterson, C.; Barth, A.; Barth, M.; Raschner, C. A new augmented eccentric loading device: Free barbell repetitions with heavy eccentric and lighter concentric loads. In Proceedings of the 7th International Conference on Strength Training, Book of Abstracts, Bratislava, Slovakia, 28–30 October 2010; pp. 180–181.
31. Stavrianidis, P.; Bhimavarapu, K. Safety instrumented functions and safety integrity levels (SIL). *ISA Trans.* **1998**, *37*, 337–351. [CrossRef]
32. King, I. *Foundations of Physical Preparation*; King Sports Publishing: Reno, NV, USA, 2000; p. 60.

33. Poliquin, C. *The Poliquin Principles Successful Methods for Strength and Mass Development*; Dayton Writer's Group: Napa, CA, USA, 1997; p. 9.
34. Siff, M.C. *Supertraining*, 6th ed.; Supertraining Institute: Denver, CO, USA, 2003; p. 11.
35. Roig, M.; O'Brien, K.; Kirk, G.; Murray, R.; Mckinnon, P.; Shadgan, B.; Reid, W.D. The effects of eccentric versus concentric resistance training on muscle strength and mass in healthy adults: A systematic review with meta-analysis. *Br. J. Sports Med.* **2009**, *43*, 556–568. [CrossRef]
36. Enoka, R.M. Eccentric contractions require unique activation strategies by the nervous system. *J. Appl. Physiol.* **1996**, *81*, 2339–2346. [CrossRef]
37. Grabiner, M.D.; Owings, T.M. MG differences between concentric and eccentric maximum voluntary contractions are evident prior to movement onset. *Exp. Brain Res.* **2002**, *145*, 505–511. [CrossRef]
38. Linnamo, V.; Strojnik, V.; Komi, P.V. EMG power spectrum and features of the superimposed M-wave during voluntary eccentric and concentric actions at different activation levels. *Eur. J. Appl. Physiol.* **2002**, *86*, 534–540. [CrossRef]
39. Hortobagyi, T.; Hill, J.P.; Houmard, J.A.; Fraser, D.D.; Lambert, N.J.; Israel, R.G. Adaptive responses to muscle lengthening and shortening in humans. *J. Appl. Physiol.* **1996**, *80*, 765–772. [CrossRef]
40. Helland, C.; Hole, E.; Iversen, E.; Olsson, M.C.; Seynnes, O.; Solberg, P.A.; Paulsen, G. Training Strategies to Improve Muscle Power. *Med. Sci. Sports Exerc.* **2017**, *49*, 736–745. [CrossRef]

Publisher's Note: MDPI stays neutral with regard to jurisdictional claims in published maps and institutional affiliations.

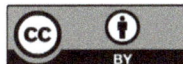

© 2020 by the authors. Licensee MDPI, Basel, Switzerland. This article is an open access article distributed under the terms and conditions of the Creative Commons Attribution (CC BY) license (http://creativecommons.org/licenses/by/4.0/).

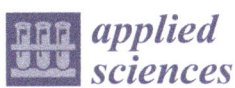 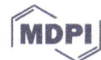

Article

The Effect of a 7-Week Training Period on Changes in Skin NADH Fluorescence in Highly Trained Athletes

Olga Bugaj [1], Krzysztof Kusy [1], Adam Kantanista [2], Paweł Korman [3], Dariusz Wieliński [4] and Jacek Zieliński [1,*]

1. Department of Athletics, Strength and Conditioning, Faculty of Sport Sciences, Poznan University of Physical Education, 61-871 Poznań, Poland; bugaj@awf.poznan.pl (O.B.); kusy@awf.poznan.pl (K.K.)
2. Department of Physical Education and Lifelong Sports, Faculty of Sport Sciences, Poznan University of Physical Education, 61-871 Poznań, Poland; kantanista@awf.poznan.pl
3. Department of Physical Therapy and Sports Recovery, Faculty of Health Sciences, Poznan University of Physical Education, 61-871 Poznań, Poland; pkorman@awf.poznan.pl
4. Department of Anthropology and Biometrics, Faculty of Sport Sciences, Poznan University of Physical Education, 61-871 Poznań, Poland; wielinski@awf.poznan.pl
* Correspondence: jacekzielinski@wp.pl; Tel.: +48-618-355-270

Received: 4 June 2020; Accepted: 24 July 2020; Published: 26 July 2020

Abstract: The study aimed to evaluate the changes of nicotinamide adenine dinucleotide (NADH) fluorescence in the reduced form in the superficial skin layer, resulting from a 7-week training period in highly trained competitive athletes ($n = 41$). The newly, non-invasive flow mediated skin fluorescence (FMSF) method was implemented to indirectly evaluate the mitochondrial activity by NADH fluorescence. The FMSF measurements were taken before and after an exercise treadmill test until exhaustion. We found that athletes showed higher post-training values in basal NADH fluorescence (pre-exercise: 41% increase; post-exercise: 49% increase). Maximum NADH fluorescence was also higher after training both pre- (42% increase) and post-exercise (47% increase). Similar changes have been revealed before and after exercise for minimal NADH fluorescence (before exercise: 39% increase; after exercise: 47% increase). In conclusion, physical training results in an increase in the skin NADH fluorescence levels at rest and after exercise in athletes.

Keywords: nicotinamide adenine dinucleotide; training; athletes; mitochondrion

1. Introduction

Skin microcirculatory function and efficiency of blood supply to the skin can impact mitochondrial activity and the changes of nicotinamide adenine dinucleotide (NADH) fluorescence in the reduced form [1]. Mitochondrial function can be indirectly evaluated by NADH fluorescence [1] that has been measured in animals [2,3] and humans [1,4] at rest and under various conditions (e.g., ischemia and temperature changes). Bugaj et al. [5] were the first to describe the time course of NADH changes in the skin in athletes at rest and after exercise. In their study, a new method of evaluating NADH fluorescence—flow mediated skin fluorescence (FMSF)—was utilized. The FMSF method is based on the ability of NADH to autofluorescence. The fluorescence measured using the FMSF method reflects the dynamics of in vivo changes in NADH levels in most superficial layers of the skin [5–7]. Bugaj et al. [5] have shown that exercise to exhaustion induces changes in skin NADH fluorescence, in other words, the values recorded after exercise were higher than those before exercise (increase in: basal NADH fluorescence 13%, maximal NADH fluorescence 7% and minimal NADH fluorescence 12%).

Nicotinamide adenine dinucleotide (NAD) is synthesized in the cytosol, mitochondria, and nucleus. This molecule is active in the cytoplasm during glycolysis and in the mitochondria during oxidative phosphorylation when adenosine-5′-triphosphate (ATP) is produced [8]. NAD occurs in two forms:

oxidized NAD$^+$ and reduced NADH. NAD takes part in many biological reactions including electron transport. The reduction of NAD$^+$ to NADH occurs almost exclusively in the mitochondria at the final stage of cellular respiration [9,10].

In the human body, there is a pool of NAD that takes reduced (NAD$^+$) and oxidized (NADH) forms, transforming into each other [8]. Importantly, the NAD pool is only constant for relatively short periods [8,11]. In the long term, the NAD amount changes depending on several factors such as age, diet, physical activity, medicaments, boosters, time of the day, etc. [11]. NAD$^+$ metabolism is complex and includes many NAD$^+$-consuming pathways as well as de novo and salvage pathways [8].

Mayevsky and Barbiro-Michaely [1] have claimed that the monitoring of the NADH level in tissue provides important information about the mitochondrial metabolic state (energy production, amount of intracellular oxygen). In addition, changes in the NAD$^+$/NADH ratio reflect cellular respiration processes in mitochondria, thus indirectly represent their function [1,5]. Studies on changes in NADH in response to physical exercise were performed on animal and human skeletal muscle samples, but not in the skin [8,9,12]. Early reports including animals did not provide a clear answer as to how NADH levels were modified by exercise [13,14]. Subsequent human research had shown that intensive exercise, unlike light exercise, shifted the NAD$^+$/NADH balance toward NADH [8,15]. Only Koltai et al. [16] have examined the influence of endurance training on changes in NAD$^+$ level in rat muscles and showed that training resulted in an increase in NAD$^+$ biosynthesis.

Studies on skeletal muscle mitochondria are valuable, but usually invasive due to the use of the biopsy technique [17,18] and expensive if transmission electron microscopy is used [19]. However, it has been suggested that physical exercise brings beneficial changes not only in skeletal muscle mitochondria, but also in skin mitochondria [20]. It has been demonstrated that physical exercise results in several beneficial mitochondrial adaptations [19,21–25]. Various changes were extensively studied in skeletal muscle mitochondria [19,21,25–27], while only one study dealt with the changes in the skin [20]. However, we do not know whether training only affects muscle mitochondria, or the adaptations also take place in skin mitochondria that are easily accessible to study because they lie superficially.

To the best of our knowledge, there is a lack of studies describing the effect of physical training on changes in NADH fluorescence in the skin. The novel, noninvasive, and cheap flow mediated skin fluorescence method can be a source of valuable information about the mitochondrial activity. Therefore, the study aimed to evaluate the changes in NADH fluorescence in the superficial skin layer resulting from a 7-week training period in highly trained competitive athletes. We hypothesize that physical training results in an increase in the NADH fluorescence levels in athletes.

2. Materials and Methods

2.1. Subjects

Forty-one highly trained athletes (28 men, 13 women), ages ranging from 18 to 35 years, participated in the study. They were members of the Polish national team or athletes taking part in national and international competitions. They represented the following sport disciplines: triathlon (Olympic distance: 1.5 km swim, 40 km bike ride, 10 km run) (seven men, four women); long-distance running (5 km, 10 km, and marathon) (six men, two women); Olympic taekwondo (six men, one woman); sprint (100 m, 200 m, and 4 × 100 m relay) (six men, one woman); canoeing (three men); and fencing (five women). Before starting the study, each participant was informed about the aim and procedures, potential risks, and the possibility to withdraw at any time without giving any reason. All athletes gave their written consent to participate in the examinations and fulfilled a questionnaire on their health status and potential contraindications. All athletes had valid health certificates issued by a physician who specialized in sports medicine, thus were eligible for training and competition. Exclusion criteria were illness symptoms, injuries, and taking drugs (temporarily or chronically). Only the data of those athletes who were present at both examinations was analyzed. The study was conducted in accordance with the Declaration of Helsinki. The Ethics Committee of the Poznan University of Medical Sciences in Poland approved the study protocol (approval no. 1017/16 issued on 5 October 2016).

2.2. Training Characteristics

All participants attended training sessions at least six times a week. During the whole 7-week period under study (general preparation phase of the one-year cycle), the athletes had on average 57 training sessions of a total duration of 71.2 h. The average duration of a single session was 84 min.

2.3. Study Design

The study was conducted in the Human Movement Laboratory of the Department of Athletics, Strength and Conditioning at the Poznan University of Physical Education (Poznań, Poland). Athletes arrived at the laboratory in the morning. During all measurements, the constant temperature was maintained (20-21 °C) by an air conditioning system. On the day of the examination, the participants could only eat a light breakfast. It was also recommended for them to avoid coffee or tea for 12 h, alcohol for 24 h, and hard exercise for 48 h before each examination. After arriving, athletes changed into their lightweight sports clothing (without watches and wristbands potentially affecting blood flow) and acclimatized to the laboratory conditions for at least 30 min. During this time, they completed the required questionnaires, and height and weight measurements were performed.

Athletes underwent the examinations twice: at the beginning of the general preparation phase and after seven weeks, at the end of this phase. Each time, the same procedure was applied: (1) initial resting blood pressure measurement; (2) resting NADH fluorescence measurement; (3) blood draw, (4) incremental exercise test; (5) second blood draw; (6) post-exercise blood pressure measurement; and (7) post-exercise NADH fluorescence measurement (3 min after the end of the test).

2.4. Incremental Exercise Test

The exercise test was conducted on the H/P Cosmos treadmill (h/p/cosmos sports & medical GmbH, Nussdorf – Traunstein, Germany). All participants were familiar with the treadmill test because they regularly (2-3 times a year) participated in similar tests. The purpose of this examination was to assess maximal oxygen uptake (VO_2max) and peak heart rate (HR).

Respiratory gases were collected and analyzed using the MetaMax 3B ergospirometer (Cortex Biophysik BmbH, Leipzig, Germany) and the MetaSoft Studio 5.1.0 software (Cortex Biophysik BmbH, Leipzig, Germany). The exercise protocol started with a 4-min warm-up at the treadmill speed of 6 km/h. Then, the treadmill accelerated by 2 km/h every 3 min. The treadmill inclination was 1% throughout the whole test. The test terminated if the athlete signaled his/her voluntary exhaustion by raising one hand. Maximal oxygen uptake was considered to be reached if the oxygen uptake (VO_2) was stabilized despite the further increase in treadmill speed. All participants were highly trained, so during the test, all of them reached a plateau in VO_2 uptake. We also checked three additional conditions to confirm reached maximal oxygen uptake: (i) HR reached at least 95% of the age-adjusted HR; (ii) cutoff blood lactate concentration ≥ 9 mmol/L for man and ≥ 7 mmol/L for women; and (iii) respiratory exchange ratio was ≥ 1.1 [28]. Heart rate was measured using the Polar H6 Bluetooth Smart monitor (Polar Electro Oy, Kempele, Finland) attached to a chest strap.

2.5. Lactic Acid Measurements

Capillary blood samples were obtained from the fingertip at rest and 2 min after the exercise test. A total of 20 µL of whole blood was drawn to a micro test tube using a capillary. Biosen C-line (EKF Diagnostics, Cardiff, UK) was used to measure the level of lactate.

2.6. Anthropometric Measure

Anthropometric measurements were performed according to standardized procedures. Body mass (kg) and height (cm) were measured with a digital measuring station Seca 285 (SECA, Hamburg, Germany). Body mass index (BMI) was calculated as body weight divided by height squared (kg/m^2).

2.7. Nicotinamide Adenine Dinucleotide Fluorescence

NADH fluorescence was measured using the AngioExpert device (Angionica, Łódź, Poland, 2016) based on the flow mediated skin fluorescence (FMSF) method. FMSF enables recording of the changes in NADH fluorescence as a function of time in response to ischemia and reperfusion in forearm skin cells. During the measurement, AngioExpert emits light at the wavelength of 460 nm [6,7]. NADH molecules have autofluorescence capability at a wavelength of 460 nm [9]. The changes in fluorescence intensity observed during the examination are produced in the most superficial skin cells (epidermis) [6,29], which is due to very shallow skin penetration by excitation light at the wavelength of 340 nm. About 90% of the recorded signal comes from the skin depth up to 0.5 mm. The activated skin region is not directly supplied with blood, but is supplied with oxygen by deeper blood vessels [6,7,29].

During the examination, each participant sat on a chair with his/her arm resting on the measuring device. Immediately before examination, systolic (SBP) and diastolic (DBP) blood pressure was measured using the Omron 3 (Omron, Kyoto, Japan) device. At the start of the FMSF examination, basal fluorescence was registered for 2 min. Then, an occlusion cuff was inflated up to the pressure of 50 mmHg above the SBP for 200 s. After this time, blood flow in the forearm was restored (cuff deflated) and the changes in NAD fluorescence were recorded for a further 3 min [7].

The following parameters related to NAD fluorescence were measured or calculated (Figure 1):

- B_{mean}—Basal fluorescence at the wavelength of 460 nm, recorded at rest at the beginning of the measurement;
- FI_{max}—The maximal increase in fluorescence above the baseline observed during forearm ischemia;
- FR_{min}—The maximal drop in fluorescence below the baseline observed during reperfusion;
- I_{max}—The relative increase in fluorescence = the difference between I_{max} and B_{mean};
- R_{min}—The relative drop in fluorescence = the difference between B_{mean} and FR_{mean};
- IR_{ampl}—The maximal range of changes in fluorescence = the sum of R_{min} and I_{max}; and
- CI_{max}—The relative (percentage) contribution of I_{max} to IR_{ampl} [7].

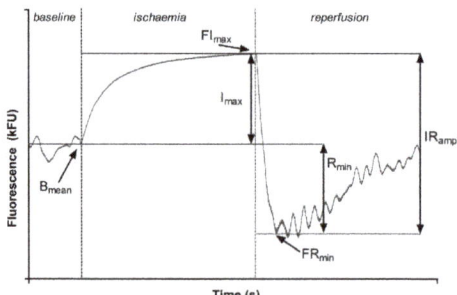

Figure 1. Parameters describing the Flow Mediated Skin Fluorescence. B_{mean}—Mean value of the basal fluorescence; FI_{max}—Maximal fluorescence during ischemia; FR_{min}—The first minimal fluorescence value during reperfusion; I_{max}—The net increase in fluorescence over the baseline during ischemia; IR_{ampl}—The amplitude of fluorescence change during ischemia and reperfusion; R_{min}—The net reduction in fluorescence below the baseline. Reprinted from Bugaj et al. [5].

The second measurement was made according to the same methodology, 3 min after the end of the treadmill test. A sample measurement of the NADH fluorescence from a 23-year-old male sprinter before and after training was shown in Figure 2.

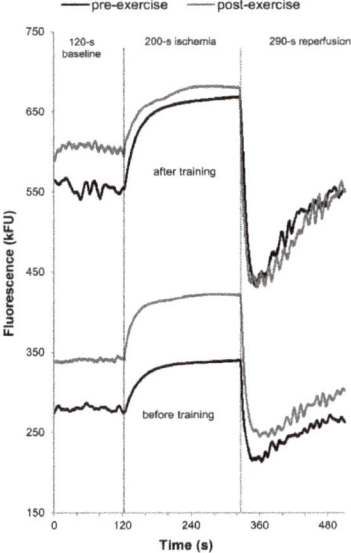

Figure 2. A sample Flow Mediated Skin Fluorescence measurement in a 23-year-old male sprinter. Changes in nicotinamide adenine dinucleotide fluorescence are shown before and after 7-weeks of training, at rest, and after cardiopulmonary exercise test until exhaustion. The first 2 min serve to determine the baseline fluorescence level. This was followed by a 200-s ischemia (increase in fluorescence) and a 290-s reperfusion (decrease in fluorescence).

3. Results

3.1. Basic Characteristics

The resting DBP, SBP, and BMI were within normal ranges. Other descriptive characteristics are presented in Table 1.

Table 1. Basic characteristics of the studied athletes.

Parameter	Before Training	After Training
Age (years)	22.4 ± 4	–
Training experience (years)	8 ± 2.3	–
Height (cm)	178.1 ± 7.3	178.1 ± 7.3
Weight (kg)	69.1 ± 10.3	69 ± 10.3
BMI (kg/m^2)	21.6 ± 2.3	21.6 ± 2.3
SBP$_{rest}$ (mmHg)	127.6 ± 14.3	119.3 ± 10.8 ***
DBP$_{rest}$ (mmHg)	69.9 ± 7.3	72.9 ± 9.3 *
SBP$_{exerc}$ (mmHg)	148 ± 18.3	139.2 ± 16.3 **
DBP$_{exerc}$ (mmHg)	74.5 ± 8.1	78.2 ± 8.1 *
VO$_2$max (mL/min/kg)	58.8 ± 8.6	59.5 ± 8.6
HR$_{peak}$ (beats/min)	191.7 ± 8	191.9 ± 8.9
LA$_{rest}$ (mmol/L)	1.2 ± 0.5	1.0 ± 0.3 **
LA$_{max}$ (mmol/L)	9.9 ± 1.5	10.2 ± 1.9

Averaged data are presented as mean ± standard deviation (SD), and results of the *t*-test for dependent samples, * $p < 0.05$, ** $p < 0.01$, *** $p < 0.001$ significantly different pre-training. BMI–body mass index; SBP–systolic blood pressure; DBP–diastolic blood pressure; rest–before cardiopulmonary exercise test; exerc–after cardiopulmonary exercise test; VO$_2$max (mL/min/kg)–maximal oxygen uptake; HR$_{peak}$–peak heart rate; LA$_{rest}$–resting lactate concentration; LA$_{max}$–maximal lactate concentration.

3.2. Measured Parameters

The values of the measured parameters are shown in Figure 3. At the first examination (before the training period), only B_{mean} significantly increased between the pre- (410.8) and post-exercise (449.3) measurements. At the second examination (after the training period), the values of all measured parameters significantly increased between resting and post-exercise condition. B_{mean} increased from 579.5 to 671.9, 16%; FI_{max} increased from 685.8 to 742.4, 8% and FR_{min} from 459.1 to 520, 13%. All measured parameters (both resting and post-exercise) significantly increased between the first and second examination.

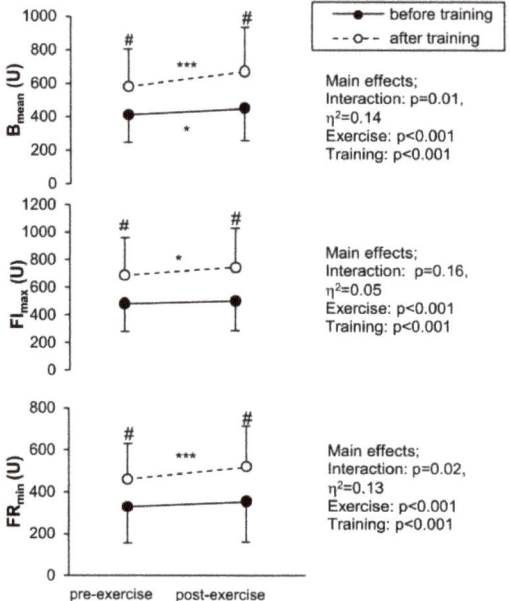

Figure 3. Measured parameters. Flow Mediated Skin Fluorescence parameters in athletes (N = 41) in two examinations, before and after the cardiopulmonary exercise test until exhaustion. B_{mean}—Changes in the mean value of the basal fluorescence; FI_{max}—Changes in maximal fluorescence during ischemia; FR_{min}—Changes in the first minimal fluorescence value during reperfusion. Values are means (SD). A two-way analysis of variance (relation between exercise and training), post-hoc Scheffe test, significant differences between pre- and post-exercise: *** $p < 0.001$, ** $p < 0.01$, * $p < 0.05$; significant differences between before and after training # $p < 0.001$, ‡ $p < 0.01$, § $p < 0.05$.

3.3. Calculated Parameters

The values of the calculated parameters are presented in Figure 4. I_{max} significantly decreased after exercise in both pre- (from 72.6 to 53.9, 26% decrease) and post-training (from 106.3 to 70.6, 34% decrease) examinations. I_{max} values were higher after than before training pre- (from 72.6 to 106.3, 46% increase) and post-exercise (from 53.9 to 70.6, 31% increase).

R_{min} significantly increased after exercise compared to resting conditions in both examinations before (from 80.3 to 94.7, 18% increase) and after training (from 120.4 to 151.9, 26% increase). The pre- and post-exercise values of R_{min} were higher after than before training (pre-exercise 50% and post-exercise 60%).

The IR_{ampl} parameter did not significantly differ between resting and post-exercise conditions in both examinations. Its pre- and post-exercise values were significantly higher after than before the training period (pre-exercise from 152.9 to 226.7, 48% increase; post-exercise from 148.6 to 222.4, 50% increase).

The values of CI$_{max}$ were significantly lower after than before exercise in both examinations (before training decreased from 0.5 to 0.4; after training decreased from 0.5 to 0.3). There were no differences observed before when compared to after training.

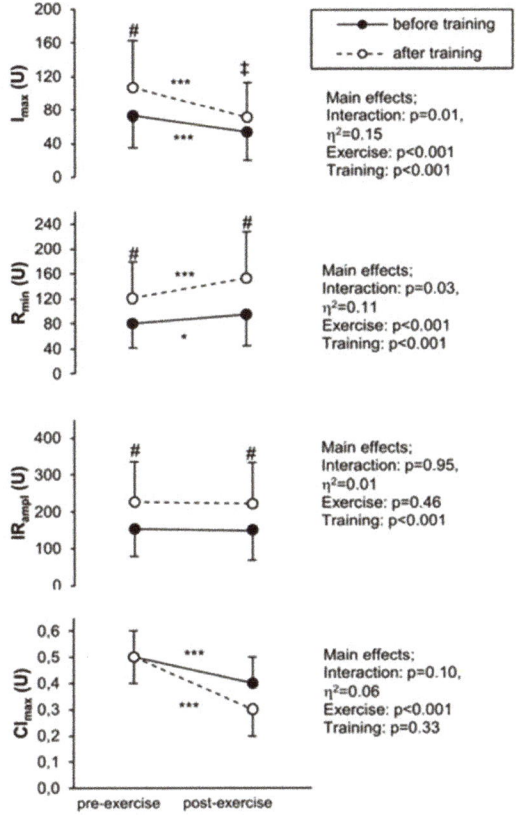

Figure 4. Calculated parameters. Flow Mediated Skin Fluorescence parameters in athletes (N = 41) in two examinations, before and after the cardiopulmonary exercise test. I$_{max}$—Changes in the net increase in fluorescence over the baseline during ischemia; IR$_{ampl}$—Changes in the amplitude of fluorescence change during ischemia and reperfusion; R$_{min}$—Changes in the net reduction in fluorescence below the baseline; CI$_{max}$ – Changes in I$_{max}$/IR$_{ampl}$ ratio. Values are means (SD). A two-way analysis of variance (relation between exercise and training), post-hoc Scheffe test, significant differences between pre- and post-exercise: *** $p < 0.001$, ** $p < 0.01$, * $p < 0.05$; significant differences between before and after training # $p < 0.001$, ‡ $p < 0.01$, § $p < 0.05$.

4. Discussion

In this study, for the first time, the changes in NADH fluorescence in epidermal cells have been investigated in highly trained athletes before and after a training period. The main and novel finding is a significant increase in NADH fluorescence after training.

4.1. The Effect of Training

In our study, an increase in NADH fluorescence after a 7-week training period in highly trained athletes was observed. It is widely known that physical training induces several adaptations including mitochondrial adaptations [22]. The measurement of NADH fluorescence may be used to indirectly evaluate the mitochondrial function and information about its metabolic status [1,5]. However, the changes in NADH fluorescence alone do not allow us to answer the question of what particular metabolic changes took place. It is known that NAD^+ and NADH are in balance (i.e., the more NAD^+, the less NADH and vice versa [8]). Therefore, the higher post-training NADH fluorescence shown in our study may indicate increased NAD turnover.

Our participants represented different sport disciplines, but the study was only conducted in the general preparation period of the annual training cycle. The main goal of this period, regardless of sports discipline, was the development of endurance capacity. VO_2max did not change after training in our athletes, which is in line with other reports [30,31] that also did not observe such changes in highly trained athletes in an annual training cycle. However, we assume that the changes occurred at the cellular respiration level. The endurance-dominant training in all athletes significantly affected the increase in the NADH fluorescence, which can be reflected by the changes in mitochondrial functions as shown in measured NADH parameters (B_{mean}, FI_{max}, FR_{min}). The post-training increase in B_{mean}, FI_{max}, and FR_{min} suggests a training-induced increase in the total NAD pool. However, there is a lack of research on training-induced changes in skin mitochondria. We can only compare our findings with those obtained from muscle mitochondria. To the best of our knowledge, the only research on training-related changes in NAD levels was performed on rat muscles. It has been found that NAD levels increased in response to endurance training [16]. There is a lack of studies on NAD changes in trained humans. The training-related changes in mitochondria have been widely described in human muscles [19,21,22,25,32]. The training-related changes in the mitochondria are probably connected with the improvement in mitochondrial biogenesis and the removal of dysfunctional mitochondria [21,22,25,32]. After training, an increase was observed in the levels of proteins related to mitochondrial biogenesis [21,25] and an improvement in mitochondrial respiratory function [19]. It is suggested that the profile of the mitochondrial changes depends on training intensity and volume. Training volume seems to affect mitochondrial content, whereas training intensity is correlated with the improvement in mitochondrial respiration [19]. It must be remembered that exercise does not necessarily imply exactly the same metabolic changes in muscle and skin mitochondria. However, intense physical activity affects mitochondrial activity and induces an increase in NADH fluorescence, which we have shown in our previous study [5]. Therefore, the observed increase in NADH fluorescence after 7-weeks of training may indirectly indicate adaptive changes in skin mitochondria.

4.2. Exercise Response

In our recent paper [5], we showed that a single bout of exercise until exhaustion induced a significant increase in skin NADH fluorescence. The results of this study are in line with our previous observations. We found that the I_{max} parameter, related to fluorescence intensity, decreased after exercise and that the R_{min} parameter increased after exercise. The likely explanation is that with limited aerobic metabolism, NADH is accumulated and the NAD^+ amount decreases because anaerobic metabolism does not allow for restoring NAD^+ from NADH to a sufficient extent [33–35].

However, some authors [36] suggest that the decrease in NADH fluorescence intensity during reperfusion not only shows the change in mitochondrial function, but also in microcirculatory and endothelial functions related to the efficiency of blood supply to the skin. Both the skin blood vessels' thermoregulatory [37–39] and endothelial [40] functions improved after training. Our study supports this view and suggests improvements in exercise tolerance based on NADH fluorescence measurement.

4.3. Practical Application

The FMSF method might be useful to evaluate metabolic adaptations related to mitochondrial function and/or microcirculatory function as the effect of training (training efficiency). This might also be used to observe the recovery after exercise when returning to the resting NADH values.

5. Conclusions

Athletes showed significant changes in NADH fluorescence in skin cells after a 7-week training period. We found that they achieved higher post-training values in basal NADH fluorescence (B_{mean}) (pre-exercise 41% increase and post-exercise 49% increase). Additionally, the maximal increase in fluorescence during occlusion (FI_{max}) and the maximal drop in fluorescence after reperfusion (FR_{min}) were higher at rest and post-exercise after training (FI_{max} 42% at rest, and 47% post-exercise, FR_{min} (39% at rest, and 47% post-exercise). In conclusion, physical training results in an increase in the skin NADH fluorescence levels at rest and after exercise in highly trained athletes. We suggest that the measurements can reflect the training-induced changes in the metabolic status of the skin mitochondria.

Author Contributions: Conceptualization, O.B. and J.Z.; Methodology, J.Z., K.K., and O.B.; Software, J.Z.; Validation, J.Z. and O.B.; Formal analysis, J.Z., D.W., and O.B.; Investigation, O.B., J.Z., D.W., K.K., A.K., and P.K.; Resources, K.K. and J.Z.; Data curation, J.Z. and O.B.; Writing—original draft preparation, O.B.; Writing—review and editing, K.K., J.Z., P.K., and A.K.; Visualization, O.B., J.Z., and A.K.; Supervision, J.Z. and K.K.; Project administration, J.Z.; Funding acquisition, J.Z. All authors have read and agreed to the published version of the manuscript.

Funding: This research was funded by ANG/ZK/2/2016 project, being a part of the project funded by the European Union from the resources of the European Regional Development Fund under the Smart Growth Operational Program, grant number POIR.01.01.01-00-0540/15.

Acknowledgments: We thank all the participants for their full cooperation.

Conflicts of Interest: The authors declare no conflict of interest.

References

1. Mayevsky, A.; Barbiro-Michaely, E. Use of NADH fluorescence to determine mitochondrial function in vivo. *Int. J. Biochem. Cell Biol.* **2009**, *41*, 1977–1988. [CrossRef]
2. Palero, J.A.; Bader, A.N.; Gerritsen, H.C. In vivo monitoring of protein-bound and free NADH during ischemia by nonlinear spectral imaging microscopy. *Biomed. Opt. Express* **2011**, *2*, 1030–1039. [CrossRef]
3. Pappajohn, D.J.; Penneys, R.; Chance, B. NADH spectrofluorometry of rat skin. *J. Appl. Physiol.* **1972**, *33*, 684–687. [CrossRef]
4. Balu, M.; Mazhar, A.; Hayakawa, C.K.; Mittal, R.; Krasieva, T.B.; König, K.; Venugopalan, V.; Tromberg, B.J. In vivo multiphoton NADH fluorescence reveals depth-dependent keratinocyte metabolism in human skin. *Biophys. J.* **2013**, *104*, 258–267. [CrossRef]
5. Bugaj, O.; Zieliński, J.; Kusy, K.; Kantanista, A.; Wieliński, D.; Guzik, P. The effect of exercise on the skin content of the reduced form of NAD and its response to transient ischemia and reperfusion in highly trained athletes. *Front. Physiol.* **2019**, *10*, 600. [CrossRef] [PubMed]
6. Katarzynska, J.; Lipinski, Z.; Cholewinski, T.; Piotrowski, L.; Dworzynski, W.; Urbaniak, M.; Borkowska, A.; Cypryk, K.; Purgal, R.; Marcinek, A.; et al. Non-invasive evaluation of microcirculation and metabolic regulation using flow mediated skin fluorescence (FMSF): Technical aspects and methodology. *Rev. Sci. Instrum.* **2019**, *90*, 104104. [CrossRef]
7. Sibrecht, G.; Bugaj, O.; Filberek, P.; Niziński, J.; Kusy, K.; Zieliński, J.; Guzik, P. Flow-Mediated Skin Flurescence method for non-invasive measurement of the NADH at 460 nm—A possibility to assess the mitochondrial function. *Postepy Biol. Komorki* **2017**, *44*, 333–352. [CrossRef]
8. White, A.T.; Schenk, S. NAD+/NADH and skeletal muscle mitochondrial adaptations to exercise. *Am. J. Physiol. Endocrinol. Metab.* **2012**, *303*, E308–E321. [CrossRef] [PubMed]
9. Mayevsky, A.; Chance, B. Oxidation-reduction states of NADH in vivo: From animals to clinical use. *Mitochondrion* **2007**, *7*, 330–339. [CrossRef] [PubMed]
10. O'Donnell, J.M.; Kudej, R.K.; LaNoue, K.F.; Vatner, S.F.; Lewandowski, E.D. Limited transfer of cytosolic NADH into mitochondria at high cardiac workload. *Am. J. Physiol. Heart Circ. Physiol.* **2004**, *286*, H2237–H2242. [CrossRef]
11. Rajman, L.; Chwalek, K.; Sinclair, D.A. Therapeutic potential of NAD-boosting molecules: The in vivo evidence. *Cell Metab.* **2018**, *27*, 529–547. [CrossRef] [PubMed]

12. Mayevsky, A.; Rogatsky, G.G. Mitochondrial function in vivo evaluated by NADH fluorescence: From animal models to human studies. *Am. J. Physiol Cell Physiol* **2007**, *292*, C615–C640. [CrossRef] [PubMed]
13. Duboc, D.; Muffat-Joly, M.; Renault, G.; Degeorges, M.; Toussaint, M.; Pocidalo, J.J. In situ NADH laser fluorimetry of rat fast- and slow-twitch muscles during tetanus. *J. Appl. Physiol.* **1988**, *64*, 2692–2695. [CrossRef] [PubMed]
14. Jobsis, F.F.; Stainsby, W.N. Oxidation of NADH during contractions of circulated mammalian skeletal muscle. *Respir. Physiol.* **1968**, *4*, 292–300. [CrossRef]
15. Sahlin, K.; Katz, A.; Henriksson, J. Redox state and lactate accumulation in human skeletal muscle during dynamic exercise. *Biochem. J.* **1987**, *245*, 551–556. [CrossRef]
16. Koltai, E.; Szabo, Z.; Atalay, M.; Boldogh, I.; Naito, H.; Goto, S.; Nyakas, C.; Radak, Z. Exercise alters SIRT1, SIRT6, NAD and NAMPT levels in skeletal muscle of aged rats. *Mech. Ageing Dev.* **2010**, *131*, 21–28. [CrossRef]
17. Boushel, R.; Gnaiger, E.; Larsen, F.J.; Helge, J.W.; Gonzalez-Alonso, J.; Ara, I.; Munch-Andersen, T.; van Hall, G.; Søndergaard, H.; Saltin, B.; et al. Maintained peak leg and pulmonary VO$_2$ despite substantial reduction in muscle mitochondrial capacity. *Scand. J. Med. Sci. Sports* **2015**, *25*, 135–143. [CrossRef]
18. Guadalupe-Grau, A.; Fernández-Elías, V.E.; Ortega, J.F.; Dela, F.; Helge, J.W.; Mora-Rodriguez, R. Effects of 6-month aerobic interval training on skeletal muscle metabolism in middle-aged metabolic syndrome patients. *Scand. J. Med. Sci. Sports* **2018**, *28*, 585–595. [CrossRef]
19. Granata, C.; Jamnick, N.A.; Bishop, D.J. Training-Induced Changes in Mitochondrial Content and Respiratory Function in Human Skeletal Muscle. *Sports Med.* **2018**, *48*, 1809–1828. [CrossRef]
20. Crane, J.D.; MacNeil, L.G.; Lally, J.S.; Ford, R.J.; Bujak, A.L.; Brar, I.K.; Kemp, B.E.; Raha, S.; Steinberg, G.R.; Tarnopolsky, M.A. Exercise-stimulated interleukin-15 is controlled by AMPK and regulates skin metabolism and aging. *Aging Cell* **2015**, *14*, 625–634. [CrossRef]
21. Busquets-Cortés, C.; Capó, X.; Martorell, M.; Tur, J.A.; Sureda, A.; Pons, A. Training and acute exercise modulates mitochondrial dynamics in football players' blood mononuclear cells. *Eur. J. Appl. Physiol.* **2017**, *117*, 1977–1987. [CrossRef] [PubMed]
22. Drake, J.C.; Wilson, R.J.; Yan, Z. Molecular mechanisms for mitochondrial adaptation to exercise training in skeletal muscle. *FASEB J.* **2016**, *30*, 13–22. [CrossRef] [PubMed]
23. Jacobs, R.A.; Lundby, C. Mitochondria express enhanced quality as well as quantity in association with aerobic fitness across recreationally active individuals up to elite athletes. *J. Appl. Physiol.* **2013**, *114*, 344–350. [CrossRef] [PubMed]
24. Jacobs, R.A.; Flück, D.; Bonne, T.C.; Bürgi, S.; Christensen, P.M.; Toigo, M.; Lundby, C. Improvements in exercise performance with high-intensity interval training coincide with an increase in skeletal muscle mitochondrial content and function. *J. Appl. Physiol.* **2013**, *115*, 785–793. [CrossRef]
25. Yan, Z.; Lira, V.A.; Greene, N.P. Exercise training-induced regulation of mitochondrial quality. *Exerc. Sport Sci. Rev.* **2012**, *40*, 159–164. [CrossRef]
26. Di Donato, D.M.; West, D.W.D.; Churchward-Venne, T.A.; Breen, L.; Baker, S.K.; Phillips, S.M. Influence of aerobic exercise intensity on myofibrillar and mitochondrial protein synthesis in young men during early and late postexercise recovery. *Am. J. Physiol. Endocrinol. Metab.* **2014**, *306*, E1025–E1032. [CrossRef]
27. Robinson, M.M.; Dasari, S.; Konopka, A.R.; Johnson, M.L.; Manjunatha, S.; Esponda, R.R.; Carter, R.E.; Lanza, I.R.; Nair, K.S. Enhanced protein translation underlies improved metabolic and physical adaptations to different exercise training modes in young and old humans. *Cell Metab.* **2017**, *25*, 581–592. [CrossRef]
28. Edvardsen, E.; Hem, E.; Anderssen, S.A. End criteria for reaching maximal oxygen uptake must be strict and adjusted to sex and age: A cross-sectional study. *PLoS ONE* **2014**, *9*, e85276. [CrossRef]
29. Dunaev, A.V.; Dremin, V.V.; Zherebtsov, E.A.; Rafailov, I.E.; Litvinova, K.S.; Palmer, S.G.; Stewart, N.A.; Sokolovski, S.G.; Rafailov, E.U. Individual variability analysis of fluorescence parameters measured in skin with different levels of nutritive blood flow. *Med. Eng. Phys.* **2015**, *37*, 574–583. [CrossRef]
30. Zarębska, E.A.; Kusy, K.; Słomińska, E.M.; Kruszyna, Ł.; Zieliński, J. Alterations in exercise-induced plasma adenosine triphosphate concentration in highly trained athletes in a one-year training cycle. *Metabolites* **2019**, *9*, 230. [CrossRef]
31. Włodarczyk, M.; Kusy, K.; Słomińska, E.M.; Krasiński, Z.; Zieliński, J. Change in lactate, ammonia, and hypoxanthine concentrations in a 1-year training cycle in highly trained athletes: Applying biomarkers as tools to assess training status. *J. Strength Cond. Res.* **2020**, *34*, 355–364. [CrossRef]

32. Wilkinson, S.B.; Phillips, S.M.; Atherton, P.J.; Patel, R.; Yarasheski, K.E.; Tarnopolsky, M.A.; Rennie, M.J. Differential effects of resistance and endurance exercise in the fed state on signalling molecule phosphorylation and protein synthesis in human muscle. *J. Physiol.* **2008**, *586*, 3701–3717. [CrossRef]
33. Finsterer, J. Biomarkers of peripheral muscle fatigue during exercise. *BMC Musculoskelet. Dis.* **2012**, *13*, 218. [CrossRef]
34. Kane, A.; Sinclair, D. Sirtuins and NADC in the development and treatment of metabolic and cardiovascular diseases. *Circ. Res.* **2018**, *123*, 868–885. [CrossRef]
35. Robergs, R.A.; Ghiasvand, F.; Parker, D. Biochemistry of exercise-induced metabolic acidosis. *Am. J. Physiol. Regul. Integr. Comp. Physiol.* **2004**, *287*, R502–R516. [CrossRef] [PubMed]
36. Hellmann, M.; Tarnawska, M.; Dudziak, M.; Dorniak, K.; Roustit, M.; Cracowski, J.L. Reproducibility of flow mediated skin fluorescence to assess microvascular function. *Microvasc. Res.* **2017**, *113*, 60–64. [CrossRef] [PubMed]
37. Charkoudian, N. Mechanisms and modifiers of reflex induced cutaneous vasodilation and vasoconstriction in humans. *J. Appl. Physiol.* **2010**, *109*, 1221–1228. [CrossRef] [PubMed]
38. Chudecka, M.; Lubkowska, A. The use of thermal imaging to evaluate body temperature changes of athletes during training and a study on the impact of physiological and morphological factors on skin temperature. *Hum. Mov.* **2012**, *13*, 33–39. [CrossRef]
39. Simmons, G.H.; Wong, B.J.; Holowatz, L.A.; Kenney, W.L. Changes in the control of skin blood flow with exercise training: Where do cutaneous vascular adaptations fit in? *Exp. Physiol.* **2011**, *96*, 822–828. [CrossRef] [PubMed]
40. Roche, D.M.; Rowland, T.W.; Garrard, M.; Marwood, S.; Unnithan, V.B. Skin microvascular reactivity in trained adolescents. *Eur. J. Appl. Physiol.* **2010**, *108*, 1201–1208. [CrossRef] [PubMed]

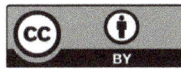

© 2020 by the authors. Licensee MDPI, Basel, Switzerland. This article is an open access article distributed under the terms and conditions of the Creative Commons Attribution (CC BY) license (http://creativecommons.org/licenses/by/4.0/).

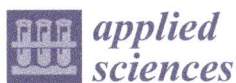

Article

Effectiveness of Positive and Negative Ions for Elite Japanese Swimmers' Physical Training: Subjective and Biological Emotional Evaluations

Goichi Hagiwara [1,*], Hirotoshi Mankyu [1], Takaaki Tsunokawa [2], Masaru Matsumoto [3] and Hirokazu Funamori [3]

1. National Institute of Fitness and Sports in Kanoya, 1 Shiromizucho, Kanoya-shi, Kagoshima 891-2393, Japan; mankyu@nifs-k.ac.jp
2. Faculty of Health and Sport Science, University of Tsukuba, 1-1-1 Tennodai, Tsukuba-shi, Ibaraki 305-8574, Japan; tsunokawa.takaaki.ke@u.tsukuba.ac.jp
3. Sharp Corporation, 3-1-72 Kitakamei-cho, Yao-shi, Osaka 581-8585, Japan; matsumoto_masaru@sharp.co.jp (M.M.); funamori.hirokazu@sharp.co.jp (H.F.)
* Correspondence: hagiwara-g@nifs-k.ac.jp; Tel.: +81-994-46-4926

Received: 21 May 2020; Accepted: 16 June 2020; Published: 18 June 2020

Abstract: The purpose of this study is to examine the subjective and objective arousal of elite swimmers during physical training under a positive and negative ion environment. The participants were 10 elite Japanese collegiate swimmers participating in the Fédération Internationale de Natation (FINA) Swimming World Cup (age: 20.80 ± 1.39, five males and five females). Each participant went through two experiments (they were subjected to both the positive and negative ion environment and the control environment) within a four-week interval. The training task was a High-Intensity Interval Training (HIIT) routine for the swimmers. The subjective arousal state was measured using a Two-Dimensional Mood Scale (TDMS). In addition, biological emotional evaluations in the form of an electroencephalogram (EEG) were conducted to assess the arousal state of the elite swimmers. The examination of the change in the arousal level at rest and during training demonstrated that both subjective and objective arousal levels were significantly higher in the positive and negative ion environment than in the control environment. In addition, the average training performance scores were also significantly higher in the positive and negative ion environment than in the control environment. This study posits that the positive and negative ion environment has a positive effect on sports training.

Keywords: training environment; sports; athletes; interval training; biological emotional evaluation; sports sciences

1. Introduction

Arousal is a human psychological state and is defined as being "worked up" or energized [1]. In addition, Oxendine [2] proposed that high levels of arousal would benefit, or be essential for, maximal performance; thus, several studies investigated the relationships between arousal and sports performance [1,3,4]. Yamazaki and Sugiyama [4] examined the relationships between subjective arousal level and sports performance and the results indicated that, among Japanese collegiate badminton players, athletes with higher arousal levels had significantly higher shot success rates. In addition, Fronso et al. [5] used an electroencephalogram (EEG) to assess the biological arousal level in Olympic athletes participating in air-pistol shooting, and investigated the relationships between arousal level and sports performance. The results demonstrated that higher levels of arousal were associated with controlled shooting performance. Although subjective evaluations about arousal level have been conducted using questionnaires [1,4,6], few studies about the biological evaluations of psychological arousal level have been attempted.

Air ions are small particles that exist in nature and are positively or negatively charged molecules or atoms in the air [7]; positively charged ions are positive ions and those negatively charged are negative ions [8]. In addition, air ions containing positive and negative ions have certain abilities such as purification of the atmosphere and deodorization [9]. Thus, several studies have been conducted on the relationship between air ions and human emotions.

Previous studies on the relationship between air ions and emotion in humans have been conducted [10]. Flory et al. [11] conducted an experiment where 18 women stayed in a high-density ion environment for over 12 consecutive days and the results indicated that the high-density negative ion environment reduced depression. In addition, other studies that examined the relationship between negative ions and depression [12–15], lower stress [16], and increased well-being [17] have been conducted. Several studies also suggest that relationships exist between positive ion environments and human emotion [10]. For instance, Gianinni et al. [18] examined the correlation between positive air ions and emotion and found that anxiety and excitement significantly increased under this condition. In addition, the relationship between positive ions and feelings of unpleasantness, irritation and anxiety has been verified [18,19].

Although there is some skepticism in the study of ions, the results of the above-mentioned studies confirm that they are connected to emotional changes. In addition, little research has been done on the relationship between positive and negative ions and the emotion and performance of athletes in the field of sports science, and no such research is found in Japan. Thus, the purpose of this study was to examine the subjective and objective arousal of elite Japanese swimmers during physical training in a positive and negative ion environment.

2. Materials and Methods

2.1. Participants and Study Design

Institutional review board approval was obtained from the corresponding author's research institute (National Institute of Fitness and Sports in Kanoya, Institutional Review Board, No.11-6). The participants were informed of the instructions and purpose of this study before the experiment.

The participants were 10 elite Japanese collegiate swimmers participating in the Fédération Internationale de Natation (FINA) Swimming World Cup (age: 20.80 ± 1.39, 5 males and 5 females). Each participant underwent two experiments within a four-week interval. Two types of experimental environment were prepared: a condition in which positive and negative ions were filled up the atmosphere in the experimental room (PNI condition), and a condition in which ions were not generated (control condition). The conditions were blinded by randomly changing the experimental environment to prevent the participants from knowing to which condition they were subjected. The details of randomization are described as follows.

The first experiment was conducted within two days. On the first day, we created a PNI condition and conducted experiments while filling the atmosphere with air ions. The participants were randomly assigned and trained in one of the two environments (in the first experiment, three female and two male athletes performed in the PNI condition). After the experiment in the PNI condition was completed, the experimental laboratory was opened for one day to stop the ionizers and release the PNI from the room. Thereafter, it was confirmed that there were no PNI and the remaining five people (three women, two men) conducted experiments in a control condition. Four weeks after the first experiment, the participants underwent the same procedure and the second experiment was conducted.

The PNI condition was delivered by six Plasmacluster^{TM} ionizers (Sharp Corporation, Sakai-shi, Osaka, Japan) and exposed the participants to positive and negative ions (147,000–164,000 PNI/cm^3). The details of the process for generating positive and negative ions were based on previous research [8]. First, molecules in the air are decomposed by applying positive and negative high voltages to each discharge brush electrode of the ion generation devices, and the devices generate positive ions and negative ions [20].

The ion concentrations were determined by an ion counter (MY1210S, Asahi System Inc., Osaka-shi, Osaka, Japan) by means of the double concentric circle tube method [20]. The room condition was a temperature of 24.0 °C ± 0.5 and humidity was 60% ± 2.0.

The experimental procedure is as follows (Figure 1). First, participants were asked to put on an EEG device for two minutes to investigate their baseline degree of arousal before training. An EEG is an electrical signal generated by the brain and can be used to measure the psychological state of humans in real time. The participants then answered a questionnaire which evaluated their subjective emotional state before the training. A training task was then assigned. The training task was a High-Intensity Interval Training (HIIT) routine for swimmers. Participants conducted eight sets of 20 s of hard exercise and 10 s of rest using a swimming ergometer (Concept2 Inc., Morrisville, VT, USA) (Figure 2). After 8 sets, participants rested for 10 min and then again performed HIIT for 20 s, with one set at maximum power. After the training task, the average load (W) for 8 sets of intervals and the maximum power set of training load (W) after a 10-min rest were evaluated. The training load was set to the load used by the participants in their daily practice. Thus, the training load was set to eight for males and six for females. Thereafter, the EEG of the participants was measured for two minutes to investigate their degree of arousal after training, after which they were required to answer a questionnaire again.

In this study, EEG was also measured during interval training but, since it was accompanied by large movements during training, accurate data could not be acquired due to noise. Therefore, the measurement values were compared for two minutes before and after training. In addition, this study used the same method as a previous study [21] that adopted two minutes to investigate the baseline degree of human emotion.

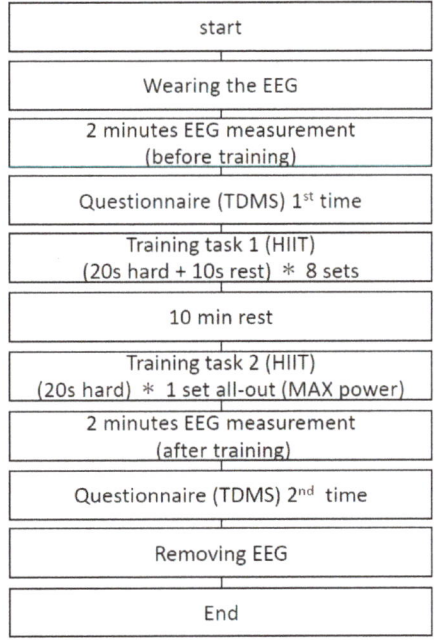

Figure 1. Experimental procedure.

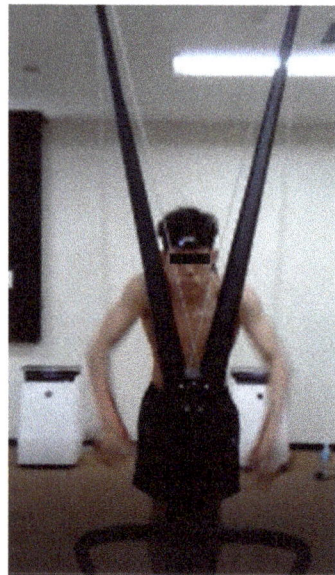

Figure 2. High Intensity Interval Training (HIIT) Training.

2.2. Emotional Evaluation

Subjective emotional evaluation was measured using a Two-Dimensional Mood Scale (TDMS) [22]. The TDMS is composed of eight items and four factors: activity, stability, comfort, and arousal. This study used the arousal score to evaluate the elite swimmers' emotional state.

A biological emotional evaluation in the form of an EEG was also conducted to assess the arousal state of the elite swimmers. In addition, the EEG measurement was used in this study because it is more easily measured in a daily living environment compared to other brain activity measurements. We adopted a simple band-type EEG device (NeuroSky Co., Ltd., Tokyo, Japan) that only measures the front polar area 1 (Fp1) lobe as defined by the international 10–20 system (Figure 3). Since Fp1 is located on the left frontal lobe, there is no need to worry about the possible noise interference caused by hair. The EEG obtained from Fp1 has been found to be suitable for obtaining data on people's psychological condition [23,24]. Thus, this study also assessed the Fp1 to estimate arousal level.

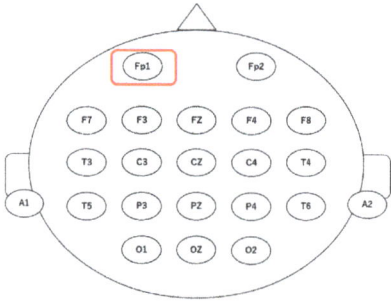

Figure 3. Measurement points of the international 10–20 system.

The electrical activity in the brain is often used as an objective evaluation index that employs biological data. Brainwaves are generally classified into four types according to their frequency range:

0.5–4 Hz: delta waves, 4–8 Hz: theta waves, 8–13 Hz: alpha waves, and 13–40 Hz: beta waves. Emotions are associated with each type [25] (Table 1).

Table 1. Type of brain wave and psychological state.

Type of Brain Wave	Frequency (Hz)	Psychological State
Delta wave	0.5–4 Hz	Non-REM sleep, unconscious
Theta wave	4–8 Hz	Sleep onset, illusion
Alpha wave	8–13 Hz	Relaxed mental state
Beta wave	13–40 Hz	Arousal

This study focused on the beta wave band. The EEG data obtained were recorded in a smartphone and the Kansei Module Logger [26]. This method produced the data output as sensitivity values were used. In addition, the Kansei Module Logger was set so that the occurrence ration of the beta wave band was defined as the arousal level, and the value was easily displayed as a value from 0 to 100. Hagiwara et al. [27] posited that the arousal level output by the Kansei Module Logger correlates with the subjective arousal level. The basic concept of Kansei Module Logger is that it calculates the power ratio between the beta wave bands. The potential difference obtained from the electrodes on the forehead and earlobe of the left Fp1 is amplified by the circuit inside the measuring instrument, digitized at 512 samples/sec, and subjected to the Hanning window processing. The power spectral analysis was then conducted using the fast Fourier transform. EEG data are analyzed every second by the fast Fourier transform, and the amplitude spectra can be obtained in the frequency range of 1–64 Hz. Thus, this study obtained delta, theta, alpha and beta waves. From the obtained power spectrum, the sum of each power in each frequency band was then calculated, and the ratio included in the total of the total power is shown as a relative numerical value. However, the sum of the power of each frequency cannot be used because the amplitude of each frequency band is different. Therefore, we took the average value of the power of each frequency band and obtained the representative value of that frequency band. The calculation method used the following Formula as a standard for analysis.

The average P_x of the x-wave power was calculated by Formula (1), where V_f is the power of the EEG at the frequency f [Hz]. Since this study concerns the beta wave band (13 Hz to 40 Hz), when $x = \beta$, it becomes (13, 40) [Hz], and the numerical value is applied to ($F^x_{max} - F^x_{min}$) in Formula (1). Next, the sum of the power averages (P_{sum}) in each frequency band is calculated by Formula (2). The ratio (R_x) included in the total power of the beta wave band was calculated in Formula (3).

$$P_x = \sum_{f=F^x_{min}}^{F^x_{max}} V_f / (F^x_{max} - F^x_{min} + 1) \tag{1}$$

$$P_{sum} = P_\delta + P_\theta + P_\alpha + P_\beta \tag{2}$$

$$R_x = P_x / P_{sum} \tag{3}$$

Based on the above calculation method, the Kansei Module Logger normalized the power ratio that can be taken in the beta band to the value of 0–100.

2.3. Analysis

For subjective data, the difference between the average value of arousal level by TDMS before and after training was used as the change value, and t-test was used to compare the PNI condition and control condition. For biological data, the difference between the average value of arousal measured before training and the average value of arousal measured after training was used as the amount of change. The paired t-test was then used to compare the difference between the PNI condition and the control condition. In the training data, the average load (W) for 8 sets of intervals and maximum power set of training load (W) after a 10-min rest were compared between the PNI condition and the control condition.

3. Results

3.1. Comparison of Changes in Arousal by TDMS before and after Training in PNI and Control Conditions

As a result of comparing the amount of change in arousal by TDMS before and after training in the PNI and the control conditions, the amount of change in the arousal level under PNI condition (M = +7.30, SD = 1.90) was found to be significantly higher than that in the control condition (M = +3.3, SD = 1.24) (t = 3.52, p < 0.01) (Figure 4).

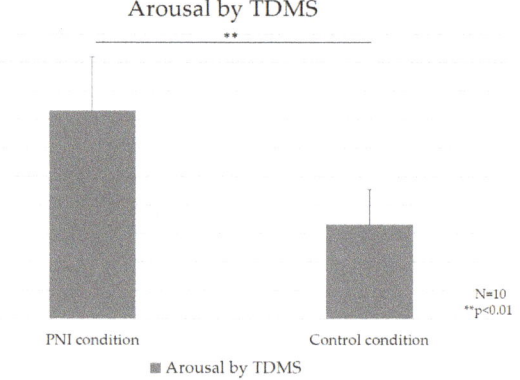

Figure 4. Comparing the amount of change in arousal by a Two-Dimensional Mood Scale (TDMS) in Positive-Negative Ions (PNI) and control conditions.

3.2. Comparison of Changes in Arousal by EEG before and after Training in the PNI and the Control Conditions

As a result of comparing the amount of change in arousal by EEG before and after training in the PNI and the control conditions, the amount of change in the arousal level under PNI condition (M = +8.16, SD = 2.14) was also found to be significantly higher than that in the control condition (M = +2.75, SD = 2.24) (t = 2.84, p < 0.05) (Figure 5).

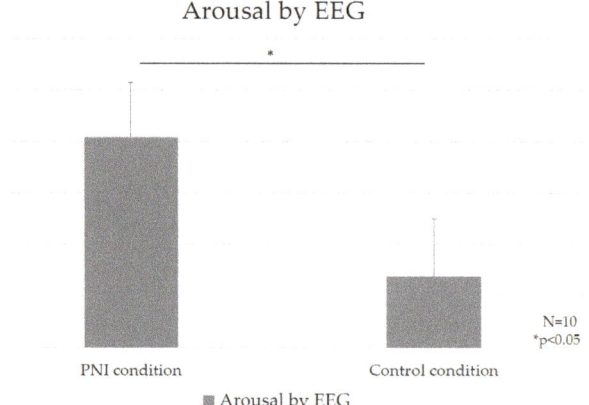

Figure 5. Comparing the amount of change in arousal by electroencephalogram (EEG) in PNI and control conditions.

3.3. Comparison of the Average Load (W) for Eight Sets of Interval Training in PNI and Control Conditions

As a result of comparing the average load (W) of interval training in the PNI and the control conditions, the average load (W) under PNI condition (M = 146.22, SD = 13.54) was shown to be significantly higher than that recorded in the control condition (M = 141.14, SD = 12.32) (t = 1.46, p < 0.10) (Figure 6).

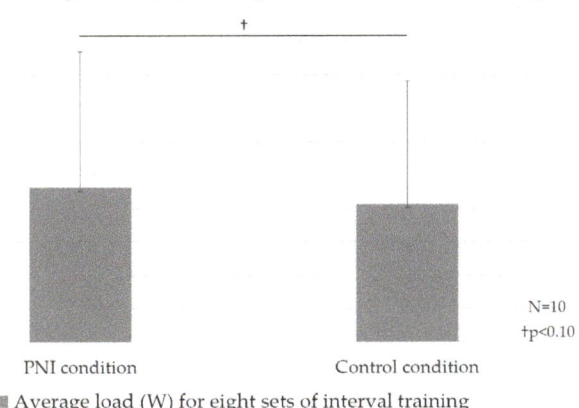

Figure 6. Comparing the average load (W) for 8 sets of interval training in PNI and control conditions.

3.4. Comparison of the Average of Training Load (W) during the Maximum Power Set in PNI and Control Conditions

As a result of comparing the average of training load (W) during the maximum power set in the PNI the and control conditions, the average load (W) under PNI condition (M = 192.78, SD = 19.36) was also found to be significantly higher than that in the control condition (M = 181.67, SD = 16.03) (t = 1.99, p < 0.05) (Figure 7).

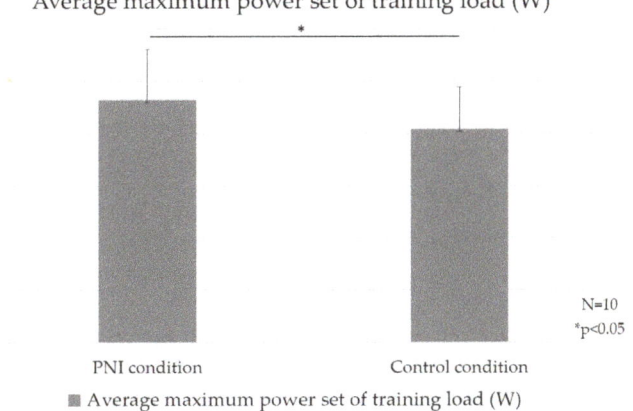

Figure 7. Comparing the average of training load (W) during the maximum power set in PNI and control conditions.

4. Discussion

This study aimed to investigate the psychological effects of both the subjective and objective arousal levels of elite Japanese swimmers during physical training under a positive and negative ion environment.

First, the results of the comparison of the subjective arousal level indicated that the PNI condition significantly improved the arousal level compared to the control condition. Previous studies [12–15] have clarified the relationship between negative ions and positive emotions by using subjective evaluation. In addition, subjective research has also shown the relationship between positive ions and emotions in previous studies [18,19]. In this study, as a result of verifying the subjective arousal level in an environment in which PNI are simultaneously generated, it is suggested that athletes may have a higher arousal level under the PNI condition. These results are considered to be new findings in the literature on PNI and emotions.

Second, the results of the comparison of the objective arousal levels obtained from EEG indicated that the PNI condition significantly improved the arousal level compared to the control condition. A few studies in the past [28,29] tried to clarify the relationship between negative ions and emotions using brain waves. Watanabe et al. [29] examined the effect of negative air ions on EEG, and the results indicated that the alpha wave tended to be higher in the negative ion condition than in the control condition. On the other hand, the results of this study indicated that the PNI condition demonstrated a significantly higher arousal level (beta band power level) than the control condition. Therefore, the results of this study differ from the previous studies that were mentioned earlier. A subjective evaluation study by Charry and Hawkinshire [19] showed that positive ions contribute to the improvement of tension. In this study, since the experiments were conducted in the environment in which positive ions were also generated, it is speculated that positive ions may affect the arousal level extracted from the EEG. As mentioned, it might demonstrate the existence of relationships between PNI conditions, and states of subjective and objective arousal. However, as mentioned previously, there is some skepticism in the study of ions; thus, it would be necessary to further study the relationships between air ions and athletes' emotions in the field of sports science.

Finally, the results of comparing the average load (W) of interval training under the PNI and the control conditions show the average load (W) under the PNI condition tended to be significantly higher than that recorded in the control condition. Moreover, the result of comparing the average of training load (W) during the maximum power set under the PNI condition was that it was recorded as significantly higher than under the control condition.

Several researches have examined the association between physical exercise and negative ions [30,31]. Ryushi et al. [30] demonstrated that, under the negative ion condition, the levels of serotonin and dopamine were decreased in the recovery period after moderate endurance exercise than those recorded under the control condition. Thus, it suggested that the negative ion condition might affect the feeling of relaxation after endurance training. This study also found that the load on the maximum power set after a 10-min rest was significantly higher, and that negative ion effects reduced dopamine and serotonin during the rest which led to a more relaxed state. There is a possibility that the PNI condition might have affected the maximum power set results for the participants.

5. Conclusions

This study suggests that the PNI condition may have a positive effect on sports training. However, there are limitations to this study. We conducted the experiments on 10 elite swimmers, but it is necessary to expand the sample size in order to generalize this study. It is thus necessary that future studies be conducted with more participants. In addition, although this study conducted the experiment twice in an environment in which the athletes were randomly switched, it is recognized that emotions may change depending on the condition of the athlete on that day. Therefore, it is suggested that conducting a longitudinal experiment on the same participants might shed more accurate findings on the matter.

Author Contributions: Conceptualization, G.H. and H.M.; methodology, G.H., H.M., and T.T.; investigation, M.M., H.F., and T.T.; writing—original draft preparation, G.H.; writing—review and editing, H.M. and T.T. All authors have read and agreed to the published version of the manuscript.

Funding: This research was funded by Sharp Corporation.

Conflicts of Interest: This study was funded by Sharp Corporation. M.M. and H.F. are employees of Sharp Corporation.

References

1. Perkins, D.; Wilson, G.V.; Kerr, J.H. The effects of elevated arousal and mood on maximal strength performance in athletes. *J. Appl. Sport Psychol.* **2001**, *13*, 239–259. [CrossRef]
2. Oxendine, J.B. Emotional arousal and motor performance. *Quest* **1970**, *13*, 23–30. [CrossRef]
3. Gould, D.; Krane, V. The arousal-performance relationship: Current status and future directions. In *Advances in Sport Psychology*; Horn, T.S., Ed.; Human Kinetics: Champaign, IL, USA, 1992; pp. 119–141.
4. Yamazaki, M.; Sugiyama, Y. Intervention effect of a motivation video for badminton athletes: Examination from watching the motivation video one hour before. *Res. J. Sport Perform.* **2009**, *1*, 275–288.
5. Fronso, S.d.; Robazza, C.; Filho, E.; Bortoli, L.; Comani, S.; Bertollo, M. Neural markers of performance states in an Olympic athlete: A EEG case study in air-pistol shooting. *J. Sports Sci. Med.* **2016**, *15*, 214–222. [PubMed]
6. Nagao, Y.; Sugiyama, Y. Influence on a collective efficacy of viewing a motivational video of a game in relation to type of video. *Res. J. Sport Perform.* **2013**, *5*, 352–368.
7. Jiang, S.Y.; Ma, A.; Ramachangran, S. Negative air ions and their effects on human health and air quality improvement. *Int. J. Mol. Sci.* **2018**, *19*, 2966. [CrossRef]
8. Yamamoto, D.; Wako, Y.; Kumabe, S.; Wako, K.; Sato, Y.; Fujishiro, M.; Yashimasa, Y.; Matsuura, I.; Ohnishi, Y. Positive and negative ions by air purifier have no effects on reproductive function or postnatal growth and development in rats. *Fundam. Toxicol. Sci.* **2015**, *2*, 101–110. [CrossRef]
9. Nishikawa, K. Air purification technology of positively and negatively charged cluster ions by plasma discharge at atmospheric pressure. *J. Plasma Fusion Res.* **2013**, *89*, 164–168.
10. Perez, V.; Alexander, D.D.; Bailey, W.H. Air ions and mood outcomes: A review and meta-analysis. *BMC Psychiatry.* **2013**, *13*, 29. [CrossRef]
11. Flory, R.; Ametepe, J.; Bowers, B. A randomized, placebo-controlled trial of bright light and high-density negative air ions for treatment of Seasonal Affective Disorder. *Psychiatry Res.* **2010**, *177*, 101–108. [CrossRef]
12. Goel, N.; Etwaroo, G.R. Bright light, negative air ions and auditory stimuli produce rapid mood changes in a student population: A placebo-controlled study. *Psychol. Med.* **2006**, *36*, 1253–1263. [CrossRef]
13. Terman, M.; Terman, J.S. Treatment of seasonal affective disorder with a high-output negative ionizer. *J. Altern. Complement Med.* **1995**, *1*, 87–92. [CrossRef]
14. Terman, M.; Terman, J.S. Controlled trial of naturalistic dawn simulation and negative air ionization for seasonal affective disorder. *Am. J. Psychiatry.* **2006**, *163*, 2126–2133. [CrossRef] [PubMed]
15. Terman, M.; Terman, J.S.; Ross, D.C. A controlled trial of timed bright light and negative air ionization for treatment of winter depression. *Arch. Gen. Psychiatry.* **1998**, *55*, 875–882. [CrossRef] [PubMed]
16. Malik, M.; Singh, K.; Singh, M. Effect of negative air ions on physiological and perceived psychological stress during computer operation. *Int. J. Environ. Health.* **2010**, *4*, 67–77. [CrossRef]
17. Lips, R.; Salawu, J.T.; Kember, P.; Probert, S.D. Intermittent exposures to enhanced air-ion concentrations for improved comfort and increased productivity? *Appl. Energy* **1987**, *28*, 83–94. [CrossRef]
18. Giannini, A.J.; Jones, B.T.; Loiselle, R.H. Reversibility of serotonin irritation syndrome with atmospheric anions. *J. Clin. Psychiatry* **1986**, *47*, 141–143.
19. Charry, J.M.; Hawkinshire, F.B. Effects of atmospheric electricity on some substrates of disordered social behavior. *J. Pers. Soc. Psychol.* **1981**, *41*, 185–197. [CrossRef]
20. Nishikawa, K.; Nojima, H. Air purification effect of positively and negatively charged ions generated by discharge plasma at atmospheric pressure. *Jpn. J. Appl. Phys.* **2001**, *40*, 835–837. [CrossRef]
21. Kanamaru, S.; Yokota, Y.; Naruse, Y.; Yairi, I. A research on quantification of the fear using EEG. In Proceedings of the 33rd Annual Conference of the Japanese Society for Artificial Intelligence, Niigata, Japan, 4–7 June 2019; pp. 1–4. [CrossRef]

22. Sakairi, Y.; Nakatsuka, K.; Shimizu, T. Development of the Two-Dimensional Mood Scale for self-monitoring and self-regulation of momentary mood states. *Jpn. Psychol. Res.* **2013**, *55*, 338–349. [CrossRef]
23. Mitsukura, Y. KANSEI Analyzing by EEG. *J. Inst. Electr. Eng. Jpn.* **2016**, *136*, 687–690. [CrossRef]
24. Hotta, M.; Kohata, Y. The evaluation of usability of EC site using electroencephalogram (EEG). In Proceedings of the 19th Japan Society of Kansei Engineering, University of Tsukuba, Tokyo, Japan, 11–13 September 2017; pp. 1–5.
25. Okubo, T.; Tamamaru, K.; Koshimizu, S. Development of the Impression Detection System by using a Portable EEG Device for Tourist Impression Analysis. *Trans. Jpn. Soc. Kansei Eng.* **2018**, *17*, 285–291. [CrossRef]
26. Littlesoftware Inc. Available online: https://hp.littlesoftware.jp (accessed on 10 May 2018).
27. Hagiwara, G.; Akiyama, D.; Tsunokawa, T.; Mankyu, H. Effectiveness of motivational videos for elite swimmers: Subjective and biological evaluations. *J. Hum. Sport Exerc.* **2019**, *14*, 178–188. [CrossRef]
28. Assael, M.; Pfeifer, Y.; Sulman, F.G. Influence of artificial air ionisation on the human electroencephalogram. *Int. J. Biometeorol.* **1974**, *18*, 306–372. [CrossRef] [PubMed]
29. Watanabe, I.; Mano, Y.; Noro, H. Effect of negative air ion in human electroencephalogram. *J. Jpn. Soc. Balneol. Climatol. Phys. Med.* **1998**, *61*, 121–126. [CrossRef]
30. Ryushi, T.; Kita, I.; Sakurai, T.; Yasumatsu, M.; Isokawa, M.; Aihara, Y.; Hama, K. The effect of exposure to negative air ions on the recovery of physiological responses after moderate endurance exercise. *Int. J. Biometeorol.* **1998**, *41*, 132–136. [CrossRef]
31. Nimmericher, A.; Holdhaus, J.; Mehnen, L.; Vidotto, C.; Loidl, M.; Barker, A.R. Effects of negative air ions on oxygen uptake kinetics, recovery and performance in exercise: A randomized, double-blinded study. *Int. J. Biometeorol.* **2014**, *58*, 1503–1512. [CrossRef]

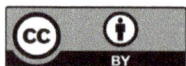

© 2020 by the authors. Licensee MDPI, Basel, Switzerland. This article is an open access article distributed under the terms and conditions of the Creative Commons Attribution (CC BY) license (http://creativecommons.org/licenses/by/4.0/).

 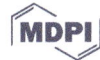

Article

Analysis of Serve and Serve-Return Strategies in Elite Male and Female Padel

Bernardino J Sánchez-Alcaraz [1], Diego Muñoz [2,*], Francisco Pradas [3], Jesús Ramón-Llin [4], Jerónimo Cañas [5] and Alejandro Sánchez-Pay [1]

1. Department of Physical Activity and Sport, Faculty of Sport Sciences, University of Murcia, C/Argentina, s/n, 30720 San Javier, Murcia, Spain; bjavier.sanchez@um.es (B.J.S.-A.); aspay@um.es (A.S.-P.)
2. Department of Didactic of Musical, Plastic and Corporal Expression, Faculty of Sports Science, University of Extremadura, Avda de la Universidad, s/n, 10003 Cáceres, Spain
3. Department of Musical, Plastic and Corporal Expression, Faculty of Human Sciences and Education, University of Zaragoza, C/Pedro Cerbuna, 12, 50009 Zaragoza, Spain; franprad@unizar.es
4. Department of Musical, Plastic and Corporal Expression, Faculty of Education, University of Valencia, Av. Dels Tarongers, 4, 46022 Valencia, Spain; jesus.ramon@uv.es
5. Department of Physical Education and Sport, Faculty of Sport Sciences, University of Granada, Carretera de Alfacar, 21, 18071 Granada, Spain; jerocanias@yahoo.com
* Correspondence: diegomun@unex.es; Tel.: +34-927-257-460

Received: 22 August 2020; Accepted: 22 September 2020; Published: 24 September 2020

Abstract: This aim of this study was to analyze serve and return statistics in elite padel players regarding courtside and gender. The sample contained 668 serves and 600 returns of serves from 14 matches (7 male and 7 female) of the 2019 Masters Finals World Padel Tour. Variables pertaining to serve (number, direction, court side and effectiveness), return of serve (direction, height, stroke type and effectiveness) and point outcome were registered through systematic observation. The main results showed that the serving pair had an advantage in rallies, under 8 shots in women and under 12 shots in men. Statistical differences according to gender and court side were found. Female players execute more backhand and cross-court returns and use more lobs than men. On the right court, serves are more frequently aimed at the "T" and more down the line returns are executed when compared to the left side. Such knowledge could be useful to develop appropriate game strategies and to design specific training exercises based on actual competition context.

Keywords: racket sports; performance analysis; game-actions; strokes

1. Introduction

Padel is a racket sport played in pairs (2 vs. 2). The court is characterized by its completely closed girth, as a small-sized grass court (20 × 10 m) surrounded by glass and metallic mesh areas on which the ball can bounce [1]. It has become a mass phenomenon in some countries, such as Spain, and is practiced in more than 35 countries around the world [2]. A professional padel circuit has been created (World Padel Tour), with tournaments in several countries. This development can be attributed to a high interaction between players and a low intensity of actions in a low level of competition [3,4]. Accordingly, the enjoyment and motivation of the players increases, inducing a greater adherence to practice [5–7].

Investigations in padel have increased in the past few years [8]. Research on padel has been mainly focused on describing the match activity and detecting effective performance indicators [9–11]. These investigations have provided primary information such as the rally length (10 to 15 s), the most common actions in offence (volley and smash) and defense (lob), and have highlighted the advantage of the net game. In addition, padel player performance has been characterized by the ratio between winning shots and errors [12]. Furthermore, previous researches have shown gender-related differences during competition [13,14]. Higher values have been observed in play time and total time in women over men players, as well as in the number and types of strokes [10]. Therefore, the players constantly try to play in offensive positions; for which they use different behaviors and technical-tactical actions, which define different styles of play [12]. The distribution of the different types of strokes, their trajectories and their efficacy stand out among these behaviours [3–5]. The results of the studies have shown that these variables may also differ depending on the gender or the side of the court on which the padel player plays [10,11]. Hence, different performance profiles of padel could exist related to gender and game-side on court [15].

However, there is an alarming lack of investigations examining players' serve and return statistics [16]. One of the most important performance indicators in racket sports is the serve [17]. In tennis, a serve directly wins the point through an ace or indirectly because of the advantage coming from the opponent's imbalance after a great serve [18]. Thus, tennis players win about 70% of points with the first serve, this percentage being higher in men's singles than in women's [17,19]. Previous studies found that serve was more determinant in tennis doubles, likely due to the presence of the server's partner covering the net [20]. Furthermore, the serve situation could influence point or game outcome in padel, since it allows players to adopt an offensive position. In this way, winners scored about 34% more points from the net than losers [9]. However, the serve in padel is different to other racket sports, because of the rules of game. In padel, the ball cannot be beaten as hard as in tennis, and the serve must be an underhand shot from a bouncing ball hit from below waist level. In addition, the effect and the side wall can affect the serve-return shot [16]. The receiver must play an accurate shot to avoid the serving pair hitting the ball into a tactically advantageous area, so they should vary the direction and height of their return of serve [15,16].

A better knowledge of players' behavior when serving or receiving is extremely useful for developing appropriate game strategies and to design specific training exercises [21]. However, at present little is known about the relationship between the serve and return of serve in padel, other than the fact that the server tends to maintain the tactical advantage until around shot five, when the advantage has dissipated [16,22]. In addition, Zhang and Zhou [23] differentiated specific serve tactics in table tennis that were associated with higher scoring rates. Furthermore, some studies highlighted the difference between first and second serves in terms of how aggressive the return could be [24]. Given that serve and return of serve are two of the most important shots in padel, the purpose of this study was to analyze serve and return statistics in elite padel players regarding court side and gender. This information could help coaches to better understand player strategies and their efficiency in padel games.

2. Materials and Methods

2.1. Sample and Variables

The study was reviewed and approved by the Ethical Committee of the University of Murcia. The sample contained 668 serves and 600 returns of serves from 14 professional matches (7 male and 7 female) of the 2019 Finals World Padel Tour. These tournaments gathered the best pairs in the world, ensuring the highest competitive level in all the matches. A total of 32 players, 16 men (mean (SD) age: 31.18 (7.27) years; height: 181.3 (4.1) cm) and 16 women (mean (SD) age: 28.66 (6.7) years; height: 168.4 (3.7) cm) performed the matches. Variables pertaining to serve and return statistics and point outcome were included in the analysis, following the methodology adopted in other similar studies [25]:

- Serve shots were analyzed regarding the serve number (1st and 2nd serve), court side (right and left), serve direction (side wall, middle and T) and effectiveness indicator (winner, error and continuity) (Figure 1).

- Return statistics were analyzed regarding the court side (right and left), stroke direction (down the line, middle and cross court), stroke height (straight and lob), stroke type (forehand and backhand) and effectiveness indicator (winner, error and continuity) (Figure 1).
- Point outcome: strokes were classified according to the winning or losing pair of the point (serving players win and returning players win).
- Total shots: number of total shots in the points were counted.

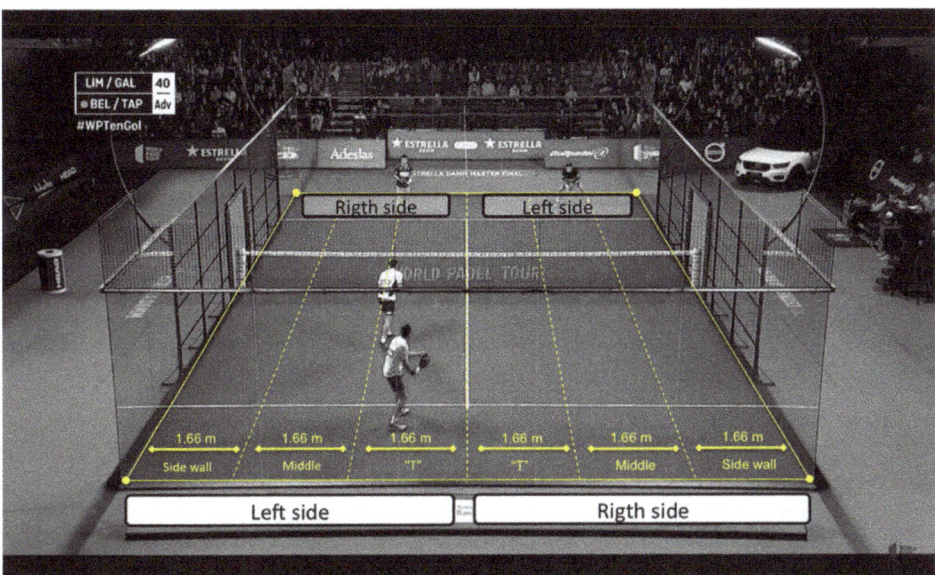

Figure 1. Illustration of court side and serve and return directions.

2.2. Procedure

The matches were downloaded from the official channel of the World Padel Tour [26]. Lince video analysis software was used to collect and register the data [27]. The Kinovea software [28] was used to place a visual grid over the video image for the serve and return directions data recording (Figure 1) and to register the feet of the serving player when impacting the ball, the place where the ball bounced after a successful serve and the direction of the ball after the returner hit it. Four observers specializing in padel (over 5 years of experience) were specifically trained to perform the recording. Observers were specifically trained in the use of the observational instrument for two weeks. The training focused on the clear identification of the variables (serve and return statistics, point outcome and total shots) and the use of the observational instrument software (Lince and Kinovea). Having completed the training process, each observer registered a training set not included in the final sample ($n = 72$ serves; $n = 68$ returns), to calculate inter-rater reliability. Consistency of records was analyzed using the free-marginal multirater Kappa [29] and the weighted Kappa [30]. The minimum score obtained was $k = 0.87$. Finally, intra-observer evaluation was done at the end of the observation process by Cohen's Kappa calculation, yielding a very good strength of agreement with scores over 0.92 [31].

2.3. Data Analysis

Descriptive analysis included means, standard deviations and frequencies. Assumptions of normality and homogeneity of variances were verified using the Kolmogorov–Smirnov test and Levene's test. Due to data not following a normal distribution, non-parametric tests were implemented [32].

Chi square analysis was performed to identify differences in serve and return statistics and point outcome between gender and court side. Column proportions were compared using Z tests on serve and return statistics according to the gender of the players and court side. A significance level of $p < 0.05$ was established which was adjusted according to Bonferroni in the Z tests. The associations among the categories of the variables were performed with corrected standardized residuals (CSR). The effect size was calculated using Cramer's V [33]. Rho Spearmen was used to know the relationship between serving point won and the number of strokes per point. IBM SPSS 25.0 Statistics for Macintosh (Armonk, NY: IBM Corp.) was used to process the data.

3. Results

3.1. Serve and Return Performances of Professional Padel Players Regarding Gender

Table 1 shows differences in serve and return statistics in relation to players' gender. With regards to serve performance, the players' gender determined the percentage of first and second serves ($\chi^2 = 5.05$; gL = 1; CRS = 2.2; $p < 0.05$). Thus, men obtained a significantly higher percentage of successful first serves than women. Furthermore, both men and women aimed more than 60% of their serves towards the side wall. Regarding return statistics, significant differences between men and women were found with regards to direction ($\chi^2 = 9.647$; gL = 2; CRS = 3.2; $p < 0.01$), height ($\chi^2 = 9.354$; gL = 2; CRS = 2.9; $p < 0.01$) and stroke type ($\chi^2 = 4.230$; gL = 1; CRS = 2.1; $p < 0.05$). Thus, women played a significantly higher proportion of backhand or cross-court returns and used the lob more when returning than men did. Finally, the point-result variable showed how men won a significantly higher percentage of points in a serve situation than women ($\chi^2 = 11.435$; gL = 1; CRS = 3.4; $p < 0.01$).

Figure 2 shows the relationship between the percentage of points won by the couple with the serve and the number of strokes per point, in relation to the players' gender. The correlation test results showed a significant relationship for male ($p < 0.001$; $r = 0.62$) and female ($p < 0.001$; $r = 0.54$) players between the percentage of points won in the serve and the number of strokes per point. Thus, the percentage of points won by the player with the serve went down as the number of strokes went up. Furthermore, with regards to gender, serving advantage was lost after the 12th stroke for men, while for women it was after the seventh stroke.

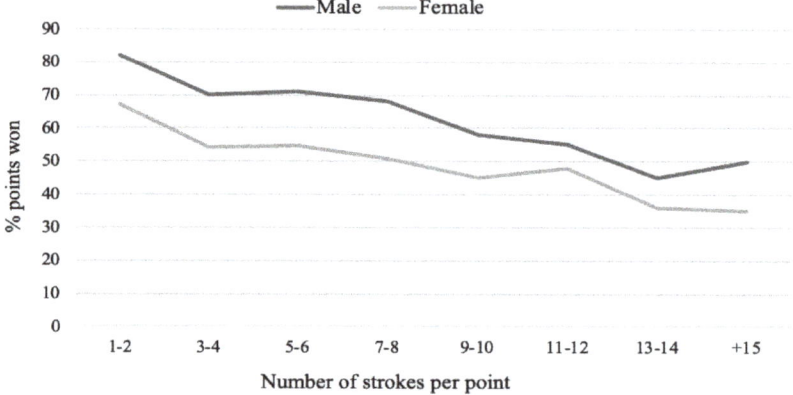

Figure 2. Percentage of points won by the serving couple with relation to the number of strokes per points: gender differences.

Table 1. Percentages for the serve and serve–return performances of the professional male and female padel players.

		Male n (%)	Female n (%)	Sig.
Serve statistics				
Serve Number				
	1st serve	378 (92.9)a	229 (87.7)b	0.025 *
	2nd serve	29 (7.1)a	32 (12.3)b	
Court side				
	Right	211 (51.8)	133 (51.0)	0.823
	Left	196 (48.2)	128 (49.0)	
Serve direction				
	Side wall	263 (64.6)	163 (62.5)	
	Middle	45 (11.1)	19 (7.3)	0.101
	T	99 (24.3)	79 (30.3)	
Effectiveness				
	Winner	0 (0.0)	0 (0.00)	
	Error	36 (8.8)	34 (13.0)	0.085
	Continuity	371 (91.2)	227 (87.0)	
Return statistics				
Stroke direction				
	Down the line	213 (57.4)a	103 (45.0)b	
	Middle	95 (25.6)	69 (30.1)	0.008 **
	Cross court	63 (17.0)a	57 (24.9)b	
Stroke height				
	Straight	242 (65.2)a	122 (53.3)b	0.009 **
	Lob	129 (34.7)a	107 (46.7)b	
Stroke type				
	Forehand	156 (42.0)a	77 (33.6)b	0.040 *
	Backhand	215 (58.0)a	152 (64.4)b	
Effectiveness				
	Winner	0 (0.0)	1 (0.4)	
	Error	20 (5.4)	9 (3.9)	0.323
	Continuity	351 (94.96)	219 (95.6)	
Point outcome				
	Serve pair win	232 (62.5)a	111 (48.5)b	0.001 **
	Returner pair win	139 (37.5)a	118 (51.5)b	

Note: n = Number; % = Percentage; * = $p < 0.05$; a, b = significant differences indicated in the Z tests for comparison of column proportions from $p < 0.05$, adjusted according to Bonferroni.

3.2. Serve and Return Performances of Professional Padel Players Regarding Court Side

Figure 3 shows serve statistics with regard to court side where said serve was played. As may be observed in the court shown above, court side significantly determined serve direction ($\chi^2 = 18.202$; gL = 2; CRS = 3.3; $p < 0.01$). It may be observed that most serves went towards the side wall, followed by the "T" and, in smaller proportion, the middle of the court. Furthermore, on the left side (ad court) players executed 12% more serves towards the side wall, whereas on the right side (deuce court) players served 14% more towards the "T." On the other hand, no significant differences were found with regards to court side for effectiveness ($\chi^2 = 1.047$; gL = 1; $p > 0.05$) and serve number ($\chi^2 = 2.972$; gL = 1; $p > 0.05$).

Figure 4 shows return statistics with regards to the player's side of the court. As may be observed, players executed around 60% of straight returns, with no significant differences regarding court side ($\chi^2 = 2.048$; gL = 2; $p > 0.05$). Furthermore, players obtained a high percentage of return effectiveness, with more than 90% of successful returns, and no difference between the right and left sides ($\chi^2 = 4.444$; gL = 2; CRS = 3.0; $p > 0.05$). Playing side significantly determined the return's direction ($\chi^2 = 28.711$; gL = 2; CRS = 7.6; $p < 0.01$). Thus, players returning from the left side executed almost 15% more down the line returns than players on the right side. Furthermore, the kind of returning stroke also showed significant differences regarding court side. Left side players executed more than 75% of their returns backhand, whereas right side players registered more balanced values, although they did execute more forehand returns. Finally, there were no significant differences between return statistics and stroke type, height or direction ($p < 0.005$).

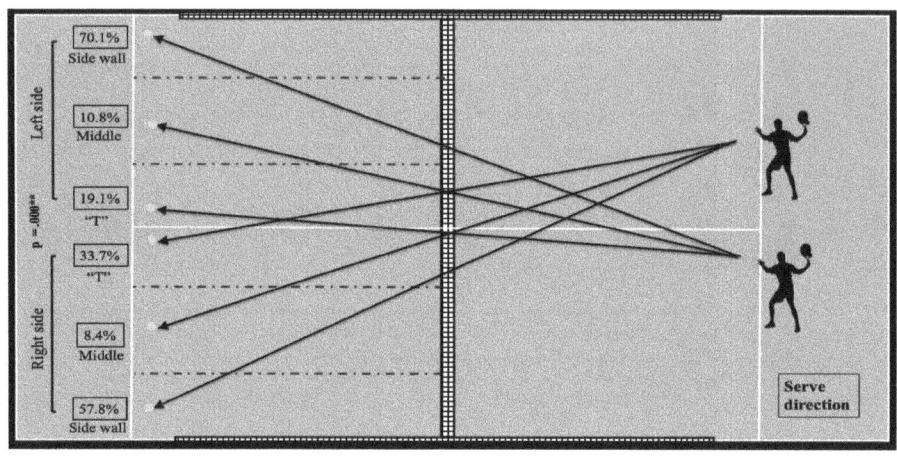

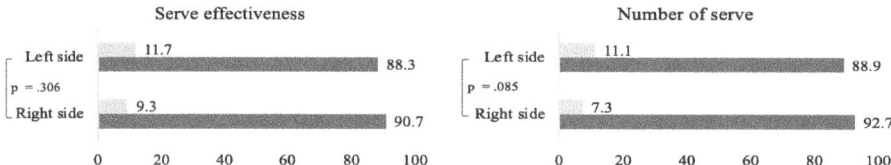

Figure 3. Serve statistics regarding court side.

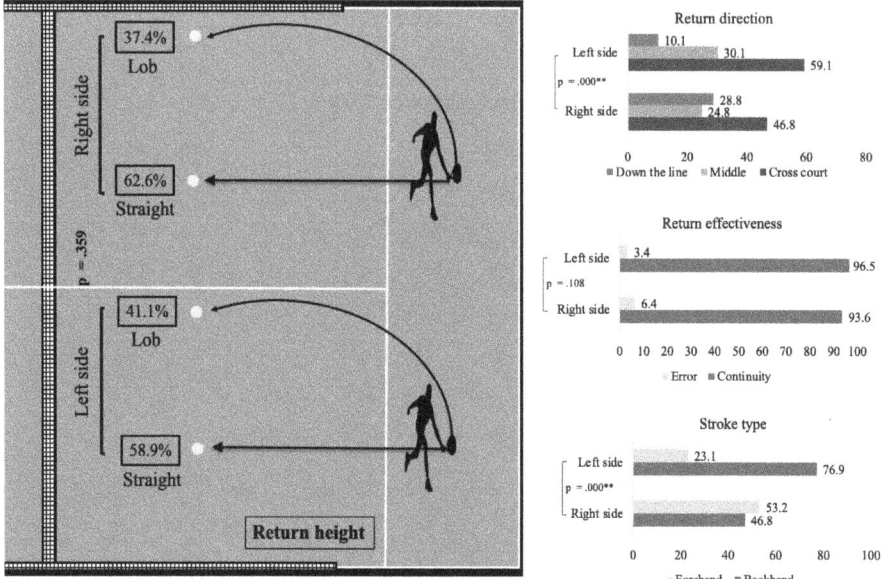

Figure 4. Serve return statistics regarding court side.

4. Discussion

This aim of this study was to evaluate the serve and return statistics in elite padel players regarding courtside and gender. The notational analysis of this research is one of the most important contributions because of the lack of previous research regarding this aspect in padel. The main results showed that the serving pair had a significant advantage in rallies, which lasted until shot 7 in women and shot 12 in men (Figure 2). Considering that serve advantage is lost after the fourth shot in tennis, this finding probably reflects the nature of padel in that it is much harder to play a winning shot, due to the court dimensions and structure, meaning that when a pair is dominating the rally, as at the start of the point when serving, it often takes more shots to finish the rally compared to tennis [16]. Regarding gender, men won a significantly higher percentage of points when serving than women (62.5% vs. 48.5%), as happens in other sports like tennis, where men obtain 14% more points with their serve than their female counterparts [34,35]. These gender differences may be due to the fact that male players are taller and can jump higher, which would enable them to sustain for a longer period of time an offensive position at the net [36,37]. However, deeper analysis and complementary variable collection is encouraged for a more relevant advance in this knowledge. In tennis, previous studies reported that men's serves had an impact on rally outcome in rallies that lasted four shots [22]. This impact of the serve was corroborated by other research, which found that the serving pair won the most rallies containing 1 to 4 shots [38]. These different results in padel suggest that the influence of service extends some way into the rally in padel because the predominance of the "serve and volley" strategy allows the serving pair to move close to the net first and adopt an offensive position [9,39]. Despite serve advantage being lost when the return players use technical actions that facilitate a change of position, such as lobs, this transition from offensive to defensive position only appears in 37% of points [40]. On the other hand, the results showed first serve effectiveness as being close to 90%. Even though there were no gender significant differences, the higher occurrence of first service faults reported by women could be due to a higher predisposition to obtain a direct point by forcing the first service [15].

With regards to serve direction, the results of this study showed how players served primarily towards the side wall, increasing that percentage on the left side (advantage), which is usually the place where more decisive points are fought. The greater distance covered by the player serving during the point [39] could explain this crossed direction of the serve towards the glass, since it would allow him to buy more time to occupy a better position at the net. Furthermore, the bounce on the side wall may complicate the return stroke, which could cause a greater number of errors, as other authors have claimed [15]. Other studies reported that the high percentage of serves to the side wall on the left side could be explained by the hand-dominance of the players [12]. Thus, since most padel players playing on the left side of the court are right-handed, servers would seek to serve towards the side wall to seek both the backhand of the return as well as the uncertainty of the wall bounce. No differences between genders were found in serve direction. Similar studies in other racket sports, such as tennis, showed that the serve aimed at the "T" was the most effective in winning the point [41]. However, on the left side of the court, better results are obtained when players serve cross-court or open [42]. It is important to highlight that some of these results regarding serve direction could be related more to players' hand dominance than court side [12], so further research is warranted.

The results of this study confirmed that the beginning of each point in professional padel seems very important and decisive for increasing the chances of winning the point. Then, serve effectiveness is directly related to the opponent's serve-return skills [17]. The results showed that a very high percentages of serve returns stayed in (around 90%), but no differences regarding gender or courtside were found. This effectiveness percentage is higher than in other racket sports such as tennis, where serve power is higher [43]. Furthermore, return height and direction in padel may allow couples in the defensive position to execute a stroke that allows them to send the attacking couple to the back of the court [11]. Previous authors showed how sending deep lobs to the corners and close to the walls will keep the rivals far from the net. However, the results of our study showed that players hit about 60% straight and 40% lob shots. These data are confirmed by a previous analysis in a national padel competition, and reflect the importance for the player serving to run toward the net and be able to approach the net to make the straight return more advantageous [16]. Furthermore, the return's height and direction showed significant differences with regards to players' gender and the side of the court. Thus, women executed more lobs and cross-court returns than men. This higher use of lobs by female players has been confirmed in previous studies that suggest a more defensive playing style among women [10,44,45]. Thus, because over-head strokes (smash and tray) are the most successful shots during a match, with a significantly higher percentage in the male category [10,46], players returning the serve have to use the lob only in comfortable positions to overcome their opponents at the net, since a poorly executed lobbed return could have as a response a winning smash from the serving players. At the national level, the lob return of serve achieved long rallies 48.8% of the time for good depth (around 5.5 m beyond the net) off first serves and 61.8% of the time off second serves, and 79.8% of the time for excellent depth (around 8.5 m beyond the net) irrespective of serve [16].

With regards to playing side, players returning the serve on the left side stroke more with their backhand than forehand, and play more straight and down the line strokes than players on the right side, corroborating the findings of Torres-Luque et al. [10], who found that about 75% of serves were directed to the backhand of players. This fact could be due to a higher game aggression of players when resting in the left side, not allowing serving players to take the lead in the point [9,47]. Furthermore, these differences in return with regards to playing side are especially important considering that 75% of the decisive points are played on the left side of the court [35].

Although this is the first study addressing serve and return statistics in professional padel, the study presents some limitations. First, contextual variables such as match status were not registered. Given the influence of situational variables on game performance [48], it would be very interesting to include such information in future research on padel. On the other hand, other variables that may affect serve and return statistics, such as serve speed or spin and players' hand dominance [12,22,43], have not been taken into account. Finally, the sample was limited, so future studies should analyze a greater number and tournaments and padel players.

5. Conclusions

The current investigation has described the advantage of serving in padel by comparing points won by servers and receiving players after a different number of shots within rallies. Given the server has a significant advantage, the aim of the return is to avoid the serving pair winning the rally quickly. This could be best achieved by good depth on lobs, regardless of the direction, and pace on straight shots, predominately aimed toward the server [16]. Statistical differences according to gender and court side were found. Female players execute more backhand and cross-court returns and use more lobs than men. On the right court, serves are more frequently aimed at the "T" and more down the line returns are executed when compared to the left side. Such knowledge may have implications for accuracy and the quality of training drills based on specific technical–tactical demands.

Author Contributions: Conceptualization, B.J.S.-A., D.M. and J.C.; methodology, B.J.S.-A., J.R.-L., F.P., A.S.-P. and D.M.; software, B.J.S.-A. and F.P.; validation, B.J.S.-A., F.P., J.R.-L. and D.M.; formal analysis, B.J.S.-A., J.C. and A.S.-P.; investigation, B.J.S.-A., J.C., J.R.-L., D.M and A.S.-P.; resources, B.J.S.-A., J.R.-L., A.S.-P. and D.M.; data curation, B.J.S.-A., J.R.-L., A.S.-P. and D.M.; writing—original draft preparation, B.J.S.-A., J.C. and D.M.; writing—review and editing, B.J.S.-A., F.P., J.R.-L., A.S.-P. and D.M.; visualization, B.J.S.-A., J.C., F.P., J.R.-L., A.S.-P. and D.M.; supervision, B.J.S.-A., F.P., J.R.-L., A.S.-P. and D.M. All authors have read and agreed to the published version of the manuscript.

Funding: This research received no external funding.

Conflicts of Interest: The authors declare no conflict of interest.

References

1. International Padel Federation. Rules of Padel. FIP, V.D. Available online: https://www.padelfip.com/wp-content/uploads/2017/06/Rules-of-Padel.pdf (accessed on 1 July 2020).
2. Courel-Ibáñez, J.; Sánchez-Alcaraz, B.J.; García, S.; Echegaray, M. Evolution of padel in spain according to practitioners' gender and age [Evolución del pádel en España en función del género y edad de los practicantes]. *Cult. Cienc. Deporte* **2017**, *12*, 39–46. [CrossRef]
3. Carrasco, L.; Romero, S.; Sañudo, B.; de Hoyo, M. Game analysis and energy requirements of paddle tennis competition. *Sci. Sports* **2011**, *26*, 338–344. [CrossRef]
4. Courel-Ibáñez, J.; Sánchez-Alcaraz, B.J.; Cañas, J. Game performance and length of rally in professional padel players. *J. Hum. Kinet.* **2017**, *55*, 161–169. [CrossRef]
5. Castillo-Rodríguez, A.; Alvero-Cruz, J.R.; Hernández-Mendo, A.; Fernández-García, J.C. Physical and physiological responses in paddle tennis competition. *Int. J. Perform. Anal. Sport* **2014**, *14*, 524–534. [CrossRef]
6. Duda, J.L. Motivation in Sport: The relevance of competence and achievement goals. In *Handbook of Competence and Motivation*; Elliot, A., Dweck, C., Eds.; Guildford Publications: New York, NY, USA, 2005; pp. 311–330.
7. Courel-Ibáñez, J.; Sánchez-Alcaraz, B.J.; Muñoz, D.; Grijota, F.J.; Chaparro, R.; Díaz, J. Gender reasons for practicing paddle tennis [Motivos de género para la práctica de pádel]. *Apunt. Educ. Fis. y Deportes.* **2018**, *133*, 116–125. [CrossRef]
8. Sánchez-Alcaraz, B.J.; Courel-Ibáñez, J.; Cañas, J. Temporal structure, court movements and game actions in padel: A systematic review [Estructura temporal, movimientos en pista y acciones de juego en pádel: Revisión sistemática]. *Retos, Nuevas Tend. Deport Educ. Física Recreación* **2018**, *33*, 221–225.
9. Courel-Ibáñez, J.; Sánchez-Alcaraz, B.J.; Cañas, J. Effectiveness at the net as a predictor of final match outcome in professional padel players. *Int. J. Perform. Anal. Sport* **2015**, *15*, 632–640. [CrossRef]
10. Torres-Luque, G.; Ramirez, A.; Cabello-Manrique, D.; Nikolaidis, P.T.; Alvero-Cruz, J.R. Match analysis of elite players during paddle tennis competition. *Int. J. Perform. Anal. Sport* **2015**, *15*, 1135–1144. [CrossRef]
11. Courel-Ibáñez, J.; Sánchez-Alcaraz, B.J.; Muñoz, D. Exploring game dynamics in padel: Implications for assessment and training. *J. Strength Cond. Res.* **2019**, *33*, 1971–1977. [CrossRef]
12. Courel-Ibáñez, J.; Sánchez-Alcaraz, B.J. The role of hand dominance in padel: Performance profiles of professional players. *Motricidade* **2018**, *14*, 33–41. [CrossRef]
13. García-Benítez, S.; Pérez-Bilbao, T.; Echegaray, M.; Felipe, J.L. The influence of gender on temporal structure and match activity patterns of professional padel tournaments. *Cult. Cienc. Deport* **2016**, *33*, 241–247. [CrossRef]
14. Sánchez-Alcaraz, B.J. Game actions and temporal structure diferences between male and female professional paddle players [Diferencias en las acciones de juego y la estructura temporal entre el pádel masculino y femenino profesional]. *Acción Mot.* **2014**, *12*, 17–22.
15. Lupo, C.; Condello, G.; Courel-Ibáñez, J.; Gallo, C.; Conte, D.; Tessitore, A. Effect of gender and match outcome on professional padel competition. *RICYDE Rev. Int. Cienc. Deport* **2018**, *51*, 29–41. [CrossRef]
16. Ramón-Llin, J.; Guzmán, J.F.; Llana, S.; Martínez-Gallego, R.; James, N.; Vučković, G. The effect of the return of serve on the server pair's movement parameters and rally outcome in padel using cluster analysis. *Front. Psychol.* **2019**, *10*, 1–8. [CrossRef] [PubMed]
17. Gillet, E.; Leroy, D.; Thouvarecq, R.; Stein, J.F. A notational analysis of elite tennis serve and serve-return strategies on slow surface. *J. Strength Cond. Res.* **2009**, *23*, 532–539. [CrossRef]
18. Reid, M.; McMurtrie, D.; Crespo, M. The relationship between match statistics and top 100 ranking in professional men's tennis. *Int. J. Perform. Anal. Sport* **2010**, *10*, 131–138. [CrossRef]
19. O'Donoghue, P. The most important points in grand slam singles tennis. *Res. Q. Exerc. Sport* **2001**, *72*, 125–131. [CrossRef]
20. Furlong, J. The service in lawn tennis: How important is it? In *Science and Racket Sports I*; Reilly, T., Hughes, M.D., Lees, A., Eds.; E &FN Spon: London, UK, 1995.
21. McGarry, T. Applied and theoretical perspectives of performance analysis in sport: Scientific issues and challenges. *Int. J. Perform. Anal. Sport* **2009**, *9*, 128–140. [CrossRef]

22. O'Donoghue, P.; Brown, E. The importance of service in Grand Slam singles tennis. *Int. J. Perform. Anal. Sport* **2008**, *8*, 70–78. [CrossRef]
23. Zhang, H.; Zhou, Z. An analytical model of the two basic situation strategies in table tennis. *Int. J. Perform. Anal. Sport* **2017**, *17*, 970–985. [CrossRef]
24. Vernon, G.; Farrow, D.; Reid, M. Returning serve in Tennis: A qualitative examination of the interaction of anticipatory information sources used by professional tennis players. *Front. Psychol.* **2018**, *9*, 1–11. [CrossRef] [PubMed]
25. Hizan, H.; Whipp, P.; Reid, M. Gender differences in the spatial distributions of the tennis serve. *Int. J. Sport Sci. Coach.* **2015**, *10*, 87–96. [CrossRef]
26. World Padel Tour Youtube Chanel. Available online: https://www.youtube.com/user/WorldPadelTourAJPP (accessed on 1 February 2020).
27. Gabin, B.; Camerino, O.; Anguera, M.T.; Castañer, M. Lince: Multiplatform sport analysis software. *Procedia-Soc. Behav. Sci.* **2012**, *46*, 4692–4694. [CrossRef]
28. Kinovea Sofware (V.08.26,). Available online: https://www.kinovea.org. (accessed on 1 February 2020).
29. Randolph, J.J. *Free-Marginal Multirater Kappa: An Alternative to Fleiss' Fixed-Marginal Multirater Kappa*; Joensuu University Learning and Instruction Symposium: Joensuu, Finlandia, 2005.
30. Robinson, G.; O'Donoghue, P.G. A weighted kappa statistic for reliability testing in performance analysis of sport. *Int. J. Perform. Anal. Sport* **2007**, *7*, 12–19. [CrossRef]
31. Altman, D.G. *Practical Statistics for Medical Research*; Chapman and Hall: London, UK, 1991.
32. Pallant, J. *SPSS Survival Manual: A Step by Step Guide to Data Analysis Using SPSS Program*; Alen & Unwin: Crows Nest, Australia, 2011.
33. Cohen, J. Statistical Power Analysis for the Behavioural Science (2nd Edition). In *Statistical Power Anaylsis for the Behavioral Sciences*; Lawrence Erlbaum: Hillsdale, NJ, USA, 1988.
34. Reid, M.; Morgan, S.; Whiteside, D. Matchplay characteristics of Grand Slam tennis: Implications for training and conditioning. *J. Sport Sci.* **2016**, *34*, 1791–1798. [CrossRef]
35. Sim, M.K.; Choi, D.G. The winning probability of a game and the importance of points in tennis matches. *Res. Q. Exerc. Sport* **2020**, *91*, 361–372. [CrossRef]
36. Sánchez-Muñoz, C.; Muros, J.J.; Cañas, J.; Courel-Ibáñez, J.; Sánchez-Alcaraz, B.J.; Zabala, M. Anthropometric and physical fitness profiles of world-class male padel players. *Int. J. Environ. Res. Public Health* **2020**, *17*, 508. [CrossRef]
37. Castillo-Rodríguez, A.; Hernández-Mendo, A.; Alvero-Cruz, J.R. Morphology of the elite paddle player—Comparison with other racket sports. *Int. J. Morphol.* **2014**, *32*, 177–182. [CrossRef]
38. Fitzpatrick, A.; Stone, J.A.; Choppin, S.; Kelley, J. A simple new method for identifying performance characteristics associated with success in elite tennis. *Int. J. Sport Sci. Coach.* **2019**, *14*, 43–50. [CrossRef]
39. Ramón-Llin, J.; Guzmán, J.F.; Belloch, S.L.; Vučković, G.; James, N. Comparison of distance covered in paddle in the serve team according to performance level. *J. Hum. Sport Exerc.* **2013**, *8*, 738–742. [CrossRef]
40. Escudero-Tena, A.; Fernández-Cortes, J.; García-Rubio, J.; Ibáñez, S.J. Use and efficacy of the lob to achieve the offensive position in women's professional padel. Analysis of the 2018 WPT finals. *Int. J. Environ. Res. Public Health* **2020**, *17*, 4061. [CrossRef]
41. Unierzyski, P.; Wieczorek, A. Comparison of tactical solutions and game patterns in the finals of two grand slam tournaments in tennis. In *Science and Racket Sports III*; Kahn, J., Lees, A., Maynard, I., Eds.; Routledge: London, UK, 2004; pp. 169–174.
42. Cui, Y.; Gómez, M.Á.; Gonçalves, B.; Sampaio, J. Performance profiles of professional female tennis players in grand slams. *PLoS ONE* **2018**, *13*, e0200591. [CrossRef]
43. O'Donoghue, P.; Ballantyne, A. The impact of speed of service in Grand Slam singles tennis. In *Science and Racket Sports III*; Lees, A., Kahn, J., Maynard, I., Eds.; Routledge: London, UK, 2008; pp. 179–184.
44. García-Benítez, S.; Courel-Ibáñez, J.; Pérez-Bilbao, T.; Felipe, J.L. Game responses during young padel match play: Age and sex comparisons. *J. Strength Cond. Res.* **2018**, *32*, 1144–1149. [CrossRef] [PubMed]
45. Muñoz, D.; Courel-Ibáñez, J.; Sánchez-Alcaraz, B.J.; Díaz, J.; Grijota, F.J.; Munoz, J. Analysis of the use and effectiveness of lobs to recover the net in the context of padel [Análisis del uso y eficacia del globo para recuperar la red en función del contexto de juego en pádel]. *Retos Nuevas Tend. Deport Educ. Física Recreación* **2017**, *31*, 19–22.

46. Priego, J.I.; Olaso, J.; Llana, S.; Pérez, P.; Gonález, J.C.; Sanchís, M. Padel: A quantitative study of the shots and movements in the high-performance. *J. Hum. Sport Exerc.* **2013**, *8*, 925–931. [CrossRef]
47. Martínez-Gallego, R.; Guzmán Luján, J.F.; James, N.; Pers, J.; Ramón-Llin, J.; Vučković, G. Movement characteristics of elite tennis players on hard courts with respect to the direction of ground strokes. *J. Sport Sci. Med.* **2013**, *12*, 275–281.
48. Gómez, M.Á.; Lago-Peñas, C.; Pollard, G. Situational variables. In *Routledge Handbook of Sports Performance Analysis*; McGarry, T., O'Donoghue, P., Sampaio, J., Eds.; Routledge: London, UK, 2003; pp. 259–269.

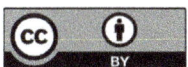

© 2020 by the authors. Licensee MDPI, Basel, Switzerland. This article is an open access article distributed under the terms and conditions of the Creative Commons Attribution (CC BY) license (http://creativecommons.org/licenses/by/4.0/).

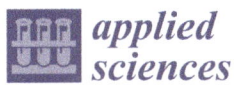 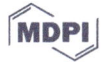

Article

Comparative Biomechanical Analysis of the Hurdle Clearance Technique of Colin Jackson and Dayron Robles: Key Studies

Milan Čoh [1], Nejc Bončina [1], Stanko Štuhec [1] and Krzysztof Mackala [2,*]

1. Faculty of Sport, University of Ljubljana, Gortanova ul. 22, 1000 Ljubljana, Slovenia; Milan.Coh@fsp.uni-lj.si (M.Č.); nejc.boncina@gmail.com (N.B.); Stanko.Stuhec@fsp.uni-lj.si (S.Š.)
2. Department of Track and Field, University School of Physical Education, Al. Ignacego Paderewskiego 35, 51-612 Wrocław, Poland
* Correspondence: krzysztof.mackala@awf.wroc.pl; Tel.: +48-71-347-3147

Received: 30 March 2020; Accepted: 6 May 2020; Published: 9 May 2020

Abstract: The purpose of the study was to compare the biomechanical parameters of the hurdle clearance technique of the fifth hurdle in the 110 m hurdle race of Colin Jackson of Great Britain (12.91 s world record was set in 1994) and Dayron Robles of Cuba (12.87 s world record was set in 2008), two world record holders. Despite the athletes having performed at different times, we used comparable biomechanical diagnostic technology for both hurdlers. Biomechanical measurements for both were performed by the Laboratory for Movement Control of the Institute of Sport, Faculty of Sport in Ljubljana. A three-dimensional video analysis of the fifth hurdle clearance technique was used. High standards of biomechanical measurements were taken into account, thus ensuring the high objectivity of the obtained results. The following program was used: the ARIEL kinematic program (Ariel Dynamics Inc., Trabuco Canyon, CA, USA). The results of the comparative analysis found minimal differences between the two athletes, which was expected given their excellence. Dayron Robles's hurdle clearance was more effective, as it was characterized by a smaller loss of horizontal center of mass (COM) velocity. Robles's hurdle clearance took 0.50 s: 0.10 s for the take-off, 0.33 s for the flight phase, and 0.07 s for the landing phase. Colin Jackson completed the hurdle clearance slightly slower, as it took him 0.54 s. Jackson's take-off phase also lasted 0.10 s, his flight phase 0.36 s, and his landing 0.08 s. The two athletes are quite different in their morphological constitution. Dayron Robles is 10 cm taller than Colin Jackson, resulting in a lower flight parabola of CM during hurdle clearance of the Cuban athlete. Dayron Robles has a more effective hurdle clearance technique compared to Jackson's achievement. It can be considered that their individual techniques of overcoming the hurdle, reached their individual highest efficiency at this time.

Keywords: hurdling; biomechanics; hurdle clearance; technique analysis

1. Introduction

The high hurdle race is one of the most technically demanding athletic events, and from a biomechanical standpoint, the hurdle race is a combination of a cyclic sprint and an acyclic clearance of ten 1.067 m high hurdles. According to Bruggemman [1], the high hurdle event can be divided into the following phases: approach run to the first hurdle, clearance of the hurdles and the rhythm between hurdles, and run-out from the last hurdle to the finishing line. Therefore, a proper hurdling technique is a complicated combination of various running and jumping kinematics [2]. Additionally the hurdler must show a high level of sprinting skill, excellent flexibility in the hip joint, coordination, balance, dynamic perception, elastic power, and a high level of technical knowledge [3,4]. Thus, athletes, coaches, and professionals are constantly looking for opportunities to improve the high hurdle performance, focusing on hurdling technique with particular emphasis on the kinematics and kinetics analysis. During the last three decades, there has been a considerable amount of references concerning the analysis of hurdling technique at different levels in order to improve performance [5–11].

One of the key elements that defines a competitive result in high hurdles is the hurdle clearance technique [11–17]. When clearing a hurdle, the loss of horizontal velocity should be minimized. This was confirmed by Amara et al. [17] and Coh et al. [18], who based on their hurdle clearance analyses, claimed that horizontal velocity is one of the most crucial factors, therefore losing it should be minimized; if not, the running time will be reduced. Additionally for the fastest possible and biomechanically effective clearance of the hurdle, the athlete's take-off distance and landing distance are essential. Furthermore, Salo and Grimshaw [19] determined the optimal ratio for an efficient hurdle clearance. The ratio applies to the dependency between the take-off of the trial leg and the landing of the lead leg and should be 60:40 in flight distance. The hurdle clearance depends on other factors, especially those that define the movement trajectory of the center of mass (COM). The correct positioning of these two points determines the optimal flight trajectory of the COM, which is reflected in the flight time, which should be as short as possible [5,9,12,20]. According to Coh et al. [18] and Bubaj et al. [21] these two situations is a prerequisite for an optimal flight path of the center of mass (COM). This optimal path results in a shorter flight time. In addition to the correct position, the kinematic–dynamic structure of the take-off and landing are important, as they directly affect the speed of hurdle clearance [7,10,16,22,23]. To sum up the above considerations after Lopez et al. [24], Li et al. [22], Park et al. [25], and Amara et al. [17], the main criteria of an optimal hurdle clearance technique include horizontal velocity, height of COM at take-off, velocity of the trail-leg, flight time, height of COM at landing, and contact time.

Over the years, with the development of technology, the ability to record and film competitions in track and field has increased significantly. There has been a considerable amount of biomechanical data concerning the kinematic analysis of hurdle races at a high level of performance such as the Olympic Games, World Championships, or international meetings [24–29]. These analyses of the specialized video recording are related to the technical aspects of single event observations where competition stress and adrenaline are imposed on athletes. There has been a limited number of studies where obtaining the kinematic parameters of 110-m male hurdlers on the basis of video techniques analyses has been carried out on two consecutive races with the same competitors–hurdlers. Therefore, researchers use various video recordings in their analyses, although sometimes there are methodological differences in data collection processes. A similar procedure was used for the analysis of hurdle races of Colin Jackson and Dayron Robles, who set high standards in this athletic discipline. They were both world record holders in their 110 m high hurdle race careers and won medals at every major international competition. Colin Jackson set the world record in the 60 m hurdle race in 1993 in Sindelfingen (Germany) with a time of 7.30 s. A year later, he improved the world record in the 110 m hurdles with a time of 12.91 s, still considered the seventh-best time in the history of this athletic discipline. Dayron Robles also improved the world record in the 110 m hurdle race (12.87 s) in 2008 in Ostrava (Czech Republic), which is considered to be the second-best result of all time in high hurdle races.

These studies were conducted to analyze comparable data held by the Laboratory for Movement Control of the Institute of Sport, Faculty of Sport in Ljubljana. Biomechanical measurements of both athletes were performed at different times, but under comparable conditions with similar measurement technologies. In both cases, a kinematic analysis of the fifth hurdle clearance technique was used. High standards of biomechanical measurements were taken into account, thus ensuring the high objectivity of the obtained results. We are aware that the study would have been even more valuable had we been able to analyze a greater number of obstacle clearances, but this was not possible due to organizational and technical constraints. The main aim of the study was to identify, analyze, and compare the essential kinematic parameters of the hurdle clearance technique at hurdle 5 of two athletes who have set the highest standards of biomechanical rationality of hurdle clearance in 110 m high hurdle races.

2. Materials and Methods

2.1. Participants

In this experiment, the participants were two world class hurdlers: Colin Jackson (body mass 75 kg, and height 182 cm) from Great Britain and Dayron Robles from Cuba (body mass 79 kg and height 191 cm). Both competitors specialized in 110 m hurdle, and were or are world record holders in 110 m hurdles. Some more personalized and anthropometric data of both athletes are shown in Table 1. The participants provided informed consent and were informed of the protocol and procedures for the study prior to the official video recording. The selection of athletes to conduct the experiment was specific and dependent on the possibility of making a video recording with its entire comprehensive procedure during an international meeting, and above all dependent on the level of participants in these competitions. Due to the fact that the experiment concerns the analysis of the hurdle technique for only two competitors, it can be qualified as a case study—the work reports scientifically sound experiments and provides a substantial amount of new information. The study was approved by the Human Ethics Committee of the University of Ljubljana.

Table 1. Basic anthropometric and biographical data of Colin Jackson (Great Britain) and Dayron Robles (Cuba).

Parameters	Colin Jackson	Dayron Robles
Date of birth	1967	1986
Body height (cm)	1.82	1.92
Body mass (kg)	75	79
Body Mass Index (BMI)	22.64	21.43
Best result (s)	12.91 *	12.87 **
Experimental result (s)	13.47	13.00
100 m best results (s)	10.29	10.71

BMI (Body Mass Index), * World Record in 1993, ** World record in 2008.

2.2. Experimental Design

The experiment design used was a comparison of dynamic and kinematic variables between two 110 m hurdles races at the segment between hurdles 4 and 5 and hurdle clearance of two world record holder. Both recordings of hurdles took place during regular international athletics competitions, although in two different places and two different years. These two conditions forced the experiment to match two different race recording methodologies. The hurdle races of Jackson and Robles were both recorded using two cameras each, although of different resolutions of 50 Hz frames per second and 100 Hz per second, respectively. From a methodological point of view, this may be a significant difference, but the conditions of variability were respected when processing data. In order to avoid the errors involved in analysis, real measurements were recalculated, taking into account the measurement error, which actually means that they corresponded (e.g., 50 Hz means 0.04 s between frames, so a hurdle clearance time of 0.5 s vs. 0.54 s represents a single frame). In both analyses the model of Dempster [30] was used for the calculation of the body's COM and the kinematic program ARIEL (Ariel Dynamics Inc., Trabuco Canyon, CA, USA) for the digitization was applied.

2.3. Procedure of Measurements—Colin Jackson

Colin Jackson's biomechanical analysis was carried out on 28 June 2002, at the International Meet in Velenje (EA Classic). His finish time was 13.47 s. The weather conditions were optimal; the outside temperature was 27 °C with a wind speed of + 0.2 m/s. Authorization to perform the experiment was approved by the Slovenian Track and Field Association. Biomechanical measurements were performed by a team of experts from the Laboratory for Movement Control of the Faculty of Sport in Ljubljana. Two synchronized cameras, namely Sony DSR-300-PK DVCAM Camcorders with Fujinon 17x lenses, were located at the main stands (the zone of hurdle 5) and operating at 50 Hz (shutter speed: 1/1000) were used to film the races. To record all kinematic parameters, the cameras were set at an angle of 120 to the direction of the moving hurdler in the segment between hurdles 4 and 5 (Figure 1). The zone of the 5th hurdle was calibrated with a calibration cube, one at the beginning of hurdle 4 and one at the end of hurdle 5. A 15-segment Dempster's model [30] and the ARIEL kinematic program (Ariel Dynamics Inc., Trabuco Canyon, CA, USA) were used to calculate the center of mass.

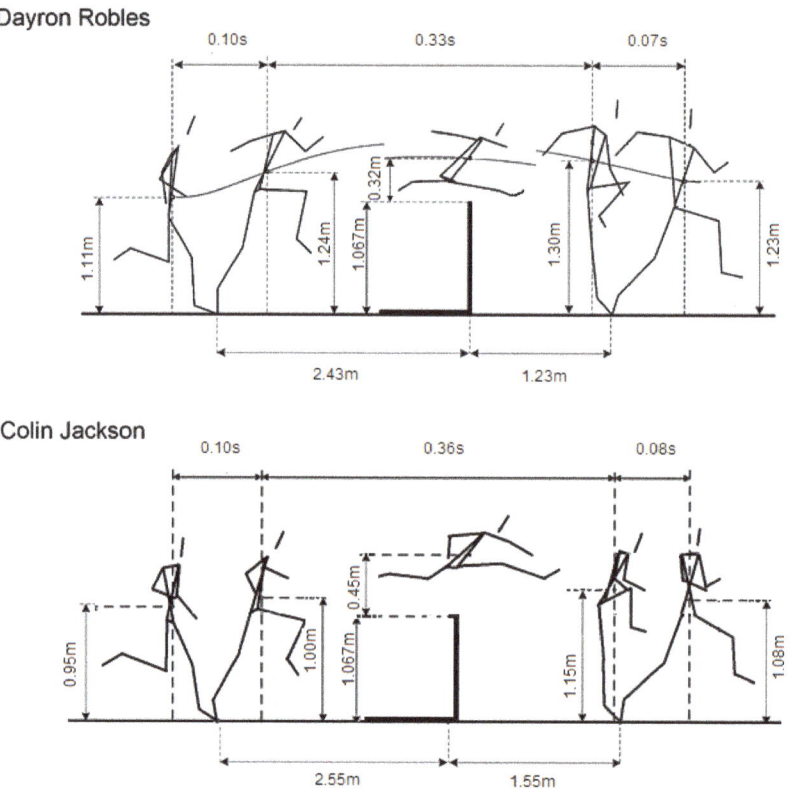

Figure 1. Comparison of biomechanical parameters of hurdle clearance.

2.4. Procedure of Measurements—Dayron Robles

Biomechanical analyses of Dayron Robles's 5th hurdle clearing technique was performed at the 2011 IAAF World Challenge—Zagreb International Race. Weather conditions were optimal; the outside temperature was 23 °C, and the wind speed was −0.2 m/s. Authorization to perform biomechanical measurements was obtained from the Technical Delegate of the European Athletics Federation and the Organizing Committee of the competition. The running track lane in the zone of the 5th hurdle was covered by two Casio high-frequency digital Casio EX-F1 512 × 384 (300 fps) sampled down to 100 fps cameras (Casio Computer Co., Ltd., Tokyo, Japan), which were interconnected and synchronized. The shutter speed of the Casio cameras was 1/300 s. The cameras were set perpendicular to the zone of the 5th hurdle (running hurdler) at an angle of 90°. The zone of the 5th hurdle was calibrated with a 2 m × 2 m × 2 m reference frame, within which eight points were measured. Data processing utilized an APAS computer system for 3D kinematic analysis (Ariel Performance Analysis System). Digitization of a 15-segment athlete body model was carried out, defined by 15 reference points [30] The point coordinates were smoothed with a 14 Hz digital filter. The center of mass (COM) was calculated from the digitized points based on Dempster's (1955) model of determination of COM via the ARIEL kinematic program (Ariel Dynamics Inc., Trabuco Canyon, CA, USA).

3. Results

The difference in body weight between competitors was only 4 kg. An even greater difference was in body height and was 10 cm in favor of Robles. Both measurements significantly differentiated hurdlers in terms of a measure of body fat (the ratio of the weight of the body in kilograms to the square of its height in meters), which was 1.21 in favor of Robles (Table 1). The time difference between those two world records is 0.04s. Jackson set his world record at the age of 26 and Robles at the age of 22. The age difference between competitors on the day of the experiment was approximately 10 years in favor of Jackson, and Robles obtained a better result by 0.47s in the 110 m performance.

Based on biomechanical analyses (Table 2), the following results were obtained: Robles's total stride length was 3.66 m, and the stride was completed in 0.33 s, while Jackson's stride length was 3.67 m, and it was slightly slower, lasting 0.36 s. During hurdle clearance, Dayron Robles reached the highest COM point at 1.38 m (0.32 m above the height of the hurdle), which corresponded to 72.2% of his body height. Colin Jackson reached the COM trajectory point at 1.52 m (0.45 m above the hurdle height), which was 83.4% of his height. The difference between the lowest COM point in the eccentric phase of the take-off was 1.11 m for Robles and 0.95 m for Jackson; and the highest COM point during the flight phase was 1.387 m for Robles and 1.517 m for Jackson. The height of the COM at the end of the concentric phase of take-off for Robles was 1.24 m and 1.08 m for Jackson.

Table 2. Biomechanical variables of the clearance of the fifth hurdle.

Variables	Colin Jackson	Dayron Robles	Difference	Δ (%)
Horizontal velocity 4 H–5 H (m/s)	9.14	9.18	0.04	0.43
Take-off (braking phase)				
Horizontal velocity of COM (m/s)	8.81	8.70	0.11	1.25
Vertical velocity of COM m/s	−0.43	−0.70	0.37	62.79
Velocity resultant of COM (m/s)	8.82	8.73	0.09	1.03
Height of COM (m)	0.95	1.11	0.16	16.84
Foot to hurdle distance (m)	2.09	2.43	0.34	16.26
Take-off (propulsion phase)				
Horizontal velocity of COM (m/s)	9.11	9.00	0.11	1.21
Vertical velocity of COM (m/s)	2.35	1.80	0.55	23.41
Velocity resultant of COM (m/s)	9.41	9.18	0.23	2.45
Height of COM (m)	1.08	1.24	0.16	14.81
Push-off angle (°)	72.9	78.7	5.80	7.95
Contact time (s)	0.10	0.10	0.0	0.0
Flight				
Flight time (s)	0.36	0.33	0.03	8.34
Height of COM above the hurdle (m)	0.45	0.32	0.13	28.89
Maximal height COM (m)	1.44	1.52	0.08	5.55
Landing (braking phase)				
Horizontal velocity of COM m/s	8.77	8.80	0.03	0.34
Vertical velocity of COM (m/s)	−1.02	−1.00	−0.02	1.97
Velocity resultant of COM (m/s)	8.84	8.86	0.02	0.22
Height of COM (m)	1.15	1.30	0.15	13.04
Foot to hurdle distance (m)	1.58	1.23	0.35	22.16
Landing (propulsion phase)				
Horizontal velocity of COM (m/s)	8.41	9.35	1.06	11.17
Vertical velocity of COM (m/s)	−1.32	−1.00	−0.32	24.25
Velocity resultant of COM (m/s)	8.53	9.40	1.13	10.19
Height of COM (m)	1.06	1.23	0.17	16.03
Contact time (s)	0.08	0.07	0.01	12.50

4. Discussion

The entire process of hurdle clearance took 0.50 s for Robles; it took 0.10 s for take-off, 0.33 s for the flight phase, and 0.07 s for the landing phase. Meanwhile, Colin Jackson completed the hurdle clearance a little more slowly, as it took him 0.54 s. Jackson also spent 0.10 s for take-off, 0.36 s for the flight phase, and 0.08 s for the landing phase. For comparison, the measurement of Amara [23]—a medium level athlete (13.90 s at 110 m hurdles) showed differences in the abovementioned parameters of 0.60 s, 0.36 s, 0.21 s, and 0.12 s (respectively for each variable). Jackson's slower clearance of the hurdle is associated with a higher rise in his COM above the hurdle and a longer landing distance over the hurdle, extending both the flight phase and the shock absorption phase. A slower hurdler [30] had a similar problem; his excessive height of the vertical COM displacement together with a high take-off angle had a negative impact on the time to clear the hurdle. The difference in the flight parabola between the two athletes can be attributed mainly to the difference in their height and the difference in their functional abilities. Based on the kinematic parameters of the parabola, we can, therefore, conclude that Dayron Robles has a more rational hurdle clearance technique (Figure 1).

The take-off distance for Robles was 2.43 m, which was 66.4% of the total clearance length over the hurdle. For Jackson, the take-off distance was 2.09 m, which was 57.0% of the total length of clearance. Jackson's landing distance was 1.58 m (43.0% of his total stride length), while Robles's was 1.23 m (33.6% of his total stride length). It can be compared with some other studies [10,30], which indicate that the optimal ratio between take-off spot and landing place should be 40–60%, which is comparable with Amara's [17] findings (i.e., 58:42). This ratio was confirmed by previous researchers [8,18,24,28,31,32], which indicated that take-off distance should range from 2.04 cm to 2.31 cm. In turn, the landing distance was shorter. We can identify two different hurdle clearance strategies. Robles has a faster hurdle clearance; his take-off is elongated, and his landing is closer to the hurdle. The duration of Robles's flight phase is 0.33 s, and that of Jackson is 0.36 s. A technical model of When [33] indicated that the optimal over the hurdle time should range between 0.30 and 0.33 s for a world class hurdler. This confirms the importance of the take-off (the angle between the top of the foot and the hip) and landing distances in high hurdler races, as was previously mentioned by Coh and Iskra [31] and Lopez at el. [24].

In the concentric phase, Robles had a take-off angle of 78.7 °, and Jackson's was 72.9 °. The COM velocity resultant during the braking phase of the take-off was 8.73 m/s for Robles and 8.82 m/s for Jackson. This velocity resultant of COM is defined as the vector sum of the vertical COM velocity (0.70 m/s for Robles, –0.43 m/s for Jackson) and horizontal COM velocity (8.70 m/s for Robles and 8.81 m/s for Jackson). It changes until the last contact of the take-off when it measured 9.18 m/s for Robles and 9.41 m/s for Jackson. Robles's vertical COM velocity at that time was 1.80 m/s, and Jackson's was 2.35 m/s; their horizontal COM velocities were 9.00 m/s and 9.11 m/s, respectively. The COM horizontal velocity during take-off thus increased by 0.30 m/s for both Robles and Jackson. The relative increase in the horizontal velocity of COM for Robles was 3.30% and 3.29% for Jackson (Figure 2). For both athletes, the duration of their take-off was the same. Robles's COM height during take-off increased by 0.13 m, equal to Jackson's (Figure 1). It is comparable with data of Amara [17], Li and Fu [34], and Lopez at el. [24], who claimed that during take-off (propulsion phase), the average height of the COM should be around 1.12 m.

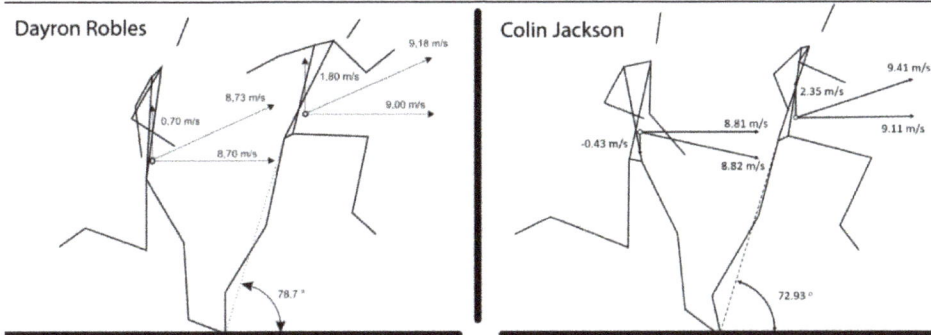

Figure 2. Comparison of the biomechanical parameters of take-off before the hurdle.

The transition between hurdle clearance and the sprint between hurdles is dependent on the landing phase. For Robles, the horizontal velocity at landing was 8.80 m/s, which means that the horizontal velocity decreased by 0.20 m/s (2.2%). For Jackson, the horizontal velocity decreased by 0.34 m/s (3.7%). During the landing phase, Robles's height of COM decreased by 0.07 m (5.4%) and 0.09 m (7.8%) for Jackson. The short duration of the landing phase (0.07 s for Robles and 0.08 s for Jackson) indicated a high level of reactive power [35] for both athletes (Figure 3), and an efficient transition to sprinting between hurdles [4,36].

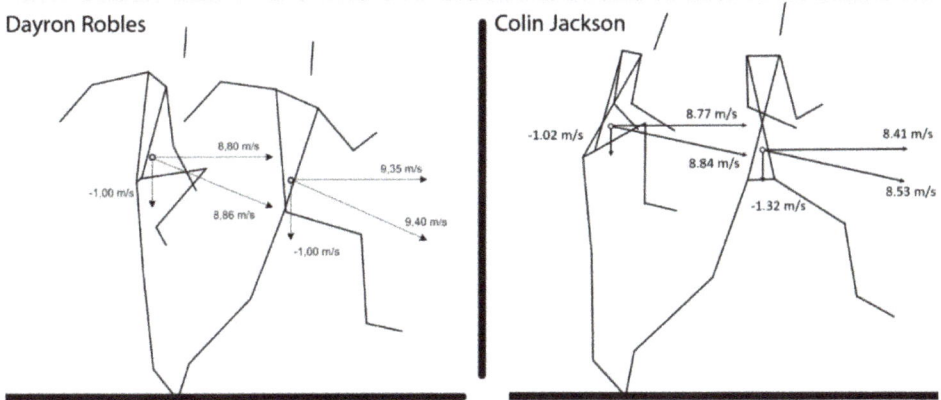

Figure 3. Comparison of the biomechanical parameters of the landing.

For Jackson, the reduction in the horizontal velocity of COM was greater than that of Robles, and the height of his center of mass (COM) was lower at landing, so it can be concluded that Robles has a slightly more biomechanically rational hurdle clearance technique. In addition, our results do not contradict the research of Amara [23], who claimed that the vertical component of COM velocity and the lead-leg/trail-leg at take-off and at flight phase constituted key factors of optimum hurdle clearance. According to Amara [17,23] and Shibayama et al. [37], in addition to the take-off angle, the knee and the hip angles are very important in high hurdles clearance, as also found in previous studies done by Coh [18,38], Xi et al. [22], Bubaj [21] and Sidhu [39]. Liu [40] just confirmed this statement and additionally indicated that the flight-phase duration is also defined by the takeoff angle, which should be lower.

5. Conclusions

In the present study, we analyzed the rationality of the 110 m hurdle clearance technique of Colin Jackson and Dayron Robles, using diagnostic technology for kinematic analysis. Both athletes have roughly the same personal record in the 110 m hurdle races (Jackson 12.91 s, Robles 12.87 s). The two hurdlers are quite different in morphological constitution, with Dayron Robles being 10 cm taller than Colin Jackson. Based on the results obtained, it can be concluded that Dayron Robles has a more effective hurdle clearance technique. It is characterized by a smaller loss of horizontal velocity of COM during clearance, a better COM flight parabola over the hurdle, and a smaller difference between the hurdle height and the height of the highest COM point, compared to Jackson's achievement. It proves that their hurdle clearance efficiencies differ but depend on the same kinematic parameters. Therefore, it can be considered that their individual technique of overcoming the hurdle their reached individual highest efficiency at this time. On this basis, we can also assume that the difference in overcoming one hurdle (the fifth) accumulated in the remaining hurdles until the end of the race, which reflects the final results of the races. Here Robles obtained a better running time in the 110 m hurdles.

6. Practical Application

From a practical point of view, based on some of the spatiotemporal parameters presented in the present analysis, there are some high hurdle common performance indicators. In order to optimize high hurdle performance with special regard to clearance hurdle movement performance, lower vertical displacement of COM, combined with right angle of take-off and short contact-time at the take-off and landing phases must be considered. These elements help improve a quick turn between horizontal and vertical velocity of forward propulsion and fast return of the trail leg at landing. To improve these indicators, appropriate training needs to be applied. It should consider high technical proficiency training and first of all activities which improve a higher rate of force development.

Author Contributions: Conceptualization, M.Č. and K.M.; Data curation, S.Š. and K.M.; Formal analysis, M.Č., N.B., S.Š. and K.M.; Investigation, M.Č., N.B. and S.Š.; Methodology, M.Č., N.B., S.Š. and K.M.; Resources, M.Č.; Software, N.B. and S.Š.; Supervision, M.Č. and K.M.; Validation, M.Č. and N.B.; Writing–original draft, M.Č., N.B. and K.M.; Writing–review & editing, M.Č. and K.M. All authors have read and agreed to the published version of the manuscript.

Funding: This research received no external funding.

Acknowledgments: The authors would like to acknowledge the involvement of the participants for their contribution to this study.

Conflicts of Interest: The authors have no conflict of interest to declare. The results do not constitute an endorsement of any product or device. The authors would like to thank the sprinters who participated in this study.

References

1. Brüggemann, G.P.; Koszewski, D.; Müller, H. *Biomechanical Research Project*; Athens 1997, Final report; Meyer & Meyer Sport: Oxford, UK, 1999; pp. 12–41.
2. Bollschweiler, L. A biomechanical Analysis of Male and Female Intermediate Hurdles and Steeplechasers. Master's Thesis, Brigham Young University, Brigham, MA, USA, 2008.
3. Salo, A.I.; Scarborough, S. Athletics: Changes in technique within a sprint hurdle run. *Sport Biomech.* **2006**, *5*, 155–166. [CrossRef]
4. Iskra, J. The most effective technical training for the 110 metres hurdles. *New Stud. Athl.* **1995**, *10*, 51–55.
5. Schluter, W. Kinematic features of the 110-meter hurdle technique (Kinematische Merkmale der 110-m Hurdentechnik). *Leistungssport* **1981**, *2*, 118–127.
6. Mero, A.; Luhtanen, P. Biomechanical examination of the hurdle race during the World Championships in Helsinki. (Biomechanische Untersuchung des Hurdenlaufs während der Weltmeisterschaften in Helsinki. *Leistungssport* **1986**, *1*, 42–43. (In German)
7. La Fortune, M.A. Biomechanical analysis of 110 m hurdles. *Track Field News* **1988**, *105*, 3355–3365.

8. McDonald, C.; Dapena, J. Linear kinematics of the men's and woman's hurdles races. *Med Sci. Sports Exerc.* **1991**, *23*, 1382–1402. [CrossRef]
9. Dapena, J. Hurdle clearance technique. *Track Field Quart Rev.* **1991**, *116*, 710–712.
10. Mclean, B. The biomechanics of hurdling: Force plate analysis to assess hurdling technique. *New Stud. Athl.* **1994**, *4*, 55–58.
11. Kampmiller, T.; Slamka, M.; Vanderka, M. Comparative biomechanical analysis of 110 m hurdles of Igor Kovač and Peter Nedelicky. *Kinesiol. Slov.* **1991**, *1–2*, 26–30.
12. Lee, J. The Kinematic analysis of the hurdling of men's 110 m hurdle. *Korean J. Sport Biomech.* **2004**, *14*, 83–98. [CrossRef]
13. Iskra, J.; Coh, M. A review of biomechanical studies in hurdle races. *Kinesiol. Slov.* **2006**, *1*, 84–102.
14. Sidhu, A.; Singh, M. Kinematical analysis of hurdle clearance technique in 110 m hurdle race. *Int. J. Behav. Soc. Mov. Sci.* **2015**, *4*, 28–35.
15. Amritpals, S.; Shamsher, S. Relationship among the Technique of Hurdle Clearance Over the DifferentHurdles in 110 m Race. *Int. J. Sci. Res.* **2015**, *4*, 1591–1594.
16. Chin-Shan, H.; Chi-Yao, C.; Kuo-Chuan, L. The wearable devices application for evaluation of 110 meter high hurdle race. *J. Hum. Sport Exerc.* **2020**, *151*, 1–9.
17. Amara, S.; Mkaouer, B.; Chaabene, H.; Negra, Y.; Hammoudi-Riahi, S.; Ben- Salah, F. Key kinetic and kinematic factors of 110-m hurdles performance. *J. Phys. Educ. Sport.* **2019**, *19*, 658–668.
18. Coh, M.; Zvan, M.; Bubanj, S. *XXIIth International Symposium on Biomechanics in Sports*; Lamontagne, M., Gordon, D., Robertson, E., Sveistrup, H., Eds.; ISBS: Ottawa, ON, Canada, 2004; pp. 311–314.
19. Salo, A.; Grimshaw, P. 3–D biomechanical analysis of sprint hurdles at different competitive level. *Med. Sci. Sports Exerc.* **1997**, *29*, 231–237. [CrossRef]
20. Lee, J.; Park, Y.; Ryu, J.; Kim, J. The kinematic analysis of the third hurdling motion of the 110 m hurdles elite. *Korean J. Sport Biomech.* **2008**, *18*, 31–39.
21. Bubaj, R.; Stankovic, R.; Rakovic, A.; Bubanj, S.; Petrovic, P.; Mladenovic, D. Comparative biomechanical analysis of hurdle clearance techniques on 110 m running with hurdles of elite and non-elite athletes. *Serb. J. Sports Sci.* **2008**, *2*, 37–44.
22. Li, X.; Zhou, J.; Li, N.; Wang, J. Comparative biomechanics analysis of hurdle clearance techniques. *Port. J. Sport Sci.* **2011**, *11*, 307–309.
23. Amara, S.; Mkaouer, B.; Chaabene, H.; Negra, Y.; Hammoudi-Riahi, S.; Ben- Salah, F. Kinetic and kinematic analysis of hurdle clearance of an African and a world champion athlete: A comparative study. *S. Afr. J. Res. Sport PH* **2017**, *39*, 1–12.
24. López, J.; Padullés, J.M.; Olsson, H.J. Biomechanical analysis and functional assessment of D. Robles, world record holder and Olympic champion in 110 m hurdles. In Proceedings of the 29th International Conference on Biomechanics in Sports, Porto, Portugal, 20–23 June 2011; Vilas-Boas, J.P., Ed.; ISBS: Porto, Portugal, 2011; pp. 315–318.
25. Park, Y.J.; Ryu, J.K.; Ryu, J.S.; Kim, T.S.; Hwang, W.S.; Park, S.K.; Yoon, S. Kinematic analysis of hurdle clearance technique for 110-m men's hurdlers at IAAF World Championships, Daegue 2011. *Korean J. Sport Biomech.* **2011**, *21*, 529–540. [CrossRef]
26. Tsiokanos, A.; Tsaopoulos, D.E.; Tsarouchas, E.; Giavroglou, A. Race pattern of Men's 110-H hurdles: Time analysis of Olympic performance. *Biol. Exerc.* **2018**, *14*, 15–36. [CrossRef]
27. Graubner, R.; Nixdorf, E. Biomechanical analysis of the sprint and hurdles events at the 2009 IAAF World Championships in Athletics. *New Stud. Athl.* **2011**, *26*, 19–53.
28. Pollitt, L.; Walker, J.; Bissas, A.; Merlino, S. Biomechanical report for the IAAF world championships 2017: 110 m hurdles men's in 2017. In *IAAF World Championships Biomechanics Research Project*; International Association of Athletics Federations: London, UK, 2018.
29. Walker, J.; Pollitt, L.; Paradisis, G.P.; Bezodis, I.; Bissas, A.; Merlino, S. *Biomechanical Report for the IAAF World Indoor Championships 2018: 60 Metres Hurdles Men*; International Association of Athletics Federations: Birmingham, UK, 2019.
30. Dempster, W.T. *Space Requirements of the Seated Operator*; USAF, WADC, Tech. Rep.; Wright-Patterson Air Force Base: Greene County, OH, USA; pp. 55–159.
31. Coh, M.; Iskra, J. Biomechanical studies of 110 m hurdle clearance technique. *Sport Sci.* **2012**, *5*, 10–14.

32. González-Frutos, P.; Veiga, S.; Mallo, J.; Navarro, E. Spatiotemporal Comparisons between Elite and High-Level 60 m Hurdlers. *Front. Psychol.* **2019**, *10*, 1–9. [CrossRef]
33. Wen, C. *The High-Grade Tutorial of Track and Field*; People's Sports Press: Beijing, China, 2003; pp. 386–389.
34. Li, J.; Fu, D. The kinematic analysis on the transition technique between run and hurdle clearance of 110 m hurdles. In *XVIIIth International Symposium on Biomechanics in Sports*; Hong, Y., Johns, D.P., Sanders, R., Eds.; ISBS: Hong Kong, China, 2000; pp. 213–217.
35. Gollhofer, A.; Kyrolainen, H. Neuromuscular control of the human leg extensor muscles in jump exercises under various stretch-load conditions. *Int. J. Sports Med.* **1991**, *12*, 34–40. [CrossRef]
36. Lee, J. Kinematic analysis of hurdling of elite 110 m hurdlers. *Korean J. Sport Biomech.* **2009**, *19*, 761–770. [CrossRef]
37. Shibayama, K.; Fujii, N.; Shimizu, Y.; Ae, M. Analysis of angular momentum in hurdling by world and Japanese elite sprint hurdlers. In *XXXth International Symposium on Biomechanics in Sports*; Bradshaw, E.J., Burnett, A., Hume, P.A., Eds.; ISBS: Melbourne, Australia, 2012; pp. 54–57.
38. Coh, M. Biomechanical analysis of Colin Jackson's hurdle clearance technique. *New Stud. Athl.* **2003**, *18*, 37–45.
39. Sidhu, A.S. Three-dimensional kinematic analysis of hurdle clearance technique. *Global J. Res. Anal.* **2016**, *4*, 4–6.
40. Liiu, Y. A Kinesiological Analysis of the Hurdling Techniques of China's 110 m Hurdlers Liu Xiang and Shi Dongpeng. Master's Thesis, Shanxi University, Shanxi, China, 2008.

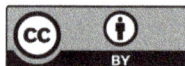

© 2020 by the authors. Licensee MDPI, Basel, Switzerland. This article is an open access article distributed under the terms and conditions of the Creative Commons Attribution (CC BY) license (http://creativecommons.org/licenses/by/4.0/).

Review

Biomechanics of Table Tennis: A Systematic Scoping Review of Playing Levels and Maneuvers

Duo Wai-Chi Wong [1], Winson Chiu-Chun Lee [2] and Wing-Kai Lam [3,4,5,*]

1. Department of Biomedical Engineering, Faculty of Engineering, The Hong Kong Polytechnic University, Hong Kong 999077, China; duo.wong@polyu.edu.hk
2. School of Mechanical, Materials, Mechatronic & Biomedical Engineering, University of Wollongong, Wollongong, NSW 2522, Australia; winson_lee@uow.edu.au
3. Guangdong Provincial Engineering Technology Research Center for Sports Assistive Devices, Guangzhou Sport University, Guangzhou 510000, China
4. Department of Kinesiology, Shenyang Sport University, Shenyang 110102, China
5. Li Ning Sports Science Research Center, Li Ning (China) Sports Goods Company, Beijing 101111, China
* Correspondence: gilbertlam@li-ning.com.cn; Tel.: +86-010-80801108

Received: 1 July 2020; Accepted: 24 July 2020; Published: 28 July 2020

Abstract: This present study aims to review the available evidence on the biomechanics of table-tennis strokes. Specifically, it summarized current trends, categorized research foci, and biomechanical outcomes regarding various movement maneuvers and playing levels. Databases included were Web of Science, Cochrane Library, Scopus, and PubMed. Twenty-nine articles were identified meeting the inclusion criteria. Most of these articles revealed how executing different maneuvers changed the parameters related to body postures and lines of movement, which included racket face angle, trunk rotation, knee, and elbow joints. It was found that there was a lack of studies that investigated backspin maneuvers, longline maneuvers, strikes against sidespin, and pen-hold players. Meanwhile, higher-level players were found to be able to better utilize the joint power of the shoulder and wrist joints through the full-body kinetic chain. They also increased plantar pressure excursion in the medial-lateral direction, but reduced in anterior-posterior direction to compromise between agility and dynamic stability. This review identified that most published articles investigating the biomechanics of table tennis reported findings comparing the differences among various playing levels and movement tasks (handwork or footwork), using ball/racket speed, joint kinematics/kinetics, electromyography, and plantar pressure distribution. Systematically summarizing these findings can help to improve training regimes in order to attain better table tennis performance.

Keywords: kinematics; kinetics; table tennis; racket

1. Introduction

Table tennis is a competitive sport which requires technical preparation, tactics, as well as mental and motor training [1]. Players with higher technical capability demonstrate good coordinated movement with controlled strike power, which yield adequate speed and spin on the ball in limited decision time [2,3]. To master the stroke, professional players have to rotate the trunk efficiently and place excellent foot drive in response to various ball conditions [2]. Whole-body coordination plays an important role in table tennis, as the biomechanics of lower extremities is closely related to the upper limb performance [4]. An incorrect technique would alter movement mechanics and thus joint loadings that are related to risk potential of injury. A retrospective study found that about one-fifth of table tennis players suffered from shoulder injuries [5]. Although numerous studies had investigated the biomechanics of table tennis maneuvers, their methods and protocols were generally inconsistent. Therefore, direct comparison across studies is not feasible. Furthermore, players of different skill levels may perform different table tennis maneuvers with unique techniques and patterns. To identify the common characteristics of higher-level players, an investigation has to be conducted properly mapping playing levels with different maneuvers. Such information can help in designing sport-specific training programs in table tennis.

Biomechanical reviews of various sports, such as football [6,7], tennis [8,9], and swimming [10–12] have identified strategies to improve sports performance and prevent injuries. While previous review articles summarized physiological demands of table tennis players [13,14], conducted match analysis [15–17], and reviewed contemporary robot table tennis [18,19], there have been no sufficient reviews on the biomechanics of table tennis. There was an article reviewing the science (including biomechanics) of major racket sports [20], however its focus was not on limb movements and the joint loading of different skill levels.

A systematic scoping review accounts for the published evidence over a broad topic by summarizing, mapping, and categorizing key concepts that underpin a particular research area using a systematic protocol [21]. Such a review looks into the literature which has demonstrated high complexity and heterogeneity. The objective of this systematic scoping review was to identify recent advances in testing protocols, variables, and biomechanical outcomes regarding table tennis maneuvers and performance. The scope of sports biomechanics in table tennis is board, which has not been comprehensively reviewed. The objectives of this review were guided by the following research questions:

1. How was the biomechanics of table tennis movements analyzed?
2. What were the biomechanical differences between higher- and lower-skilled players?
3. What were the biomechanical differences among various table tennis maneuvers?

The principle focus or concept of this review pertained the categorization of biomechanical variables while the primary context was to summarize the playing skill levels and maneuvers. This study can contribute to the field of sports science by identifying key ideas for performance improvement and identify research gaps in table tennis.

2. Materials and Methods

The searches of the scoping review were designed and conducted by the first author. The first author and the third author conducted the abstract and full-text screening, and data extraction. Any disagreements were resolved by seeking consensus with the second author, and all authors conducted a final check of the review. Electronic literature searches of electronic databases, including ISI Web of Science (excluding patents, from 1970), Scopus (from 1960), and PubMed (from 1975), were performed on 13 July 2020.

The searches were conducted using the keywords "table tennis" AND the terms "biomechan*" or "kinematics" or "kinetics" in the topic field, but NOT "catalyst", "catalysis", "enzyme", "biochemistry", "oxidase", "acid", "biochemistry", "colorimetric", or "nanocomposite" to rule out a similar topic in biochemistry. The titles, abstracts, and then full-text of the papers were screened based on the following inclusion criteria: (1) published in English; (2) research article in peer-reviewed journals; (3) biomechanical studies on table tennis with experiments involving adult players; (4) original research articles either case-control or longitudinal studies investigating playing levels or differences in maneuvers. Studies were excluded if the articles (1) did not consider any table tennis moves, (2) considered participants with disability, musculoskeletal problems, or rehabilitation, (3) only considered physical, psychological attributes or tactics, (4) were not original peer-reviewed articles, (5) studied table tennis robots, or (6) used simulations or theoretical models. The searching selection process is summarized in Figure 1. There was no disagreement among authors in the selection of studies eligible for the review. The following information was extracted: bibliographic details, sample size, characteristics of participants, inclusion and exclusion criteria of studies, and experimental settings.

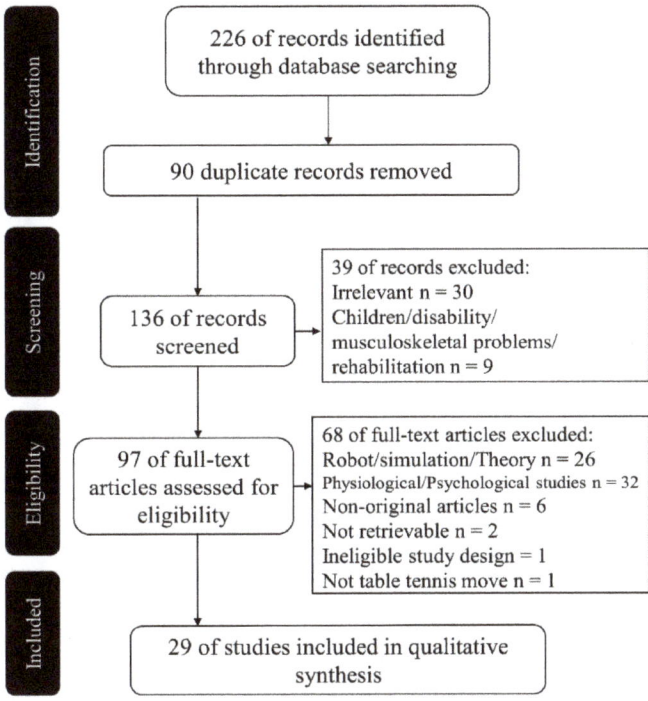

Figure 1. Flowchart of the systematic search and selection process.

3. Results

3.1. Search Results

An initial search identified 226 studies. After pooling the results and removing duplicates, 136 articles were screened for titles and abstracts. Finally, there were 29 studies successfully meeting the eligibility criteria (Figure 1). The studies were excluded because they were irrelevant (n = 30); they involved players with disabilities, musculoskeletal problems, or children (n = 9); they used robotic players, simulations or theoretical calculations (n = 26); they ocused on psychological issues, tactics, decision-making, coaching, cardiopulmonary or metabolic assessments (n = 32); they were survey, conference paper, review, and expert comment papers (n = 6). One study did not fall into the inclusion criteria of study design whilst another study did not examine any table tennis move. The full-text of one article could not be retrieved because it was too old and the journal was closed down [22]. One study was not retrievable with the given digital object identifier (DOI) [23].

The participant characteristics and study designs of the 29 included articles are summarized in Tables 1 and 2, respectively. In brief, participant characteristics, test protocols, and outcome variables of each article were summarized according to playing levels (n = 12), movement tasks (handwork, n = 6; footwork, n = 4; ball/serve against, n = 8) and other factors (n = 4) to identify performance determinants. Six included studies considered multiple factors on different servings with handwork [1,2] or playing level [24,25], racket mass with ball frequency [26], and footwork with footwear [27]. Furthermore, the categorization of dependent and independent variables are mapped in Figure 2. Key findings of the included studies related to playing levels and maneuvers are provided in Tables 3 and 4.

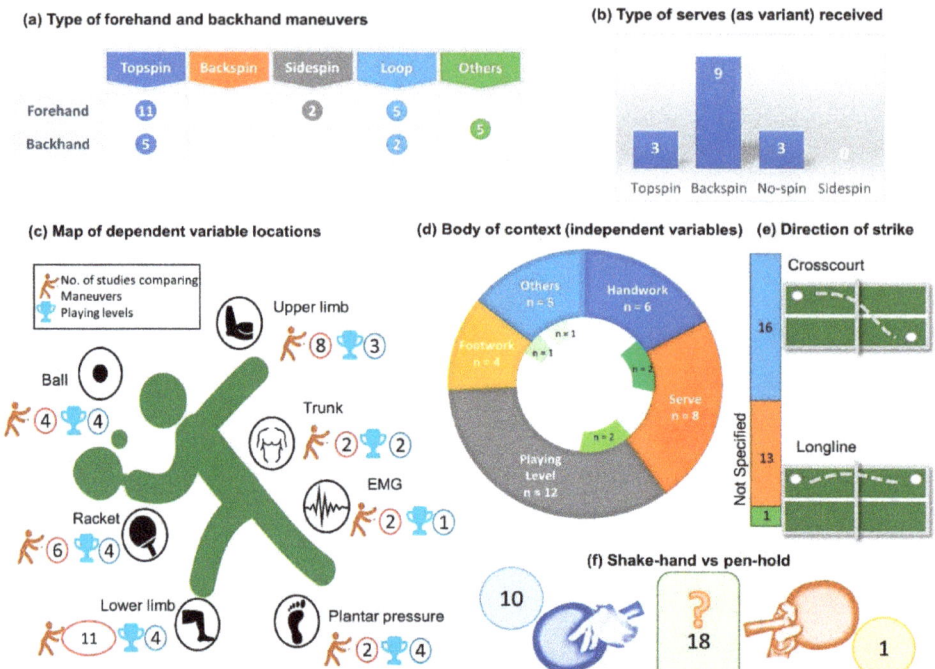

Figure 2. A scoping review map summarizing: (**a**) types of forehand and backhand maneuvers; (**b**) types of serves (as variant) to hit back; (**c**) map of dependent variables comparing the number of studies between topics on maneuvers and playing levels; (**d**) body of context (independent variables), the n-values in the interior circle denote number of studies with multiple independent variables between or within the factors stated on the exterior circle; (**e**) direction of strike; and (**f**) shake-hand vs pen-hold.

3.2. Classification of Movement Stage/Phase

While some included studies adopted the maximum or average values of performance outcome of strokes, the majority of the studies divided stroke into movement sub-phases or targeted to selected instants for subsequent analysis. Typically, the stroke was classified into backswing and forward-swing phases, targeted on the specific time points at the termination, backward-end and forward-end [1,3,28–34]. A few included studies [2,24,26,33,35,36] focused on the instant at ball impact which was used to determine the velocity of the racket and ball, while some other included studies investigated the biomechanics at pre-impact and post-impact stages [24,36–38], and over a longer period of time before and after the instant of ball contact [1,2,38,39]. Some included studies endeavored that pelvic and hip rotations were correlated with the racket velocity at impact and thus focused on the starting time of the pelvic forward rotation [36,37]. To sum up, the included studies often investigated the biomechanical parameters at the instant of ball or racket impact as well as the maximum or average value during the time before and after the ball impact.

3.3. Ball and Racket Performance

Eight included studies examined the effects of ball and racket mechanics as well as serve techniques on table-tennis performance [1,2,24–26,33,35,37], and some of these studies also compared the influences of different handworks [1,2] and playing levels [24,25]. Common variants included the type of ball spin [1,2,33,35,37,39] and the spin rate [24,25]. Moreover, seven included studies investigated ball, racket, and serve as outcome measures instead of variants [31,38,40–45].

Ball speed, accuracy, and repeatability were suggested to be the key indicators of playing level. Ball speed and accuracy were significantly correlated with player ranking in a competition [43]. Higher-level players produced higher ball speed and accuracy, which could be due to significantly shorter duration and variability of duration in the forward swing phase [31,32,38,41]. However, Iino and Kojima [24] found that racket speed at impact was not significantly different between playing levels (advanced vs. intermediate), although players with higher-level can rotate the trunk effectively to produce a greater racket acceleration at ball impact. Yet, Iino and Kojima [24] imposed a stringent significance level using a Bonferroni correction. Similarly, Belli et al. [40] found that while there was only a slight difference in ball speed comparing higher and lower-level players, players with higher-level demonstrated higher accuracy of ball target placement and made fewer errors in training and competition. On the other hand, inexperienced players showed higher inconsistency in ball speed and accuracy during within- and between-day trials [43]. Compared to the intermediate players, advanced players showed smaller variance of joint angle that affected the racket vertical angle during forehand topspin stroke [41]. Furthermore, a lower variability in the racket orientation and movement direction could be the reason for more successful returns and higher accuracy of the ball bounce location [38]. An uncontrolled manifold analysis suggested that higher-level players exploited higher degree of redundancy to maintain a similar racket angle at ball impact [41]. In brief, higher-level players exhibited higher accuracy and reproducibility on ball and racket mechanics but may not necessarily produce higher ball speed than lower-level players.

Compared to the topspin serves, returning backspin serves demonstrated significantly higher resultant and vertical racket velocities at ball impact [35,37], which could be contributed greatly by the wrist extension [35]. A possible explanation for this is that backspin serves tend to be treated back-low owing to the spin, resulting in a greater upward velocity of the shoulder joint center [37]. Moreover, peak shoulder torques in all directions, as well as elbow valgus torques, were significantly larger against backspin, in addition to the peaks of upper trunk right axial rotation and extension velocities [37]. Returning a spinning ball also alters the moving distance and velocity of the racket in the upward-downward direction, as compared to an ordinary stroke or a stroke with higher power. Hitting back a backspin serve could be more demanding than a topspin serve.

In addition, biomechanical differences between returning light and heavy backspin serves were assessed by two included articles from the same research group [24,25]. They produced different rates of ball backspin (11.4 vs. 36.8 revolutions/s) for light and heavy spin conditions. The heavy spin would direct the racket face to be more open [24]. Furthermore, their results found higher maximum loading at elbow and shoulder joints which might result in higher work done at the racket arm [25]. However, higher-level players showed a higher amount of energy transfer of the elbow for a light spin compared to intermediate players, but the opposite was true for the heavy spin [25], implying significant interaction effect between ball spin and playing level. The influence of racket mass and ball frequency were investigated by Iino and Kojima [26], who suggested that a heavier racket could impose higher demand on wrist extension torque, but did not influence trunk and racket arm kinematics and kinetics. A frequent ball serve could result in a lower racket speed at impact possibly since the pelvis and upper trunk rotations were not responsive enough. Table tennis players managed to identify the differences in ball spin, frequency, and mass, and accommodated by tilting the racket face angle and adjusting the power output of upper extremity.

Table 1. Participant characteristics of reviewed studies.

Author (Year)	Participants Information Sample Size; Age (years); Height (cm); Weight (kg)	Group/Level *	Inclusion Criteria (IC)/Exclusion Criteria (EC)
Bankosz and Winiarski (2017) [1]	n = 12F; 20.0 (5.5); 167.2 (6.9); 55.3 (6.2)	Players in high-level sports training and performance	IC: 1st 16 in their category of age; EC: NS
Bankosz and Winiarski (2018) [2]	n = 10F; 16.0 (2.5); 165 (6); 54.4 (3.2)	Junior elite players	IC: Top 16 junior players EC: NS
Bankosz and Winiarski (2018) [39]	Junior, n = 4F; 18.0 (0.5); 167.7 (5.7); 52.0 (3.6) Senior, n = 6F; 24.8 (3.2); 168.3 (6.3); 64.5 (2.4)	Junior and senior high sport skill players	IC: Top 16 TT players in Poland. EC: NS
Bankosz and Winiarski (2020) [33]	n = 7M; 23 (2); 178 (3); 76.5(8)	Top-ranked international players	IC: Top 10 TT players in Poland. EC: NS
Belli et al. (2019) [40]	Local, n = 9M; 24.3 (2.6); 174.6 (3.3); 68.1 (5.7); Regional, n = 10M; 23.9 (1.8); 176.9 (2.1); 79.8 (3.1)	Local group: 2.2 (0.3) yExp, 3.2 (0.5) hrWTR egional group: 7.5 (0.9) yExp, 10.0 (0.9) hrWT	IC: Local: low experience, w/o participation in tournaments; Regional: <5 years training, completed regional and national tournament
Fu et al. (2016) [3]	Intermediate, n = 13M; 21.2 (1.6); 175.2 (2.4); 69.1 (4.1); Superior, n = 13M; 20.1 (0.9); 174.8 (2.5); 66.9 (5.1)	National level Intermediate: (Div. II) 10.2 (1.9) yExp Superior: (Div. II) 13.4 (1.2) yExp	IC: NS EC: Previous lower extremity and foot disease or deformity, injury in the last 6 months
Ibrahim et al. (2020) [44]	n = 16M; 21.5 (1.27); 168 (56); 61.59 (8.60)	Collegiate players, min 3 yExp	IC: right-handed and shake-hand grip EC: NS
Iino et al. (2008) [35]	n = 11M; 21.1 (4.4); 171 (7); 66.3 (8.1)	International and collegiate players	IC: Shakehand grip attacking players EC: NS
Iino and Kojima (2009) [24]	Intermediate, n = 8M 20.6 (1.5); 170 (8); 59 (5.7) Advanced, n = 9M 20.6 (1.2); 171 (6); 66.2 (9.5)	Intermediate 7.4 (1.8) yExp Advanced 11.2 (0.8) yExp	IC: Intermediate: not qualified for national tournaments, Division III collegiate Advanced: qualified for national tournaments, Division I collegiate EC: NS
Iino and Kojima (2011) [25]	Intermediate, n = 8M 20.6 (1.5); 170 (8); 59 (5.7) Advanced, n = 9M 20.6 (1.2); 171 (6); 66.2 (9.5)	Intermediate 7.4 (1.8) yExp Advanced 11.2 (0.8) yExp	IC: Intermediate: Div. III collegiate Advanced: Div. I collegiate EC: NS
Iino and Kojima (2016) [26]	n = 8M 20.6 (1.3); 170 (4); 63.1 (5.7)	Advanced players 13.0 (1.7) yExp	IC: Div. I collegiate team in Kanto Collegiate TT League in Japan; Offensive players; use shake hands grip rackets; EC: NS
Iino and Kojima (2016) [37]	n = 10M 20.6 (1.3); 171 (5); 61.6 (5.7)	Advanced skill players 12.8 (2.4) yExp	IC: Qualified for national level TT competitions in high school or college; EC: NS
Iino et al. (2017) [41]	Intermediate, n = 8M 20.9 (0.9); 173 (7); 62.5 (6.3); Advanced, n = 7M 20.4 (1.3); 172 (7); 65.3 (5.4)	Intermediate (Div. III) 7.8 (1.0) yExp Advanced (Div. I) 11.3 (2.2) yExp	IC: Intermediate: not qualified for national tournaments Advanced: qualified for national tournaments EC: NS
Iino (2018) [36]	n = 18M; 20.7 (1.1); 171 (5); 64.0 (7.6)	Advanced players 12.2 (2.2) yExp	IC: Div. I or II collegiate players EC: NS
Lam et al. (2019) [4]	n = 15M; 23.6 (2.2); 180 (4); 72.3 (6.2)	Div. I players	IC: NS; EC: lower extremity injury in the last 6 months
LeMansec et al. (2016) [43]	Inexperience, n = 18M 19.5 (0.9); 176.9 (5.9); 69 (6.4); Advanced, n = 14M; 30.7 (11.3); 178.3 (6.2); 74 (12.3); Expert, n = 20M; 28.4 (6.7); 178.9 (6.2); 74.5 (9.7)	Inexperience Advanced: 13.4 (5.6) yExp 4.1 (2.3) hrWT Expert: 19.8 (6.8) yExp 10.4 (7.9) hrWT	IC: Inexperience: students w/o experience in TT; not ranked in the Federation of TT; Advanced: participated in regional championship; Expert: participated in National or international competition; EC: NS
LeMansec et al. (2018) [46]	n = 14M; 27.1 (4.9); 177.5 (5.3); 73.5 (8.4)	National level players 4.7 (1.9) hrWT	IC: Official competition players in the national championship EC: Lower limb pain in last 2 years

Table 1. Cont.

Author (Year)	Participants Information Sample Size; Age (years); Height (cm); Weight (kg)	Group/Level *	Inclusion Criteria (IC)/Exclusion Criteria (EC)
Malagoli Lanzoni et al. (2018) [45]	n = 7M; 22.2 (3.2); 177.4 (4.2); 72.9 (11)	Competitive player: 10.2 (2.5) yExp	IC: 1st and 2nd national league players and ranked among 1st 200; EC: Consume caffeine last 4 h
Meghdadi et al. (2019) [47]	Healthy, n = 30M; 24 (2.59); 176 (7.81); 74 (5.82); Syndromic, n = 30M; 25 (2.29); 174 (7.06); 75 (5.50)	National-level players: Healthy: 5 (2.11) yExp; Syndromic: 6 (1.97) yExp	IC: top 100 list of Federation and active in League; right-handed. Syndromic: impingement on dominant side; EC: History of shoulder dislocation, surgery, occult/overt instability, symptoms on cervical spine, rotator cuff tendinitis, documented injuries/pathology to shoulder
Qian et al. (2016) [28]	Intermediate, n = 13M 21.2(1.6); 175.2(2.4); 69.1 (4.1); Superior, n = 13M 20.1 (0.9); 174.8 (2.5); 66.9 (5.1)	Intermediate (Div. III) 10.2 (1.9) yExp Superior (Div. I) 13.4 (1.2) yExp	IC: NS EC: Lower extremity and foot disease or deformity, injury for the last 6 months
Shao et al. (2020) [34]	Amateur, n = 11M; 20.8 (0.6); 174.2 (1.4); 62.4 (3.5) Prof., n = 11M; 21.6 (0.4); 173.5 (1.7); 63.7 (4.2)	Amateur: university students: 0.4 (0.2) yExp; Prof.: Div. I players: 14.2 (1.4)	IC: right-handed, Prof.: Div. I players; EC: any previous lower limb injuries and surgery or foot disease for at least 6 months
Sheppard and Li (2007) [38]	Novice, n = 12(NS); 22.2 (5.6); NS; NS; Expert, n = 12(NS); 21.7 (2.9); NS; NS	Novice: university population; Expert: table tennis club and sports center players	IC: right-handed, normal or corrected vision; Expert: at least years of experience and play at least 2 h per week; EC: no physical impairment
Wang et al. (2018) [29]	Amateur, n = 10M Elite, n = 10M NS; NS; NS	NS	IC: NS; EC: lower extremity, foot diseases/deformity; Injury in the past 6 months
Yan et al. (2017) [27]	n = 8M; 21.9 (1.1); 173.1 (4.2); 62.8 (2.7)	Collegiate players	IC: right-handed, second grade EC: no history of serious injury to lower limb; did not engage in vigorous exercise 24 h before experiment
Yu et al. (2018) [30]	n = 10F 21.6 (0.3); 164 (3); 54.2 (2.8)	Advanced 15.8 (1.7) yExp	IC: Div. I players EC: NS
Yu et al. (2019) [48]	n = 12M; 20.64 (1.42); 174 (3); 67.73 (3.31)	Elite national level players	EC: No previous lower limb injuries and surgeries or foot diseases
Yu et al. (2019) [32]	Beginners, n = 9M; 22.7 (1.62); 175 (4.6); 73.7 (3.1); Prof., n = 9M; 25.5 (1.24); 175 (5.3); 74.6 (2.5)	University TT team Beginners: 0.45 (0.42) yExp; Prof.: 14.8 (1.57) yExp	EC: free from any previous lower limb injuries, surgeries or foot diseases in the past 6 months.
Zhang et al. (2016) [31]	Novice, n = 10M 23.1 (4.1); NS; NSExpert, n = 10M 24.1 (1.6); NS; NS	Novice: university population Expert: prof. from TT teams and clubs	IC: NS EC: Novice: w/o formal training
Zhou (2014) [42]	n = 18M 22.3 (1.8); 172.7 (5.1); 64.6 (5.8)	Physical education major	IC: Played table tennis for more than 5 years EC: NS

* The names of the level or group are adopted from the included studies. Numbers in brackets denote standard deviation. M: male; F: female; Number in bracket denotes standard deviation. NS: not specified; yExp: year of experience; Div: division; h: hours; hrWT: hours per week training; TT: table tennis; Prof.: professionals; w/: with; w/o: without.

3.4. Upper Limb Biomechanics

There were eight included studies targeting handwork as the variant, while two of them co-variated with different serves (Table 2). Higher racket speed and faster ball rotation were the key attributes of attacking shots and this could be determined by the kinematics/kinetics of upper extremity as well as the efficiency of energy transfer through the upper arm [25,49]. Higher-level players showed significantly larger maximum shoulder internal rotation, elbow varus, and wrist radial deviation torques, in addition to the maximum joint torque power at shoulder joint in both internal and external rotation directions [25]. Higher angular velocity of the wrist joint contributed to a higher ball and racket speed during drop shot services, while that also produced higher racket speed during long shot services [44].

Moreover, higher-level players rotated the lower trunk efficiently contributing to higher racket speed at ball impact [24]. Meanwhile, the racket horizontal velocity at ball impact was related to the hip axial rotation torque at the playing side (i.e., racket side), while the racket vertical velocity was correlated with backward tilt torques and upward hip joint forces [36]. In contrast, players with shoulder impingement syndrome had sub-optimal coordination and movement patterns of the shoulder girdle [47]. These players significantly reduced muscle activity of the serratus anterior and supraspinatus, which was compensated by increasing overall muscle activity and early activation of upper trapezius [47]. Whole-body coordination and movement would play an important role in driving a speedy ball impact.

Comparing forehand and backhand strokes, racket speed during ball impact was similar but presented differences in the upward and forward velocity components [1]. Forehand stroke lasts slightly longer duration for whole movement cycle and individual phases, and noticeably longer total traveling distance of the racket. This could be because forehand had greater body involvement while the arm and trunk range of motion (RoM) in backhand stroke is limited. Forehand stroke may produce more energy, whilst a longer backswing phase in the high-force condition may generate higher force and longer contact time with the balls [1]. The racket velocity produced by forehand and backhand strokes could be different. During forehand stroke, racket velocity was correlated with the angular velocities of internal arm rotation and shoulder adduction, whereas the racket velocity was correlated with the angular velocities of arm abduction and shoulder rotation during a backhand stroke [2].

A longline forehand topspin produced larger ball rotation, compared to the crosscourt topspin shot. At the instant of the maximum velocity of racket in a forehand topspin stroke, players put their racket more inclined whilst maintaining a more flexed knee and elbow posture, in addition to a more pronounced trunk rotation [45]. Other maneuvers including loop, flick, fast break, and curling ball were also studied [35,42,46]. Compared to curving balls, Zhou et al. [42] suggested that fast breaking significantly reduced racket speed during ball impact. While the flick maneuver was specified as an attack when the ball is closed to the net, there were no detailed explanations on the moves of the fast break and curling ball in which we believed that they could be the flick/drop shot and topspin/sidespin loop maneuvers, respectively. On the other hand, Le Mansec et al. [46] demonstrated that aggressive strokes required greater muscle activities. During smash, biceps femoris, gluteus maximus, gastrocnemius, and soleus muscles were highly activated. Forehand topspin with more power or spin produced significantly higher muscle activation of biceps femoris and gluteus maximus muscles compared to other maneuvers, including backhand top, forehand smash, and flick.

3.5. Lower Limb Biomechanics

Four included studies investigated different footwork targeting side versus cross-step [4], long versus short chasse step [48], stepping directions and friction [27], and squatting [30], as shown in Tables 1 and 4, while one study compared players of different levels performing a cross-step [34]. Lam et al. [4] identified that both side-step and cross-step footwork produced significantly higher ground reaction force, knee flexion angle, knee moment, ankle inversion and moment compared with one-step footwork, in addition to a significant higher peak pressure on the total foot, toe, first, second and fifth metatarsal regions. On the other hand, long and short chasse steps during a forehand topspin stroke were compared [48]. Long chasse steps produced an earlier muscle activation for vastus medialis, quicker angular velocity, and larger ankle and hip transverse RoM, whereas larger ankle coronal RoM and hip sagittal RoM compared with the short chasse steps [48]. A stable lower limb support base is another important attribute to tackle serve. Yu et al. [30] compared a squat serve with stand serve and found that squat serve produced larger angles and velocities of hip flexion, adduction, knee flexion, and external rotation and ankle dorsiflexion, whereas standing serve produced a higher force-time integral in the rearfoot region. Different stepping angle and footwear friction could also influence the center of mass and kinematics of knee joint, respectively [27]. Different footwork imposed different lower limb kinematics requirements for table tennis players.

Table 2. Study characteristics of reviewed studies.

Author (Year)	Variant (s)	Maneuvers/Conditions	Type of Parameters
Bankosz and Winiarski (2017) [1]	Handwork (2) × power/serve (3)	Handwork: 1. Forehand crosscourt topspin 2. Backhand crosscourt topspin Handwork power and serve: a. Strength, speed and rotation of 75% max, against no-spin serve; b. Strength, speed and rotation of 75% max, against backspin serve; c. Strength and speed close to max, against no-spin serve;	Racket kinematics
Bankosz and Winiarski (2018) [2]	Handwork (2) × power/serve (3)	Handwork: 1. Forehand crosscourt topspin 2. Backhand crosscourt topspin Handwork power and serve: a. Force, velocity and rotation of 75%, against no-spin serve; b. Force, velocity and rotation of 75%, against backspin serve; c. Force, velocity close to max, against no-spin serve;	Racket kinematics, upper and lower limb kinematics
Bankosz and Winiarski (2018) [39]	Power/serve (3)	Forehand crosscourt topspin a. Force, velocity and rotation of 75%, against no-spin serve; b. Force, velocity and rotation of 75%, against backspin serve; c. Force, velocity close to max, against no-spin serve;	Racket kinematics, lower limb kinematics
Bankosz and Winiarski (2020) [33]	Serve (2)	Forehand crosscourt topspin 1. against a topspin ball 2. against a backspin ball	Upper limb, lower limb and trunk kinematics
Belli et al. (2019) [40]	Level (2)	Forehand or backhand offensive stroke chosen by players against backspin ball 100–120 cm from net and 30 cm away from either left or right side at 25 km/h with frequency of 54 balls per min	Ball speed, accuracy, performance index
Fu et al. (2016) [3]	Level (2)	Forehand crosscourt loop	PP
Ibrahim et al. (2020) [44]	Handwork (2)	1. Forehand drop shot 2. Long shot	Ball and racket kinematics, upper limb kinematics
Iino et al. (2008) [35]	Serve (2)	Backhand crosscourt loop 1. Against topspin serve 2. Against backspin serve	Ball kinematics, Upper limb kinematics
Iino and Kojima (2009) [24]	Level (2) × Serve (2)	Forehand crosscourt topspin as hard as possible 1. Against light backspin ball 2. Against heavy backspin ball	Ball and racket kinematics, trunk and upper limb kinematics
Iino and Kojima (2011) [25]	Level (2) × serve (2)	Forehand crosscourt topspin at max effort 1. Against light backspin ball 2. Against heavy backspin ball	Kinetics of upper limb
Iino and Kojima (2016) [26]	Racket mass (3) × ball frequency (2)	Backhand topspin at max effort Racket mass (153.5 g, 176 g, 201.5 g) Ball projection frequency (75 and 35 ball per minutes)	Racket kinematics, Upper limb and trunk kinematics and kinetics
Iino and Kojima (2016) [37]	Serve (2)	Backhand crosscourt topspin at max effort 1. Against topspin serve 2. Against backspin serve	Upper limb kinetics
Iino et al. (2017) [41]	Level (2)	Forehand crosscourt topspin 1. Intermediate players 2. Advanced players	Kinematics and variability of trunk, upper limb and racket kinematics
Iino (2018) [36]	Correlation study	Forehand crosscourt topspin at max effort	Racket kinematics/kinetics and pelvis kinetics

Table 2. Cont.

Author (Year)	Variant (s)	Maneuvers/Conditions	Type of Parameters
Lam et al. (2019) [4]	Footwork (3)	Forehand crosscourt topspin 1. One-step; 2. Side-step; 3. Cross-step	GRF, knee and ankle kinematics and kinetics, PP
LeMansec et al. (2016) [43]	Level (3)	Forehand crosscourt topspin 1. Inexperience players 2. Advanced players 3. Expert players	Ball speed and accuracy
LeMansec et al. (2018) [46]	Handwork (5)	1. Backhand top; 2. Flick (a close to net attack); 3. Forehand spin (topspin with more spin less power); 4. Forehand top (topspin with more power less spin); 5. Smash	Lower limb muscle EMG
Malagoli Lanzoni et al. (2018) [45]	Handwork (2)	1 Forehand longline topspin 2. Forehand crosscourt topspin	Racket, upper and lower limb kinematics
Meghdadi et al. (2019) [47]	Healthy vs. syndromic (2)	Forehand topspin loop	EMG, muscle onset and offset time
Qian et al. (2016) [28]	Level (2)	Forehand topspin loop	Lower limb kinematics and kinetics, PP
Shao et al. (2020) [34]	Level (2)	Forehand loop using a cross-step with maximal power against topspin	Lower limb kinematics, PP
Sheppard and Li (2007) [38]	Level (2)	1. Forehand return aimed for speed 2. Forehand returns aimed for speed with accuracy 3. Forehand returns aimed for accuracy Note: the three conditions were not independent factors of the study	Ball speed and accuracy, racket kinematics
Wang et al. (2018) [29]	Level (2)	Backhand crosscourt loop	Lower limb kinematics and kinetics, EMG
Yan et al. (2017) [27]	Footwork (2) × Footwear (3)	Footwork: 1. 180° step 2. 45° step Sole-ground friction: a. Low; b. Medium; c. High	CoM, Lower limb kinematics
Yu et al. (2018) [30]	Footwork (2)	Stroke NS 1. Stand serve 2. Squat serve	Lower limb kinematics and kinetics, PP
Yu et al. (2019) [48]	Footwork (2)	Forehand loop 1. Short chasse step 2. Long chasse step	Lower limb kinematics, EMG
Yu et al. (2019) [32]	Level (2)	Chasse step movement and forehand loop with maximal power against topspin	Foot kinematics, PP
Zhang et al. (2016) [31]	Level (2)	Forehand crosscourt stroke 1. Novice players 2. Expert players	Accuracy, Racket kinematics
Zhou (2014) [42]	Handwork (2)	1. Fast break 2. Curling ball	Racket speed

NS: not specified; CoM: centre of Mass; w/: with; w/o: without; PP: plantar pressure distribution; EMG: electromyography.

Comparing the lower limb biomechanics among players with various playing levels, Qian et al. [28] and Wang et al. [29] reported distinct findings for respective forehand and backhand crosscourt loops. When executing forehand topspin loop, higher-level players increased knee external rotation, hip flexion and decreased ankle dorsiflexion during backward end phase, and increased hip extension and internal rotation, decreased ankle and knee internal rotation during forward end phase. There was an overall increase in the ankle sagittal RoM as well as hip sagittal and coronal RoM [28]. When performing backhand crosscourt loop against backspin ball, higher-level players increased ankle dorsiflexion, eversion and external rotation, increased knee flexion and abduction and increased hip flexion, adduction, and external rotation at the beginning of backswing, as well as increased ankle dorsiflexion, knee flexion, reduced hip flexion but increased abduction at the end of swing [29]. During cross-step footwork, higher-level players executed superior foot motor control, as indicated by a smaller RoM of foot joints and higher relative load on the plantar toes, lateral forefoot and rearfoot regions [34]. They also demonstrated smaller forefoot plantarflexion and abduction during cross-step end phase but larger forefoot dorsiflexion and adduction during forward end phase [34]. Effective coordination of lower limb facilitates better upper body rotation in higher-level players [39].

Bańkosz and Winiarski [33] compared inter- and intra-individual variabilities of kinematic parameters. They reported that both variabilities could be quite high, but players attempted to minimize variability at critical moments, such as the instant of ball impact. Higher inter-individual variability could also imply that the technique of coordination movement is rather individual. Adopting or imitating a particular training regime has to pay more attention.

Plantar pressure was also used to evaluate foot loading among different playing levels. When performing forehand loop during backward end phase, higher-level players displayed larger plantar pressure excursion in the medial-lateral direction but smaller in the anterior-posterior direction, accompanied by increased contact areas at midfoot and rearfoot regions while decreased contact area at lesser toe region [3,28]. During forward end phase, higher-level and intermediate players decreased similarly the plantar pressure excursion in the anterior-posterior direction. The contact areas were increased at midfoot, rearfoot, and forefoot regions while decreased at the hallux region [3,28]. The change of plantar pressure excursion and contact area could reflect the strategy compromising dynamic stability and agility in different directions.

Table 3. Key findings of included studies comparing playing levels.

Author (Year)	Outcome Measures	Key Findings of Higher–Level Compared to Lower-Level Players
Belli et al. (2019) [40]	Ball speed; accuracy score, performance index (average speed × accuracy/100); percentage error for ball toward target zone	↑ Accuracy score; ↑ Performance index; ↓ Percentage error.
Fu et al. (2016) [3]	ML and AP excursion; Contact area for big toe, lesser toes, medial forefoot, lateral forefoot, midfoot and rearfoot	During backward end: ↑ ML excursion; ↓ AP excursion; ↑ Contact area for midfoot and rearfoot; ↓ Contact area for lesser toes; During forward end:↓ AP excursion; ↑ Contact area for midfoot, rearfoot, medial forefoot and lateral forefoot; ↓ Contact area for big toe
Iino and Kojima (2009) [24]	Ball speed before and after impact; Racket speed, face angle, path inclination and height at ball impact; Time required to reach 25% of racket speed at impact and max racket acceleration; Contributions to racket speed by: Max lower trunk axial rotation; mid hip linear; lower trunk lateral bending, flexion/extension, axial rotation; upper trunk axial rotation relative to lower trunk; shoulder linear relative to upper trunk; shoulder abduction, flexion, internal rotation; elbow flexion/extension; forearm supination/pronation; wrist palmar/dorsi flexion, radial/ulnar deviation	↑ Max racket acceleration; ↑ Contribution of lower trunk axial rotation to racket speed

Table 3. Cont.

Author (Year)	Outcome Measures	Key Findings of Higher–Level Compared to Lower–Level Players
Iino and Kojima (2011) [25]	Max joint torques of: shoulder adduction, flexion, internal rotation; elbow varus, flexion; wrist dorsiflexion and radial deviation; Max joint torque power of shoulder adduction, flexion, positive and negative internal rotation, elbow flexion, wrist dorsiflexion, and radial deviation; Net work done by shoulder adduction and internal rotation; Positive and negative work done by shoulder internal rotation torque; Max rate of energy transfer by: shoulder addiction and internal rotation; elbow varus and flexion; wrist radial deviation Amount of energy transfer by: shoulder adduction, flexion, internal rotation; elbow varus and flexion; wrist radial deviation; Max rate of energy transfer and amount of energy transfer through shoulder, elbow and wrist joints; Increase in mechanical energy of racket arm;Mechanical energy transferred to racket arm; Energy transfer ratio of racket arm.	↑ Normalized max joint torques of shoulder internal rotation, elbow varus, and wrist radial deviation; ↑ Max joint torque power of shoulder internal rotation in both positive and negative directions; ↑ Negative work done by shoulder internal rotation torque; ↑ Max rate of energy transfer for shoulder internal rotation, elbow varus and wrist radial deviation.
Iino et al. (2017) [41]	Racket speed at ball impact; Standard deviation of racket face angle in vertical and horizontal directions; Total, controlled and uncontrolled variable variance for racket race angle in vertical and horizontal directions; Ratio of uncontrolled to controlled variance	↑ Racket speed at ball impact; ↓ Controlled variance for horizontal angle of racket surface.
LeMansec et al. (2016) [43]	Ball speed; accuracy; performance index (average speed × accuracy/100)	Elite ↑ ball speed, accuracy and performance index than advanced players Advanced ↑ Ball speed, accuracy and performance index than inexperienced players.
Qian et al. (2016) [28]	Joint angle of ankle, knee and hip in all planes at backward-end (BE) and forward-end (FE); RoM of ankle, knee and hip joint in all planes.ACR of ankle, knee and hip in all planes during forward–swing phase; Contact area in big toe, other toes, medial and lateral forefoot, midfoot and rearfoot regions during BE and FE.	↑ Ankle RoM in sagittal plane; ↑ Hip RoM in sagittal and transverse planes; ↓ Knee RoM in sagittal plane. ↑ ACR of ankle and hip in all planes;During BE, ↑ Hip angle in sagittal plane; ↑ Knee angle in transverse plane; ↓ Contact area in other toes; ↑ Contact area in midfoot and rearfoot;During FE, ↑ Hip angle in sagittal (−) and transverse (−) planes; ↓ Knee angle in transverse (−) plane. ↓ Contact area in big toe; ↑ Contact area in medial and lateral forefoot, midfoot and rearfoot.

Table 3. Cont.

Author (Year)	Outcome Measures	Key Findings of Higher–Level Compared to Lower–Level Players
Shao et al. (2020) [34]	Duration for backswing phase, forward-swing phase and whole cycle;HTA, FTA in all planes and XFA in sagittal plane at BE and FE; RoM and ACR of HTA, FTA in all planes and XFA in sagittal plane at backswing phase;PP at backswing and forward-swing phases and relative load during entire motion of hallux, other toes, medial, central and lateral forefoot, medial and lateral midfoot, medial and lateral rearfoot regions	↓ Backswing phase but ↑ forward swing phase and total duration; ↓ FTA in sagittal (−) and transverse planes at BE; ↑ XFA in sagittal plane at BE;↓ HTA in frontal plane at FE; ↑ FTA in sagittal and transverse (−) planes but ↓ in frontal plane at FE; ↓ XFA in sagittal plane at FE;↓ RoM of HTA and FTA but ↑ XFA in sagittal plane at backswing phase; ↓ RoM of HTA in sagittal and frontal but ↑ in transverse plane at forward–swing; ↑ RoM of XFA in transverse plane at forward–swing;↑ ACR in all joints and planes at backswing phase; ↑ ACR in all joints and planes at forward–swing phase except HTA in frontal plane;↑ PP of lateral forefoot and medial rearfoot but ↓ lateral forefoot, central forefoot, medial forefoot, other toes, hallux at backswing phase;↑ PP if lateral rearfoot, lateral forefoot, other toes but ↓ central forefoot, hallux at forward swing phase; ↑ relative load of other toes, lateral forefoot, medial rearfoot, lateral rearfoot but ↓ hallux, medial forefoot
Sheppard and Li (2007) [38]	Frequency of successful returns, ball speed, ball bounce location accuracy; Racket speed, position, direction of motion, orientation; and Variability of racket speed, acceleration, horizontal and vertical direction of motions, orientation; at the −200, −150, −100, −50, 0, +50 ms relative to the moment of ball contact	↑ successful returns, ball speed, ball bounce location accuracy; Significant interaction between playing level and time on the overall ball kinematics variables (MANOVA) ↑ racket speed, rightward direction, downward oriented; ↓ variability on racket horizontal direction of motion and orientation
Wang et al. (2018) [29]	Hip, knee and ankle joint angles and ACRs in all planes at beginning of backswing and end of swing phases. Standardized average, mean power frequency and median frequency for EMG of rectus femoris and tibialis anterior for both limbs.	↑ Rate of angular change for knee and hip in all planes; ↑ Rate of angular change for ankle in sagittal but ↓ in horizontal; ↑ MPF mean power frequency for all muscles; At beginning of backswing ↑ Ankle dorsiflexion; eversion; external rotation; ↑ Knee flexion; abduction; ↑ Hip flexion, adduction and external rotation;At end of swing ↑ Ankle dorsiflexion; knee flexion; ↓ Hip flexion, ↑ abduction.

Table 3. Cont.

Author (Year)	Outcome Measures	Key Findings of Higher–Level Compared to Lower–Level Players
Yu et al. (2019) [32]	Duration for backswing phase, forward-swing phase and whole cycle; HTA, FTA in all planes and XFA in sagittal plane at backswing and forward-swing phases; RoM and ACR of HTA, FTA in all planes and XFA in sagittal plane at backswing and forward-swing phases; PP and relative load of hallux, other toes, medial, central and lateral forefoot, medial and lateral midfoot, medial and lateral rearfoot at backswing and forward-swing phases.	↓ Backswing phase but ↑ forward swing phase and total duration; ↓RoM of HTA, HFA in all planes ↑RoM of XFA in sagittal plane ↑ Relative load for other toes, lateral forefoot; ↓ Relative load for medial forefoot and medial rearfoot. During backswing phase, ↑ HTA in sagittal and transverse (−); ↓ HTA in frontal; ↓ FTA in all planes (−) ↑ XFA in sagittal (−); ↑ ACR of HTA in sagittal and frontal;↑ ACR of RTA in frontal;↓ ACR of XFA in sagittal ↑ Lateral forefoot, medial and lateral rearfoot; ↓ PP for hallux, medial and central forefoot; During forward-swing phase, ↑ HTA in sagittal and transverse (−); ↑ HFA in frontal and transverse; ↑ XFA in sagittal (−) ↑ ACR of FTA in y direction; ↑ PP for other toes, central and lateral forefoot; ↓ PP for hallux.
Zhang et al. (2016) [31]	Accuracy; Duration and variability of duration for each phase (preparatory, backswing, forward–swing, follow through)	↑ Accuracy; ↓ Variability of duration for forward-swing and follow through phases;

ACR: angular changing rate; AP: anteroposterior; BE: backward-end; EMG: electromyography; FE: forward-end; FTA: right forefoot to hindfoot angle; HTA: right hindfoot to tibia angle; ML: mediolateral; PP: peak pressure; RoM: range of motion; XFA: right hallux to forefoot angle. (−) in negative direction/value. The increase/decrease of (−) refer to the absolute magnitude; ↑: significantly higher/larger/increase; ↓: significantly lower/smaller/decrease.

4. Discussion

There was evidence suggesting that higher-level table tennis players produced higher ball accuracy, performance index, and trial-to-trial repeatability in both training and competition. Meanwhile, it was generally perceived that ball and racket velocities were deterministic to playing level since high velocities make the opponent difficult to return the ball. In particular, the maximum racket speed at the moment of impact was regarded as the most important playing technique [1]. However, the current evidence did not come into a consensus that higher-level players necessarily produce higher ball or racket speed. Shoulder joint seems to play an important role to coordinate an effective stroke, as indicated by the effective use of elbow flexion torque, while the power of wrist joint is important during drop shot or long shot services. On the other hand, lower extremities facilitated momentum generation for increased racket velocity. In fact, leg–hip–trunk kinetics accounted for more than half of the energy and muscle force generation in racket sports [28]. Apart from a shorter period of swinging time, the increase in hip flexion and knee external rotations for higher-level players would potentially facilitate a more efficient muscle output to maximize racket velocity through the kinetic chain [28,29], in addition to larger hip and ankle angular velocities [28] which could be correlated with an increased ball speed after ball impact [50]. It should be noted that body coordination movement varies across individuals and trials but players attempted to reproduce movement during critical instants [33]. This was known as functional variability such that players could adapt to the conditions and requirements of the tasks and compensated for the changes with other movement parameters [51]. An optimal training model of body movement could be different among athletes.

Techniques in footwork could play an important role in compromising between dynamic stability and agility to recover back to the ready position for next moves or strokes. Less experienced players tended to have a larger peak ankle dorsiflexion and anterior center of pressure but lesser contact area, which indicated a poorer support base and stability [3,28]. Additionally, a shorter center of pressure in the anterior–posterior direction in higher level players facilitates quicker responses to resume to a neutral position for the next move [3,28]. However, it should be noted that higher level players exhibited larger ankle RoM during the match which may inherit the risk of ankle sprain [28,29].

Regarding the methodological quality, more than half of the included studies did not reveal clearly the source of population and sampling method. There was also a lack of blinding. Although blinding the maneuver conditions seemed to be impossible since the participants needed to be acknowledged for the tasks they performed, it could be accomplished by counting successive returns from delivering random serves by the coaches or serving robots [30,40]. Furthermore, the implementation of a randomized cross-over design across various interventions and maneuvers is necessary to avoid carry-over effects. Future studies can investigate how technologies can improve training outcomes. For instance, augmented reality (AR) technology with different filmed footages of different balls and gaze information can be modulated with artificial intelligence program to simulate the virtual opponent with the matched playing levels. Such simulations would provide a steppingstone towards individualized training solutions. On the other hand, several studies investigated a large number of outcome variables which was not well justified. While a full biomechanical profile with a large number of outcome variables were endeavored, statistical analyses were performed without corrections for multiple or multivariate comparisons. This may fall into the trap of data dredging or p-hacking [52] and those research may confine to exploratory studies [53].

There are some limitations when interpreting our findings. A systematic scoping review covered a vast volume of literature over a topic and thus offered an overview picture within the discipline [21]. However, due to the heterogeneity and breadth of the included studies, the established data framework did not attempt to answer a single research question which shall be put forward by a systematic review. It is also not possible to conduct meta-analysis to estimate overall determinants on playing levels, movement tasks, and equipment because of the diversity of objectives and designs across the included studies. In fact, the amount of literature required for a subset study was insufficient to formulate a focused research question for a traditional systematic review. For example, only two included studies were comparing upper limb kinematics of forehand topspin among different player levels in our review. In other words, it is pragmatically demanding to call for more research to establish the map over biomechanical variables, maneuvers, and playing levels, and reinforce key ideas on the determinants of performance using a unified study design and protocol.

Additionally, there was potential publication or language bias since some relevant articles were excluded for being published in Chinese, despite the fact that China is one of the dominating countries in the table tennis sports [16]. Summarizing information from the Chinese literature can enhance the impact of table tennis research but may require considerable effort in screening, translation, and interpretation. Furthermore, we found that there was a lack of literature on backspin maneuvers, longline maneuvers, strikes against sidespin ball, and pen-hold players that warrant further investigations.

Table 4. Key findings of included studies comparing different movement tasks.

Author (Year)	Outcome Measures	Key Findings
Bankosz and Winiarski (2017) # [1]	Time parameters (total time, duration of forward, hit-to-forward end, backward phases, time to reach max velocity (resultant and direction components) of racket); Distance parameters (resultant and direction components of distance travelled by racket during whole cycle, forward, hit-to-forward end, backward phases); Velocity parameters of racket (resultant and direction components of mean, max and at impact).	Forehand stroke ↓ total duration than against a spin serve and more power ball. Backhand stroke ↓ total duration than against a spin Strokes with more power produced ↑ velocity and distance parameters in AP direction; strokes against spin produced ↑ velocity and distance parameters in vertical direction; Forehand stroke (against spin and more power), produced ↑ velocity and distance parameters than backhand stroke.
Bankosz and Winiarski (2018) # [2]	Max racket velocity, racket velocity at ball impact, time to reach max racket velocity, time to reach racket velocity at ball impact; Angular velocity (max, min, at impact) for wrist, elbow, shoulder, pelvis, hip, knee and ankle; Multiple regression on racket velocity and angular velocity parameters of body segments.	For maximum-effort forehand topspin, racket velocity was correlated with hip flexion velocity on playing side, hip extension velocity on opposite site, and ankle flexion velocity on playing side; For maximum-effort backhand stroke, racket velocity was correlated with shoulder joint angular velocities on playing side, flexion velocity of ankle and adduction velocity of hip on opposite side.
Bankosz and Winiarski (2018) # [39]	Racket speed at impact; RoM of ankle, knee, hip, wrist, elbow and elbow joints in all planes during forward, hit-to-forward end, backward phases.	Diff forehand topspin types produced different RoM; ↑shot power accompanied by ↑rotation of upper body, pelvis and shoulders, flexion and rotation in shoulder, elbows and knees.
Bankosz and Winiarski (2020) # [33]	Lumbar, chest, hips, knees, shoulders, elbows and wrists angles and inter-individual coefficient of variation at ready, backswing, contact and forward instants; Above data for exemplary players and intra-individual coefficient of variation; Acceleration of hand at contact instant.	↑ intra-individual variability and high range of inter-individual variability; ↑ variability was observed in abduction/adduction of hip joints, wrist joints, thoracic and lumbar spines; Slightly ↑ variability when hit against a backspin compared to that against a topspin; ↑ variability at ready instants than other instants;
Ibrahm et al. (2020) [44]	Horizontal velocity of ball and racket head; Mean angular velocity of shoulder, elbow and wrist joints; Correlation between horizontal velocity of ball and racket head, and body segmental angular velocity at impact.	In forehand drop shot, Ball horizontal velocity correlated with racket head horizontal velocity positively; Wrist radial deviation velocity positively correlated with horizontal ball and racket head velocity; In long shot, Wrist radial deviation velocity and palmar flexion angular velocity positively correlated with horizontal racket head velocity.
Iino et al. (2008) [35]	Ball speed before and after impact; Magnitude, direction components of upper arm flexion, abduction, external rotation, elbow extension, forearm supination, wrist ulnar deviation and dorsiflexion at impact; Contributions to forward and upward racket velocities.	Against topspin, compared to against backspin: ↑ Upward component of elbow extension (−); ↓ Upward component of wrist dorsiflexion; ↑ Contribution to racket upward velocity by elbow extension (−), ↓ wrist dorsiflexion and racket tip linear.
Iino and Kojima (2016) [26]	Racket speed, face angle and path inclination at ball impact; Racket trajectory length; Ball impact location; Max pelvis axial rotation velocity; Upper trunk axial rotation velocity relative to pelvis, shoulder flexion velocity, external rotation velocity, elbow extension velocity, wrist dorsiflexion velocity at impact; Peak torque for shoulder, elbow and wrist; Shoulder, elbow and wrist angular velocities at instants of their matching peak joint torque.	No significant interaction between racket mass and ball frequency on all variables. Higher ball frequency, compared to lower ball frequency: ↓ Racket speed at impact; significantly more forward impact location; ↓ Max pelvis axial rotation velocity, upper trunk axial rotation velocity relative to pelvis at impact; Large racket mass, compared to small racket mass: ↑ Peak wrist dorsiflexion torque.

Table 4. Cont.

Author (Year)	Outcome Measures	Key Findings
Iino and Kojima (2016) [37]	Racket resultant, horizontal and vertical velocity at impact; Max shoulder joint center velocity in rightward and upward; Max angular velocity of upper trunk in extension and axial rotation; Peak joint torque for shoulder, elbow and wrist; Torque work by shoulder and elbow; Amount of energy transfer by joint torque and force components; Energy transfer ratio of racket arm.	Against backspin, compared to against topspin ↑ Resultant and vertical; but ↓ horizontal racket velocity; ↑ Max shoulder center velocity in upward direction; ↑ Max angular velocity of upper trunk in both extension and axial rotation; ↑ Peak shoulder flexion, external rotation torque and elbow valgus torque; ↑ Torque work by shoulder flexion/extension; but ↓ shoulder internal rotation and elbow extension;↑ Energy transfer through shoulder joint in rightward, upward, flexion/extension torque, abduction torque; ↑ Sum of energy transferred through shoulder; ↑ Mechanical energy of racket arm; ↑ Energy transfer ratio of racket arm;
Iino (2018) [36]	Correlation coefficients with horizontal (hV) and vertical velocities (vV) of racket at impact on: peak pelvis angular velocities in axial rotation and backward tilt; lateral flexion, axial rotation and backward tilt of playing side hip and forward tilt of non-playing side hip;Torque and force of both hips; Posterior tilt torques and vertical forces at both hips;Axial rotation torques at both hips; Total work done on pelvis.	Peak pelvis angular velocity in axial rotation direction was significantly correlated with hV and vV (−); Forward tilt of non-playing side hip was significantly correlated with hV and vV (−); Axial rotation torque of playing side hip was significantly correlated with hV; Axial rotation torque of non-playing side hip was significantly correlated with hV and vV(−); Posterior tilt torques and vertical forces at both hips was significantly correlated vV; Axial rotation torques at both hips was significantly correlated with hV.
Lam et al. (2019) [4]	Max vGRF and hGRF; Max knee flexion angle and moment; Max ankle inversion angle, angular velocity and moment; PP; Pressure time integral for plantar regions: total foot, toe, 1st MT, 2nd MT, 3rd–4th MT, 5th MT, medial and lateral midfoot and heel.	One-step, compared to both side-step and cross step: ↓ Max hGRF and vGRF; ↓ Max knee flexion and moment; ↓ Max ankle inversion, angular velocity and moment. and max ankle inversion angular velocity; ↓ PP for total foot, toe, 1st MT, 2nd MT, 5th MT. Side-step, compared to cross-step only: ↓ Max hGRF and vGRF; ↓ Max knee flexion and max ankle inversion angular velocity; ↓ PP for total foot and 1st MT. One-step, compared to cross-step only: ↓ PP for medial midfoot, medial heel and lateral heel
LeMansec et al. (2018) [46]	EMG muscle activity level of vastus lateralis, vastus medialis, rectus femoris, soleus, gastrocnemius lateralis, gastrocnemius medialis, biceps femoris, gluteus maximus Global level (average level) of EMG for all muscles	Comparing 5 maneuvers: Backhand top (BT), flick (FL), forehand spin (FS), forehand top (FT), smash (SM): Global level of EMG BT ↑ all others; FL ↑ FS, FT, SM; FS↑ SM; For EMG of vastus lateralis and vastus medialis FS ↑ B, FL, SM; FT ↑ SM For rectus femorisFS and FT ↑ BT, FL, SM; For soleus and gastrocnemius lateralis BT ↓ FL, FT; SM ↑ all others For gastrocnemius medialis SM ↑ all others; FL ↑ BT, FS; FT ↑ BT, FS; For gluteus maximusFS, FT, SM ↑ BT, FL For biceps femoris FS, FT, SM ↑ BT, FL; FL ↑BT

Table 4. Cont.

Author (Year)	Outcome Measures	Key Findings
Malagoli Lanzoni et al. (2018) [45]	Angle of racket in all planes; Average feet-table angle; Max, min angle and moment of max velocity of racket (MMV) for angulation of: shoulders-table, shoulder-racket, pelvis-table, elbow and left/right knees	Cross-court, compared to long-line was: ↓ Racket angle in axial direction (z); ↓ Average feet-table angle; ↓ Max and min shoulder-table; ↓ Max but ↑ MMV of shoulder-racket angles; ↓ Max, min and MMV of pelvis-table angles; ↑ Elbow MMV; ↓ Right knee MMV
Meghdadi et al. (2019) [47]	Muscle activity; muscle onset; offset time instant for: supraspinatus, upper trapezius, lower trapezius, serratus anterior, biceps brachii, anterior deltoid	Shoulder impingement syndrome group, compared to healthy group ↓ muscle activity of supraspinatus and serratus anterior; ↑ muscle activity of upper trapezius; Significantly later muscle onset time for serratus anterior but significantly earlier muscle onset time for upper trapezius
Yan et al. (2017) [27]	Buffer time; CoM in AP and ML directions; Right knee angle at peak GRF	180° step compared to 45° step ↑ CoM in AP direction (A or P direction not specify); Higher sole-ground friction ↓ right knee angle at peak GRF.
Yu et al. (2018) [30]	Duration from initiation to backward-end, from backward-end (BE) to forward-end (FE), from forward-end to initial ready position (RP)Hip, knee and ankle angle at RP, BE and FE in three planes. Force-time integral in big toe, other toes, medial forefoot, lateral forefoot, midfoot and rearfoot	Squat serve, compared to standing serve: In sagittal plane ↑ hip angle at RP, BE and FE; ↑ knee angle at BE and FE; ↓ ankle angle at RP but ↑ at BE and FE; In frontal plane ↑ hip angle (–) at BE and FE; ↓ knee angle at BE and FE;In transverse plane ↑ hip angle at FE; ↑ knee angle at BE and FE; ↓ force-time integral in rearfoot
Yu et al. (2019) [48]	RoM of hip, knee and ankle joint in three planes. Hip, knee and ankle joint in three planes at take-off (T1) and backward-end (BE) instants. ACR of hip, knee ankle in three planes.	Long chasse steps, as compared to short chasse steps: ↑ RoM of hip in sagittal and transverse planes; ↑ RoM of knee in coronal plane; ↑ RoM of ankle in coronal and transverse planes; ↑ ACR of hip in sagittal plane; ↓ ACR of knee but ↑ that of ankle joint in coronal plane; ↑ ACR of hip and ankle in transverse plane; During T1, long chasse steps, compared to short chasse steps: ↓ hip angle in sagittal and transverse planes; ↓ knee angle in transverse plane; ↑ ankle angle in sagittal plane but ↓ in coronal and transverse planes (–); During BE, long chasse steps, compared to short chasse steps: ↓ hip angle in sagittal plane; ↑ knee angle in coronal plane but ↓ in transverse; ↑ ankle angle in sagittal plane
Zhou et al. (2014) [42]	Racket speed at ball contact, during backswing and follow through; percentage duration of backswing, attack and follow through phases	Curving ball, compared to fast break: ↑ racket speed at ball contact

ACR: angular changing rate; AP: anterior-posterior; BE: backward-end; CoM: center of mass; EMG: electromyography; FE: forward-end; hGRF: horizontal ground reaction force; hV: horizontal velocity; MMV: maximum velocity of the racket; MT: metatarsal; PP: peak pressure; RoM: Range of Motion; RP: ready position; T1: take-off; vGRF: vertical ground reaction force; vV: vertical velocity. (–) in negative direction/value. ↑: significantly higher/larger/increase; ↓: significantly lower/smaller/decrease of the absolute magnitude. # Only highlighted key findings were summarized in the table since these studies included too many outcome variables and/or pairwise comparison results to be listed.

5. Conclusions

A systematic scoping review of published studies specific to the biomechanics of table tennis maneuvers was conducted to categorize biomechanical variables within the domain of playing levels and maneuvers. This review could serve as the first scoping review to provide a clear overview about table tennis research in the past decades. Recent research on table tennis maneuvers targeted the differences between playing levels and between maneuvers using parameters which included ball and racket speed, joint kinematics and kinetics, electromyography, and plantar pressure distribution.

Different maneuvers underlined changes on body posture and lines of movement which were accommodated particularly by racket face angle, trunk rotation, knee and elbow joints, and different contributions of muscles. Key findings regarding determinants of playing levels were summarized to offer practical implications as follows:

- Higher-level players produced ball striking at higher accuracy and repeatability but not necessarily of higher speed.
- Strengthening shoulder and wrist muscles could enhance the speed of strike.
- Whole-body coordination and footwork were important to compromise between agility and stability for strike quality.
- Personalized training shall be considered since motor coordination and adaptation vary among individuals.

Moreover, this scoping review found that while most investigations focused on the upper and lower limb biomechanics of table tennis players performing different maneuvers, fewer studies looked into trunk kinematics and EMG. Furthermore, our study identified research gaps in backspin maneuvers and longline maneuvers, strikes against sidespin, and pen-hold players that warrant future investigations.

Author Contributions: Conceptualization, D.W.-C.W., and W.-K.L.; methodology, D.W.-C.W.; validation, W.C.-C.L.; formal analysis, D.W.-C.W., W.C.-C.L., and W.-K.L.; data curation, D.W.-C.W., and W.C.-C.L.; writing–original draft preparation, D.W.-C.W.; writing–review and editing, W.C.-C.L. and W.-K.L.; visualization, D.W.-C.W. All authors have read and agreed to the published version of the manuscript.

Funding: This research received no external funding.

Conflicts of Interest: This is to declare that W.L.K. is an employee of Li Ning Sports Goods Company Limited. While the company sold table tennis rackets and garments, there is no direct connection and conflict of interest to this review article.

References

1. Bańkosz, Z.; Winiarski, S. The kinematics of table tennis racquet: Differences between topspin strokes. *J. Sports Med. Phys. Fit.* **2017**, *57*, 202–213.
2. Bańkosz, Z.; Winiarski, S. Correlations between angular velocities in selected joints and velocity of table tennis racket during topspin forehand and backhand. *J. Sports Sci. Med.* **2018**, *17*, 330. [PubMed]
3. Fu, F.; Zhang, Y.; Shao, S.; Ren, J.; Lake, M.; Gu, Y. Comparison of center of pressure trajectory characteristics in table tennis during topspin forehand loop between superior and intermediate players. *Int. J. Sports Sci. Coach.* **2016**, *11*, 559–565. [CrossRef]
4. Lam, W.-K.; Fan, J.-X.; Zheng, Y.; Lee, W.C.-C. Joint and plantar loading in table tennis topspin forehand with different footwork. *Eur. J. Sport Sci.* **2019**, *19*, 471–479. [CrossRef]
5. Kondrič, M.; Matković, B.; Furjan-Mandić, G.; Hadžić, V.; Derviševič, E. Injuries in racket sports among Slovenian players. *Coll. Antropol.* **2011**, *35*, 413–417. [PubMed]
6. Lees, A.; Asai, T.; Andersen, T.B.; Nunome, H.; Sterzing, T. The biomechanics of kicking in soccer: A review. *J. Sports Sci.* **2010**, *28*, 805–817. [CrossRef]
7. Kellis, E.; Katis, A. Biomechanical characteristics and determinants of instep soccer kick. *J. Sports Sci. Med.* **2007**, *6*, 154.
8. Abrams, G.D.; Sheets, A.L.; Andriacchi, T.P.; Safran, M.R. Review of tennis serve motion analysis and the biomechanics of three serve types with implications for injury. *Sports Biomech.* **2011**, *10*, 378–390. [CrossRef]
9. Bahamonde, R. Review of the biomechanical function of the elbow joint during tennis strokes. *Int. SportMed J.* **2005**, *6*, 42–63.

10. Vantorre, J.; Chollet, D.; Seifert, L. Biomechanical analysis of the swim-start: A review. *J. Sports Sci. Med.* **2014**, *13*, 223.
11. Psycharakis, S.G.; Sanders, R.H. Body roll in swimming: A review. *J. Sports Sci.* **2010**, *28*, 229–236. [CrossRef] [PubMed]
12. Costa, M.J.; Bragada, J.A.; Marinho, D.A.; Silva, A.J.; Barbosa, T.M. Longitudinal interventions in elite swimming: A systematic review based on energetics, biomechanics, and performance. *J. Strength Cond. Res.* **2012**, *26*, 2006–2016. [CrossRef] [PubMed]
13. Kondrič, M.; Zagatto, A.M.; Sekulić, D. The physiological demands of table tennis: A review. *J. Sports Sci. Med.* **2013**, *12*, 362. [PubMed]
14. Zagatto, A.M.; Kondric, M.; Knechtle, B.; Nikolaidis, P.T.; Sperlich, B. Energetic demand and physical conditioning of table tennis players. A study review. *J. Sports Sci.* **2018**, *36*, 724–731. [CrossRef]
15. Fuchs, M.; Liu, R.; Malagoli Lanzoni, I.; Munivrana, G.; Straub, G.; Tamaki, S.; Yoshida, K.; Zhang, H.; Lames, M. Table tennis match analysis: A review. *J. Sports Sci.* **2018**, *36*, 2653–2662. [CrossRef] [PubMed]
16. Zhang, H.; Zhou, Z.; Yang, Q. Match analyses of table tennis in China: A systematic review. *J. Sports Sci.* **2018**, *36*, 2663–2674. [CrossRef]
17. Straub, G.; Klein-Soetebier, T. Analytic and descriptive approaches to systematic match analysis in table tennis. *Ger. J. Exerc. Sport Res.* **2017**, *47*, 95–102. [CrossRef]
18. Zheng, K.; Cui, P. Review on the promoting robot table tennis. *Mach. Tool Hydraul.* **2009**, *8*, 238–241.
19. Mülling, K.; Kober, J.; Kroemer, O.; Peters, J. Learning to select and generalize striking movements in robot table tennis. *Int. J. Robot. Res.* **2013**, *32*, 263–279. [CrossRef]
20. Lees, A. Science and the major racket sports: A review. *J. Sports Sci.* **2003**, *21*, 707–732. [CrossRef]
21. Peters, M.D.; Godfrey, C.M.; Khalil, H.; McInerney, P.; Parker, D.; Soares, C.B. Guidance for conducting systematic scoping reviews. *Int. J. Evid. Based Healthc.* **2015**, *13*, 141–146. [CrossRef]
22. Neal, R.J. The mechanics of the forehand loop and smash shots in table tennis. *Aust. J. Sci. Med. Sport* **1991**, *23*, 3–11.
23. Wang, Z.P.; Rong, K. Sports Biomechanics Analysis of the Backhand Chop in Table Tennis. *Res. J. Biotechnol.* **2017**, *12*, 102–110.
24. Iino, Y.; Kojima, T. Kinematics of table tennis topspin forehands: Effects of performance level and ball spin. *J. Sports Sci.* **2009**, *27*, 1311–1321. [CrossRef] [PubMed]
25. Iino, Y.; Kojima, T. Kinetics of the upper limb during table tennis topspin forehands in advanced and intermediate players. *Sports Biomech.* **2011**, *10*, 361–377. [CrossRef] [PubMed]
26. Iino, Y.; Kojima, T. Effect of the racket mass and the rate of strokes on kinematics and kinetics in the table tennis topspin backhand. *J. Sports Sci.* **2016**, *34*, 721–729. [CrossRef]
27. Yan, X. Effects of friction property on biomechanics of lower limbs of table tennis players. *Acta Tech. CSAV* **2017**, *62*, 29–36.
28. Qian, J.; Zhang, Y.; Baker, J.S.; Gu, Y. Effects of performance level on lower limb kinematics during table tennis forehand loop. *Acta Bioeng. Biomech.* **2016**, *18*, 149–155.
29. Wang, M.; Fu, L.; Gu, Y.; Mei, Q.; Fu, F.; Fernandez, J. Comparative study of kinematics and muscle activity between elite and amateur table tennis players during topspin loop against backspin movements. *J. Hum. Kinet.* **2018**, *64*, 25–33. [CrossRef]
30. Yu, C.; Shao, S.; Baker, J.S.; Gu, Y. Comparing the biomechanical characteristics between squat and standing serves in female table tennis athletes. *PeerJ* **2018**, *6*, e4760. [CrossRef]
31. Zhang, Z.; Halkon, B.; Chou, S.M.; Qu, X. A novel phase-aligned analysis on motion patterns of table tennis strokes. *Int. J. Perform. Anal. Sport* **2016**, *16*, 305–316. [CrossRef]
32. Yu, C.; Shao, S.; Baker, J.S.; Awrejcewicz, J.; Gu, Y. A comparative biomechanical analysis of the performance level on chasse step in table tennis. *Int. J. Sports Sci. Coach.* **2019**, *14*, 372–382. [CrossRef]
33. Bańkosz, Z.; Winiarski, S. Kinematic Parameters of Topspin Forehand in Table Tennis and Their Inter- and Intra-Individual Variability. *J. Sports Sci. Med.* **2020**, *19*, 138–148. [PubMed]
34. Shao, S.; Yu, C.; Song, Y.; Baker, J.S.; Ugbolue, U.C.; Lanzoni, I.M.; Gu, Y. Mechanical character of lower limb for table tennis cross step maneuver. *Int. J. Sports Sci. Coach.* **2020**. [CrossRef]
35. Iino, Y.; Mori, T.; Kojima, T. Contributions of upper limb rotations to racket velocity in table tennis backhands against topspin and backspin. *J. Sports Sci.* **2008**, *26*, 287–293. [CrossRef] [PubMed]

36. Iino, Y. Hip joint kinetics in the table tennis topspin forehand: Relationship to racket velocity. *J. Sports Sci.* **2018**, *36*, 834–842. [CrossRef]
37. Iino, Y.; Kojima, T. Mechanical energy generation and transfer in the racket arm during table tennis topspin backhands. *Sports Biomech.* **2016**, *15*, 180–197. [CrossRef]
38. Sheppard, A.; Li, F.X. Expertise and the control of interception in table tennis. *Eur. J. Sport Sci.* **2007**, *7*, 213–222. [CrossRef]
39. Bańkosz, Z.; Winiarski, S. The evaluation of changes of angles in selected joints during topspin forehand in table tennis. *Mot. Control* **2018**, *22*, 314–337. [CrossRef]
40. Belli, T.; Misuta, M.S.; de Moura, P.P.R.; Tavares, T.d.S.; Ribeiro, R.A.; dos Santos, Y.Y.S.; Sarro, K.J.; Galatti, L.R. Reproducibility and Validity of a Stroke Effectiveness Test in Table Tennis Based on the Temporal Game Structure. *Front. Psychol.* **2019**, *10*, 427. [CrossRef]
41. Iino, Y.; Yoshioka, S.; Fukashiro, S. Uncontrolled manifold analysis of joint angle variability during table tennis forehand. *Hum. Mov. Sci.* **2017**, *56*, 98–108. [CrossRef]
42. Zhou, J. Biomechanical study of different techniques performed by elite athletes in table tennis. *J. Chem. Pharm. Res.* **2014**, *6*, 589–591.
43. Le Mansec, Y.; Dorel, S.; Nordez, A.; Jubeau, M. Sensitivity and reliability of a specific test of stroke performance in table tennis. *Int. J. Sports Physiol. Perform.* **2016**, *11*, 678–684. [CrossRef] [PubMed]
44. Ibrahim, N.; Abu Osman, N.A.; Mokhtar, A.H.; Arifin, N.; Usman, J.; Shasmin, H.N. Contribution of the arm segment rotations towards the horizontal ball and racket head velocities during forehand long shot and drop shot services in table tennis. *Sports Biomech.* **2020**. [CrossRef]
45. Malagoli Lanzoni, I.; Bartolomei, S.; Di Michele, R.; Fantozzi, S. A kinematic comparison between long-line and cross-court top spin forehand in competitive table tennis players. *J. Sports Sci.* **2018**, *36*, 2637–2643. [CrossRef] [PubMed]
46. Le Mansec, Y.; Dorel, S.; Hug, F.; Jubeau, M. Lower limb muscle activity during table tennis strokes. *Sports Biomech.* **2018**, *17*, 442–452. [CrossRef] [PubMed]
47. Meghdadi, N.; Yalfani, A.; Minoonejad, H. Electromyographic analysis of shoulder girdle muscle activation while performing a forehand topspin in elite table tennis athletes with and without shoulder impingement syndrome. *J. Shoulder Elb. Surg.* **2019**, *28*, 1537–1545. [CrossRef]
48. Yu, C.; Shao, S.; Awrejcewicz, J.; Baker, J.S.; Gu, Y. Lower Limb Maneuver Investigation of Chasse Steps Among Male Elite Table Tennis Players. *Medicina* **2019**, *55*, 97. [CrossRef]
49. Poizat, G.; Thouvarecq, R.; Séve, C. A descriptive study of the rotative topspin and of the striking topspin of expert table tennis players. In *Science and Racket Sports III: The Proceedings of the Eighth International Table Tennis Federation Sports Science Congress and The Third World Congress of Science and Racket Sports*; Kahn, J.-F., Lees, A., Maynard, I., Eds.; Routledge: Abingdon-on-Thames, UK, 2004; p. 126.
50. Seeley, M.K.; Funk, M.D.; Denning, W.M.; Hager, R.L.; Hopkins, J.T. Tennis forehand kinematics change as post-impact ball speed is altered. *Sports Biomech.* **2011**, *10*, 415–426. [CrossRef]
51. Komar, J.; Seifert, L.; Thouvarecq, R. What Variability tells us about motor expertise: Measurements and perspectives from a complex system approach. *Mov. Sport Sci.-Sci. Mot.* **2015**, *89*, 65–77. [CrossRef]
52. Downs, S.H.; Black, N. The feasibility of creating a checklist for the assessment of the methodological quality both of randomised and non-randomised studies of health care interventions. *J. Epidemiol. Community Health* **1998**, *52*, 377–384. [CrossRef] [PubMed]
53. Frane, A.V. Planned Hypothesis Tests Are Not Necessarily Exempt from Multiplicity Adjustment. *J. Res. Pract.* **2015**, *11*, 2.

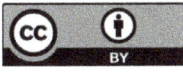

© 2020 by the authors. Licensee MDPI, Basel, Switzerland. This article is an open access article distributed under the terms and conditions of the Creative Commons Attribution (CC BY) license (http://creativecommons.org/licenses/by/4.0/).

 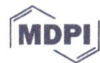

Article

Lower Back Complaints in Adolescent Competitive Alpine Skiers: A Cross-Sectional Study

Attilio Carraro [1,*], Martina Gnech [2], Fabio Sarto [3,*], Diego Sarto [2], Jörg Spörri [4,5] and Stefano Masiero [6]

1. Faculty of Education, Free University of Bolzano, 39042 Bressanone (Bolzano), Italy
2. School of Human Movement Sciences, University of Padova, 35122 Padova, Italy; gnechmartina@gmail.com (M.G.); centrostudi@diegosarto.it (D.S.)
3. Department of Biomedical Sciences, University of Padova, 35131 Padova, Italy
4. Sports Medical Research Group, Department of Orthopaedics, Balgrist University Hospital, University of Zurich, 8006 Zurich, Switzerland; joerg.spoerri@balgrist.ch
5. University Centre for Prevention and Sports Medicine, Department of Orthopaedics, Balgrist University Hospital, University of Zurich, 8006 Zurich, Switzerland
6. Department of Neurosciences, Section of Rehabilitation, University of Padova, 35128 Padova, Italy; stef.masiero@unipd.it
* Correspondence: attilio.carraro@unibz.it (A.C.); fabio.sarto.2@phd.unipd.it (F.S.); Tel.: +39-0472-01439 (A.C.); +39-0498275309 (F.S.)

Received: 7 October 2020; Accepted: 19 October 2020; Published: 22 October 2020

Abstract: Background: Little is known about lower back complaints in adolescent competitive alpine skiers. This study assessed their prevalence and severity (i.e., intensity and disability) with respect to sex, category, discipline preference, and training attributes. Methods: 188 competitive skiers aged 15 to 18 years volunteered in this study. Data collection included (i) questions on participants' demographics, sports exposure, discipline preferences, and other sports-related practices; (ii) the Nordic Musculoskeletal Questionnaire on lower back complaints; and (iii) the Graded Chronic Pain Scale. Results: As many as 80.3% and 50.0% of all skiers suffered from lower back complaints during the last 12 months and 7 days, respectively. A total of 50.7% reported their complaints to be attributable to slalom skiing, and 26% to giant slalom. The majority of complaints were classified as low intensity/low disability (Grade I, 57.4%) and high intensity/low disability complaints (Grade II, 21.8%). The Characteristic Pain Intensity was found to be significantly related to the skiers' years of sports participation, number of competitions/season, and number of skiing days/season. Conclusion: This study further supports the relatively high magnitudes of lower back-related pain in adolescent competitive alpine skiers, with a considerable amount of high intensity (but low disability) complaints, and training attributes being a key driver.

Keywords: alpine skiing; athletes' health; epidemiology; spine; musculoskeletal injuries

1. Introduction

Competitive alpine skiing is a popular yet high-risk sport. At all competition levels, health problems are frequent [1–7]. In particular, lower back has been reported to be one of the most affected body regions for overuse complaints [8]. Adolescent competitive alpine skiers are also known to suffer from relatively high rates of radiographic abnormalities in the thoracolumbar spine [9]. Specifically, degenerative disc changes were observed to be more prevalent in adolescent competitive alpine skiers than in age-matched controls [10]. Moreover, a recent study found such disc degenerations (particularly disc dehydration and disc protrusion) to be significantly more prevalent in symptomatic than in asymptomatic athletes [11]. However, little is known about the prevalence of lower back complaints in adolescent skiers with respect to severity (i.e., intensity and disability). Additionally, the role of discipline preference is widely unexplored as of yet.

The link between lower back pain and physical activity has been described as a U-shaped relationship, whereas increased risk was found for both sedentary subjects and those practicing strenuous physical activities [12]. According to this association, athletes may be considered a high-risk population, mainly due to the training and competition loads they are subjected to. Moreover, as a result of their musculoskeletal and spinal immaturity and excessive height growth, adolescent athletes are especially vulnerable [11,13].

From a biomechanical perspective, the following factors may contribute to overloading of the lower back structures in alpine ski racing [14]: (a) repetitive and heavy mechanical loads, particularly when accompanied by insufficient recovery between the training sessions [15]; (b) unphysiological postures (i.e., frontal bending, lateral bending, and torsion), associated with high ground reaction forces (up to 2.89 times the body weight) [16]; and (c) excessive exposure to low-frequency whole-body vibrations [17–20]. Since all of these factors are typical characteristics of alpine skiing-specific sports exposure, studying the relations between training attributes and lower back complaints is of superior importance.

Therefore, the aims of this study were: (1) to describe the demographics, sports exposure, and other sports- or warm-up-related practices of adolescent competitive alpine skiers; (2) to assess the prevalence of lower back complaints in this specific cohort with respect to sex, category, and discipline preference; (3) to explore their lower back complaints severity (i.e., intensity and disability); and (4) to investigate the potential relations with training attributes.

2. Materials and Methods

2.1. Study Design and Setting

This study was designed as a cross-sectional observation and was based on a structured and customized questionnaire package. Data were collected in the participants' sport clubs facilities at the end of the competition season. Questionnaires were spread physically. A member of the research team introduced the questionnaires to the participants, explaining all the questionnaire items and scales. Subsequently, the participants filled the questionnaires independently and individually.

2.2. Participants and Recruitment

Participants were included if they were members of ski clubs associated with the FISI (Italian Winter Sports Federation) Veneto region section and competed in the categories under 16 (U-16) and under 18 (U-18) years old. There were no study exclusions. All the ski clubs associated with the FISI Veneto region were contacted and invited to take part in the study. Finally, 188 adolescent competitive alpine skiers (110 males and 78 females) volunteered for the purpose of the current study; 128 belonged to the category U-16 and 60 to the U-18. The entire study sample represented about 70% of all U-16 and U-18 competitive alpine skiers affiliated to the FISI clubs in that region. The Ethics Committee of the Department of Biomedical Sciences of the University of Padua approved the study (HEC-DSB/02-19). Prior to the study, all the participants and their parents or legal representatives provided written informed consent. The participants did not receive any reward for their participation in the study.

2.3. Assessment Methods and Parameters

The questionnaire package comprised four parts: (1) questions on participants' demographics, sports exposure (years of sports participation, number of competitions/season, number of skiing days/season, number of athletic preparation days/season) and other sports- or warm-up-related practices; (2) the Nordic Musculoskeletal Questionnaire (NMQ), Italian version [21,22]; (3) specific questions on how their skiing discipline (e.g., Slalom—SL; Giant Slalom—GS; Super-G—SG;

or Downhill (DH)) was related to the occurrence of lower back complaints; (4) the Graded Chronic Pain Scale (GCPS), Italian version [23,24].

The NMQ aimed on investigating the time prevalence of musculoskeletal complaints in the lower back during the last 12 months and 7 days, respectively, as well as on whether these complaints resulted in any restrictions while carrying out normal activities or whether they required medical attention or not. Questionnaire completion was supported by a body map displaying the pain area. The GCPS was used to grade the severity of the lower back complaints. The underlying methodology consists of seven questions related to pain intensity items and disability items with respect to the 6 months preceding the questionnaire. Answers were provided on a scale from 0 (e.g., "no pain" or "no interference/change") to 10 (e.g., "pain as bad it could be" or "unable to carry on any activity/extreme change") [23]. Based on these scale points, as well as on a specific scoring system, the Characteristic Pain Intensity (0–100), Disability Score (0–100), and Disability Points (0–3) were calculated and, subsequently, were assigned to five severity grades, as described in Von Korff et al. [23]: Grade 0 (pain-free); Grade I (low disability—low intensity); Grade II (low disability, high intensity); Grade III (high disability, moderately limiting); and Grade IV (high disability—severely limiting).

2.4. Statistical Analysis

Participant demographics, sports exposure, and training/competition/other sports practices were expressed as the mean ± SD and percentage proportions, respectively. NMQ-related measures and GCPS-based classifications were expressed as the absolute number and percentage of participants affected. The GCPS scores were described as the mean ± SD. All the measures were presented for the entire sample and the subgroups based on sex (female and male) and competition category (U-16 and U-18). Prevalence was additionally described with respect to the discipline to which they were perceived as being attributable. Pearson's Chi-squared tests were used to assess the potential sex and category differences in measures with percentage proportions at $p < 0.05$. Independent sample t-tests were used to evaluate the sex and category differences in interval scaled measures at $p < 0.05$. Pearson's correlation analysis was performed on GCPS items and scores, as well as on the relationship between GCPS scores, years of sports participation, number of competitions/season, number of skiing days/season, and number of athletic preparation days/season. For any correlation analysis, statistical significance was set at $p \leq 0.05$.

3. Results

3.1. Participant Demographics, Sports Exposure and Training/Competition/Other Sports Practices

Male participants were characterized as follows: age: 16.1 ± 1.1 y; weight: 65 ± 10 kg; height: 1.74 ± 0.08 m; BMI: 21.5 ± 2.3 kg/m^2; years of sports participation: 8.1 ± 2.4 y. The group of female participants had the following characteristics: age: 16 ± 1 years; weight: 56.2 ± 6.4 kg; height: 1.65 ± 0.05 m; BMI: 20.7 ± 1.9 kg/m^2; years of sports participation: 7.1 ± 2.9 y. Over the past competition (i.e., winter) season, the participants reported a mean of 85.4 ± 47.2 days (3.5 ± 1.3 days/week) of ski training and participated in 17.2 ± 12.0 competitions on average. Independent sample t-tests revealed no significant differences between the sexes. However, there were significant differences in the number of skiing days/season (t (186) = 2.18, $p = 0.029$) and the number of competitions in the last season (t (186) = 7.22, $p < 0.001$) between the U-16 and U-18 categories, with athletes in the U-18 category who performed more skiing days and competitions. Most participants (62.8%) declared that they practiced one or more sports other than alpine skiing, 83.5% reported that they participated in specific athletic preparation programs, and 78.3% declared that they regularly warm-up before skiing. The Chi-squared tests revealed, however, no significant sex or category differences in these variables at $p < 0.05$.

3.2. Prevalence of Lower Back Complaints

An overview of the NMQ-related results is presented in Table 1. A total of 80.3% of all participants reported having suffered from lower back complaints during the last 12 months, and 50.0% during the last 7 days. As many as 28.2% reported that they have been restricted in normal activities (e.g., job and leisure activities) during the last 12 months, and 27.7% indicated that their lower back complaints required medical attention during the last 12 months. Except for lower back complaints during the last 7 seven days, which were more frequent in females, there were found no sex or category differences. Interestingly, 50.7% of the participants reported their lower back complaints being attributed to performing SL, 26.0% to GS, and 7.3% to SG; meanwhile, no participants attributed their lower back complaints to DH skiing. A remarkable season period-related difference in the frequency patterns of lower back complaints was found between the competition period and the off-season period. During the off-season period, only 3.3% reported their lower back complaints to last longer than two weeks, while during the competition period this percentage proportion was more than six times higher (21.3%).

Table 1. Overview of the Nordic Musculoskeletal Questionnaire (NMQ)-based results and differences between sexes and categories.

NMQ Measure	Overall $n = 188$	Male $n = 110$	Female $n = 78$	$\chi^2(df), p$	U-16 $n = 128$	U-18 $n = 60$	$\chi^2(df), p$
Lower back complaints during the last 12 months	(151) 80.3%	(89) 80.9%	(62) 79.5%	n.s.	(103) 80.5%	(48) 80%	n.s.
Lower back complaints during the last 7 days	(94) 50%	(42) 42.7%	(47) 60.3%	5.61(1) 0.018	(65) 50.8%	(29) 48.3%	n.s.
Restricted in normal activities during the last 12 months	(53) 28.2%	(31) 28.2%	(22) 28.2%	n.s.	(36) 28.1%	(17) 28.3%	n.s.
Required medical attention during the last 12 months	(52) 27.7%	(33) 30%	(19) 24.4%	n.s.	(35) 27.3%	(17) 28.3%	n.s.

All NMQ-related measures are expressed as absolute numbers and the percentage proportion on the overall group/subgroups (number of affected skiers/number of skiers per group × 100). Levels of significance for sex and category differences are based on Pearson chi-square tests. n.s.: not significant at $p < 0.05$; U-16: under 16 years; U-18: under 18 years.

3.3. Severity of Lower Back Complaints

The GCPS-related results are summarized in Table 2. The mean value of Characteristic Pain Intensity was 37.53 ± 18.0 and the Disability Score was 13.27 ± 14.59 on average. There were no significant sex or category differences at $p < 0.05$. Most participants (57.4%) suffered from low intensity—low disability complaints (Grade I), and 21.8% from high intensity—low disability complaints (Grade II). Again, there were no significant differences between males and females, or between U-16 and U-18 skiers.

Table 2. Overview of the Graded Chronic Pain Scale (GCPS) scores and differences between sexes and categories.

GCPS Score	Overall $n = 188$	Male $n = 110$	Female $n = 78$	t(df), p	U-16 $n = 128$	U-18 $n = 60$	t(df), p
Characteristic Pain Intensity	37.53 ± 18.0	28.30 ± 21.98	32.26 ± 22.11	n.s.	30.62 ± 22.71	28.50 ± 20.70	n.s.
Disability Score	13.27 ± 14.59	11.29 ± 15.22	9.61 ± 12.32	n.s	11.51 ± 15.06	8.64 ± 11.59	n.s
GCPS Classification				χ^2			χ^2
Grade 0 Pain free	(39) 20.7%	(23) 20.9%	(16) 20.5%	n.s.	(27) 21.1%	(12) 20%	n.s.
Grade I Low intensity-Low disability	(108) 57.4%	(64) 58.2%	(44) 56.4%	n.s.	(70) 54.7%	(38) 63.3%	n.s.
Grade II High intensity-Low disability	(41) 21.8%	(23) 20.9%	(18) 23.1%	n.s.	(31) 24.2%	(10) 16.7%	n.s
Grade III High Disability-Moderately Limiting	—	—	—	—	—	—	—
Grade IV High Disability-Severely Limiting	—	—	—	—	—	—	—

GCPS scores are expressed as mean ± SD. GCPS classifications are expressed as absolute numbers and the percentage proportion of the overall group/subgroups (number of affected skiers/number of skiers per group × 100). Levels of significance for sex and category differences are based on independent sample t-tests and Pearson chi-square tests, respectively. n.s.: not significant at $p < 0.05$; U-16: under 16 years; U-18: under 18 years.

3.4. Relationship between Different Severity Measures, as well as between Severity and Training Attributes

We found a medium-correlation Characteristic Pain Intensity and Disability Score ($r = 0.62$, $p < 0.01$). Moreover, the average lower back complaint intensity, as well as the intensity at the time of filling out the questionnaire, positively correlated with the worst pain intensity experienced within the last 6 months ($r = 0.63$, $p < 0.01$; $r = 0.47$, $p < 0.01$, respectively).

The results of the correlation analysis between the GCPS scores and different training attributes are highlighted in Table 3. There were small yet significant correlations between the Characteristic Pain Intensity and the training attributes "years of sports participation", "number of competitions/season", and "number of skiing days/season". Moreover, an additional independent *t*-test showed a significant difference ($t (186) = 2.12$, $p = 0.035$, $d = 0.31$) in the lower back complaint severity (i.e., GCPS—Characteristic Pain Intensity) between skiers who exclusively practiced alpine skiing and those who also practiced other sports, with the first group reporting higher intensities.

Table 3. Correlation between the Grading Chronic Pain Scale scores and questions on sports exposure.

	Characteristic Pain Intensity	Disability Score
Years of sports participation	0.28 **	0.15 *
Number of competitions/season	0.21 **	−0.02
Number of skiing days/season	0.27 **	0.12
Number of athletic preparation days/season	0.03	−0.09

Level of significance based on Pearson correlation analysis: * $p < 0.05$, ** $p < 0.01$.

4. Discussion

The main findings of this study were: (1) as many as 80.3% of all participating adolescent skiers suffered from lower back complaints during the last 12 months (50.0% during the last 7 days; 28.2% with restrictions in normal activities; and 27.7% requiring medical attention); (2) 50.7% of the participants reported their lower back complaints being attributable to SL, and 26.0% to GS; (3) despite the fact that the majority of the participants experienced lower back complaints of a low intensity/low disability (Grade I, 57.4%), a considerable portion suffered from a high intensity/low disability complaints (Grade II, 21.8%); (4) there were small yet significant correlations between the Characteristic Pain Intensity and the training attributes "years of sports participation", "number of competitions/season", and "number of skiing days/season".

4.1. Prevalence of Lower Back Complaints with Respect to Sex, Category and Discipline Preference

The current study found relatively high rates of lower back complaints in adolescent competitive alpine skiers. Indeed, 50.0% and 80.3% of the participants displayed lower back complaints in the last 7 days and 12 months, respectively. These values are considerably higher than those was previously reported for other populations. For example, a 12 months lower back pain prevalence of between 49.8% and 65.0% was observed in previous studies in elite athletes of different sports [25–27]. A 7 days lower back pain prevalence between 19.4% and 25.3% was reported for endurance athletes [25]. Previous works found a 12 months lower back complaints prevalence ranging from 20.5% to 57.0% in non-athletic adolescents [25,28,29], while a 7 days lower back complaints prevalence of about 20.0% was reported for young non-athletes [25].

The higher prevalence of lower back complaints observed in the present study compared to other athletic (and non-athletic) adolescents suggests that competitive alpine skiers are especially prone for lower back complaints. Indeed, in the sport of alpine ski racing, repetitive and heavy mechanical loads, high ground reaction forces, and the exposure to low-frequency whole-body vibrations have been shown to adversely affect the spinal structures while skiing [14,16,17]. Moreover, in young skiers, the immaturity of the musculoskeletal system may exacerbate the damage experienced by the spine during the practice of this sport [13].

Despite these plausible sports-related adverse loading patterns, only a few studies, however, have investigated the occurrence of lower back complaints in competitive alpine skiers. Moreover, due to focusing on a different age group and reporting other time prevalence measures or absolute injury rates, most of them are not directly comparable to the results of the current study [3,4,6,8,11]. The only study directly comparable to our investigation reported similar magnitudes of current low back pain (67.0%) in ski high school athletes aged 15–19 years [30].

Noteworthy, in our study, a higher 7 days lower back complaints prevalence was observed in females with respect to males (60.3% vs. 42.7%). These results are in agreement with previous works and, on the one hand, may be explained by a different pain threshold and symptom perception between males and females [31,32]. On the other hand, this sex difference may also be explained by the different anatomical characteristics of the female body (e.g., greater spine flexibility), as well as the different pubertal growth and hormonal states [33,34].

Furthermore, our study revealed that, during the 12 months prior to data collection, 28.2% of the participants were restricted in carrying out normal daily life activities, while 27.2% needed to see a physician. This latter percentage is similar to the magnitudes found in previous studies (range between 24.0 and 33.0%) including large cohorts of children and adolescents [35,36].

Interestingly, we found different skiing disciplines to have different perceived impacts on lower back complaints. Indeed, 50.7% attributed their lower back complaints to SL, while 26.0% reported to have suffered them in connection with GS and 7.3% with SG. None of the participants attributed their lower back complaints to DH. A possible explanation is that, in SL, there are more pronounced and larger ground reaction force peaks (approximately plus 20.0%) after gate passage than in GS [37].

Regarding the prevalence of lower back complaints according to the annual programming period, we found that the prevalence of lower back complaints lasting less than 7 days was 86.0% in the off-season and 33.3% in the competition season. Conversely, the frequency of lower back complaints lasting more than two weeks changed from 3.3% in the off-season to 21.3% in the period of the competition season. This fact may suggest that more severe lower back complaints emerge from skiing rather than from off-snow training [3].

4.2. Severity of Lower Back Complaints with Respect to Intensity and Disability

Another aim of this work was to study the severity (i.e., pain intensity and disability) of lower back complaints in adolescent competitive alpine skiers. Despite the fact that most of the participants (57.4%) reported low intensity—low disability complaints (Grade I of the GCPS), 21.8% showed high intensity—low disability complaints (Grade II). These findings showed that a considerable part of the participants suffered from a relatively high severity of lower back complaints already at a relatively young age (15–18 y). However, the pain resulted in being of low disability, which is in agreement with previous studies in adolescent athletes [25,38]. One potential explanation for this finding may be the consideration that the cohort of the current study consisted of relatively young athletes, who may not have suffered from an extensive accumulation of adverse loadings over time yet.

4.3. Relationship between Lower Back Complaints Severity and Training Attributes

The current study revealed small yet significant correlations between Characteristic Pain Intensity and the training attributes "years of sports participation", "number of competitions/season", and "number of skiing days/season". These findings further support our current understanding of the development of lower back overuse injuries, according to which an accumulation of adverse loadings on the athletes' spine is a key driver for inducing pain [16]. However, the present sample was homogeneous with respect to training attributes, since the participants of our study belonged to ski clubs of the same region. Therefore, the results of this study may be specific to our cohort and should be interpreted with caution.

4.4. Methodological Considerations

Despite providing valuable new insights into the prevalence and severity of lower back complaints in adolescent competitive alpine skiers, this study has some limitations that one should be aware of. First, the retrospective nature of the NMQ and GCPS methodologies may cause them to suffer from a recall bias. Recent and more severe complaints are more likely to be remembered than older and less severe ones. Second, the background and experience of the participants filling out the questionnaires may influence the outcomes. Third, other potential cofounders for lower back complaints, such as smoking, hours of sleep per night, and psychosocial factors (depression, stress, poor academic performance, poor competitive results, etc.), were not evaluated in this study.

5. Conclusions

This study provides a new set of data regarding the prevalence and severity of lower back complaints in a sample of adolescent competitive alpine racers. It further supports the relatively high magnitudes of lower back-related pain, with a considerable amount of high intensity but low disability complaints. Interestingly, more low back complains were reported during SL and GS than other skiing disciplines. Moreover, this study further highlights an accumulation of adverse loadings on the athletes' spine being a key driver for developing pain conditions. Accordingly, adolescent competitive alpine skiers should be particularly protected by rigorous prevention strategies already before reaching adolescence.

Author Contributions: Conceptualization, A.C., D.S., and S.M.; investigation, M.G.; resources, D.S. and M.G.; data curation, A.C., F.S., and M.G.; writing—original draft preparation, F.S., M.G. and J.S.; writing—review and editing A.C., J.S., and S.M. All authors have read and agreed to the published version of the manuscript.

Funding: This research received no external funding.

Acknowledgments: The authors would like to thank the participants for their kind participation and their coaches, ski clubs, and the FISI Veneto Committee for supporting and facilitating the completion of this study.

Conflicts of Interest: The authors declare no conflict of interest.

References

1. Flørenes, T.W.; Bere, T.; Nordsletten, L.; Heir, S.; Bahr, R. Injuries among male and female World Cup alpine skiers. *Br. J. Sports Med.* **2009**, *43*, 973–978. [CrossRef] [PubMed]
2. Bere, T.; Flørenes, T.W.; Nordsletten, L.; Bahr, R. Sex differences in the risk of injury in World Cup alpine skiers: A 6-year cohort study. *Br. J. Sports Med.* **2014**, *48*, 36–40. [CrossRef] [PubMed]
3. Schoeb, T.; Peterhans, L.; Fröhlich, S.; Frey, W.O.; Gerber, C.; Spörri, J. Health problems in youth competitive alpine skiing: A 12-month observation of 155 athletes around the growth spurt. *Scand. J. Med. Sci. Sports* **2020**. [CrossRef] [PubMed]
4. Fröhlich, S.; Helbling, M.; Fucentese, S.F.; Karlen, W.; Frey, W.O.; Spörri, J. Injury risks among elite competitive alpine skiers are underestimated if not registered prospectively, over the entire season and regardless of whether requiring medical attention. *Knee Surgery Sport. Traumatol. Arthrosc.* **2020**. [CrossRef]
5. Müller, L.; Hildebrandt, C.; Müller, E.; Oberhoffer, R.; Raschner, C. Injuries and illnesses in a cohort of elite youth alpine ski racers and the influence of biological maturity and relative age: A two-season prospective study. *Open Access J. Sport. Med.* **2017**, *8*, 113–122. [CrossRef]
6. Alhammoud, M.; Racinais, S.; Rousseaux-Blanchi, M.P.; Bouscaren, N. Recording injuries only during winter competitive season underestimates injury incidence in elite alpine skiers. *Scand. J. Med. Sci. Sport.* **2020**, *30*, 1177–1187. [CrossRef]
7. Westin, M.; Alricsson, M.; Werner, S. Injury profile of competitive alpine skiers: A five-year cohort study. *Knee Surgery Sport. Traumatol. Arthrosc.* **2012**, *20*, 1175–1181. [CrossRef] [PubMed]

8. Hildebrandt, M.C.; Raschner, A.C. Traumatic and overuse injuries among elite adolescent alpine skiers: A two-year retrospective analysis. *Int. Sport. J.* **2013**, *14*, 245–255.
9. Rachbauer, F.; Sterzinger, W.; Eibl, G. Radiographic Abnormalities in the Thoracolumbar Spine of Young Elite Skiers. *Am. J. Sports Med.* **2001**, *29*, 446–449. [CrossRef]
10. Witwit, W.A.; Kovac, P.; Sward, A.; Agnvall, C.; Todd, C.; Thoreson, O.; Hebelka, H.; Baranto, A. Disc degeneration on MRI is more prevalent in young elite skiers compared to controls. *Knee Surg. Sport. Traumatol. Arthrosc.* **2018**, *26*, 325–332. [CrossRef]
11. Peterhans, L.; Fröhlich, S.; Stern, C.; Frey, W.O.; Farshad, M.; Sutter, R.; Spörri, J. High Rates of Overuse-Related Structural Abnormalities in the Lumbar Spine of Youth Competitive Alpine Skiers: A Cross-sectional MRI Study in 108 Athletes. *Orthop. J. Sport. Med.* **2020**, *8*, 1–10. [CrossRef]
12. Heneweer, H.; Vanhees, L.; Picavet, H.S.J. Physical activity and low back pain: A U-shaped relation? *Pain* **2009**, *143*, 21–25. [CrossRef]
13. Meyer, M.; Laurent, C.; Higgins, R.; Skelly, W. Downhill ski injuries in children and adolescents. *Sport. Med.* **2007**, *37*, 485–499. [CrossRef]
14. Spörri, J.; Kröll, J.; Supej, M.; Müller, E. Reducing the back overuse-related risks in alpine ski racing: Let's put research into sports practice. *Br. J. Sports Med.* **2019**, *53*, 2–3. [CrossRef]
15. Soligard, T.; Schwellnus, M.; Alonso, J.M.; Bahr, R.; Clarsen, B.; Dijkstra, H.P.; Gabbett, T.; Gleeson, M.; Hägglund, M.; Hutchinson, M.R.; et al. How much is too much? (Part 1) International Olympic Committee consensus statement on load in sport and risk of injury. *Br. J. Sports Med.* **2016**, *50*, 1030–1041. [CrossRef]
16. Spörri, J.; Kroll, J.C.H.; Fasel, B.; Muller, E. Potential Mechanisms Leading to Overuse Injuries of the Back in Alpine Ski Racing A Descriptive Biomechanical Study. *Am. J. Sports Med.* **2015**, *43*, 2042–2048. [CrossRef]
17. Spörri, J.; Kröll, J.; Fasel, B.; Aminian, K.; Müller, E. The Use of Body Worn Sensors for Detecting the Vibrations Acting on the Lower Back in Alpine Ski Racing. *Front. Phyisiol.* **2017**, *8*, 522. [CrossRef]
18. Supej, M.; Ogrin, J.; Holmberg, H. Whole-Body Vibrations Associated With Alpine Skiing: A Risk Factor for Low Back Pain? *Front. Phyisiol.* **2018**, *9*, 204. [CrossRef]
19. Supej, M.; Ogrin, J. Transmissibility of whole-body vibrations and injury risk in alpine skiing. *J. Sci. Med. Sport* **2019**, *22*, S71–S77. [CrossRef]
20. Tarabini, M.; Saggin, B.; Scaccabarozzi, D. Whole-body vibration exposure in sport: Four relevant cases. *Ergonomics* **2015**, *58*, 1143–1150. [CrossRef]
21. Kuorinka, I.; Jonsson, B.; Kilbom, A.; Vinterberg, H.; Biering-Sørensen, F.; Andersson, G.; Jørgensen, K. Standardised Nordic questionnaires for the analysis of musculoskeletal symptoms. *Appl. Ergon.* **1987**, *18*, 233–237. [CrossRef]
22. Gobba, F.; Ghersi, R.; Martinelli, S.; Richeldi, A.; Clerici, P.; Grazioli, P. Traduzione in lingua italiana e validazione del questionario standardizzato Nordic IRSST per la rilevazione di disturbi muscoloscheletrici. *Med. del Lav.* **2008**, *99*, 424–443.
23. Von Korff, M.; Ormel, J.; Keefe, F.J.; Dworkin, S.F. Clinical Section Grading the severity of chronic pain. *Pain* **1992**, *50*, 133–149. [CrossRef]
24. Salaffi, F.; Stancati, A.; Grassi, W. Reliability and validity of the Italian version of the Chronic Pain Grade questionnaire in patients with musculoskeletal disorders. *Clin. Rheumatol.* **2006**, *25*, 619–631. [CrossRef] [PubMed]
25. Bahr, R.; Andersen, S.O.; Løken, S.; Fossan, B. Low Back Pain Among Endurance Athletes With and Without Specific Back Loading—A Cross-Sectional Survey of Cross-Country Skiers, Rowers, Orienteerers, and Nonathletic Controls. *Spine* **2004**, *29*, 449–454. [CrossRef]
26. Schulz, S.S.; Lenz, K.; Büttner-Janz, K. Severe back pain in elite athletes: A cross-sectional study on 929 top athletes of Germany. *Eur. Spine J.* **2016**, *25*, 1204–1210. [CrossRef]
27. Fett, D.; Trompeter, K.; Platen, P. Back pain in elite sports: A cross-sectional study on 1114 athletes. *PLoS ONE* **2017**, *12*, e0180130. [CrossRef]
28. Masiero, S.; Carraro, E.; Celia, A.; Sarto, D.; Ermani, M. Prevalence of nonspecific low back pain in schoolchildren aged between 13 and 15 years. *Acta Pædiatrica* **2008**, *97*, 212–216. [CrossRef]
29. Kędra, A.; Czaprowski, D. Epidemiology of back pain in children and youth aged 10–19 from the area of the southeast of Poland. *Biomed Res. Int.* **2013**, *2013*. [CrossRef]
30. Bergstrøm, K.A.; Brandseth, K.; Fretheim, S.; Tvilde, K.; Ekeland, A. Back injuries and pain in adolescents attending a ski high school. *Knee Surgery Sport. Traumatol. Arthrosc.* **2004**, *12*, 80–85. [CrossRef]

31. Keogh, E.; Eccleston, C. Sex Differences in Adolescent Chronic Pain and Pain-Related Coping. *Pain* **2006**, *12*, 275–284. [CrossRef] [PubMed]
32. Mingheli, B.; Raul, O.; Nunes, C. Non-specific Low Back Pain in Adolescents From the South of Portugal: Prevalence and Associated Factors. *J. Orthop. Sci.* **2014**, *19*, 883–892. [CrossRef]
33. Shehab, D.K.; Al-Jarallah, K.F. Nonspecific low-back pain in Kuwaiti children and adolescents: Associated factors. *J. Adolesc. Heal.* **2005**, *36*, 32–35. [CrossRef]
34. Balanguè, F.; Damidot, P.; Nordin, M.; Parnianpour, M.; Waldburger, M. Cross-sectional Study of the Isokinetic Muscle Trunk Strength Among School Children. *Spine* **1993**, *18*, 1199–1205. [CrossRef] [PubMed]
35. Masiero, S.; Carraro, E.; Sarto, D.; Bonaldo, L.; Ferraro, C. Healthcare service use in adolescents with non-specific musculoskeletal pain. *Acta Paediatr.* **2010**, *99*, 1224–1228. [CrossRef]
36. Watson, K.D.; Papageorgiou, A.C.; Jones, G.T.; Taylor, S.; Symmons, D.P.M.; Silman, A.J.; Macfarlane, G.J. Low back pain in schoolchildren: Occurrence and characteristics. *Pain* **2002**, *97*, 87–92. [CrossRef]
37. Spörri, J.; Kröll, J.; Fasel, B.; Aminian, K.; Müller, E. Course Setting as a Prevention Measure for Overuse Injuries of the Back in Alpine Ski Racing. *Orthop. J. Sport. Med.* **2016**, *4*, 1–8. [CrossRef]
38. Müller, J.; Müller, S.; Stoll, J.; Fröhlich, K.; Otto, C.; Mayer, F. Back pain prevalence in adolescent athletes. *Scand. J. Med. Sci. Sports* **2017**, *27*, 448–454. [CrossRef]

Publisher's Note: MDPI stays neutral with regard to jurisdictional claims in published maps and institutional affiliations.

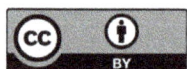

© 2020 by the authors. Licensee MDPI, Basel, Switzerland. This article is an open access article distributed under the terms and conditions of the Creative Commons Attribution (CC BY) license (http://creativecommons.org/licenses/by/4.0/).

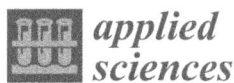 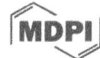

Article

Effects of Backpack Loads on Leg Muscle Activation during Slope Walking

Yali Liu [1], Ligang Qiang [2], Qiuzhi Song [1], Mingsheng Zhao [1] and Xinyu Guan [3,*]

1. Department of Mechanical and Engineering, Beijing Institute of Technology, Haidian, Beijing 100081, China; buaaliuyali@126.com (Y.L.); qzhsong@bit.edu.cn (Q.S.); 18351898665@163.com (M.Z.)
2. Robot Research Institute, Guizhou Aerospace Control Technology co., LTD, Economic and Technological Development District, Guiyang 550000, China; qiangligang123@163.com
3. Division of Intelligent and Biomechanical System, State Key Laboratory of Tribology, Tsinghua University, Haidian, Beijing 100086, China
* Correspondence: guanxinyu@mail.tsinghua.edu.cn

Received: 15 June 2020; Accepted: 13 July 2020; Published: 16 July 2020

Abstract: Hikers and soldiers usually walk up and down slopes with a load carriage, causing injuries of the musculoskeletal system, especially during a prolonged load journey. The slope walking has been reported to lead to higher leg extensor muscle activities and joint moments. However, most of the studies investigated muscle activities or joint moments during slope walking without load carriage or only investigated the joint moment changes and muscle activities with load carriages during level walking. Whether the muscle activation such as the signal amplitude is influenced by the mixed factor of loads and grades and whether the influence of the degrees of loads and grades on different muscles are equal have not yet been investigated. To explore the effects of backpack loads on leg muscle activation during slope walking, ten young male participants walked at 1.11 m/s on a treadmill with different backpack loads (load masses: 0, 10, 20, and 30 kg) during slope walking (grade: 0, 3, 5, and 10°). Leg muscles, including the gluteus maximus (GM), rectus femoris (RF), hamstrings (HA), anterior tibialis (AT), and medial gastrocnemius (GA), were recorded during walking. The hip, knee, and ankle extensor muscle activations increased during the slope walking, and the hip muscles increased most among hip, knee, and ankle muscles (GM and HA increased by 46% to 207% and 110% to 226%, respectively, during walking steeper than 10° across all load masses (GM: $p = 1.32 \times 10^{-8}$ and HA: $p = 2.33 \times 10^{-16}$)). Muscle activation increased pronouncedly with loads, and the knee extensor muscles increased greater than the hip and ankle muscles (RF increased by 104% to 172% with a load mass greater than 30 kg across all grades (RF: $p = 8.86 \times 10^{-7}$)). The results in our study imply that the hip and knee muscles play an important role during slope walking with loads. The hip and knee extension movements during slope walking should be considerably assisted to lower the muscle activations, which will be useful for designing assistant devices, such as exoskeleton robots, to enhance hikers' and soldiers' walking abilities.

Keywords: muscle activations; electromyography; slope walking; backpack loads

---

Highlights

- Hip extensor muscle activations increase most during slope walking;
- Muscles increased pronouncedly during slope walking with backpack loads;
- Knee extensor muscle activations increased most with increasing backpack loads.

1. Introduction

Hiking is a popular exercise providing benefits, including the acceleration of calorie consumption and the burning of fat tissue [1,2]. Hiking on slopes and with backpack loads can cause pain and injuries of the musculoskeletal system, especially during a prolonged load journey [3–5].

Walking with load carriage leads to high energetic consumptions and joint moments. Many studies have explored the energetics and kinematics with different backpack loads during level walking [6–10]. Karen et al. [6] analyzed the energy cost of walking with and without a backpack load and pointed out that the load increased the oxygen uptake at a constant rate. Raymond et al. [7] further analyzed the effects of load masses added to the legs on energetics and biomechanics. They summarized that the metabolic rate increased with the load mass and the kinematics and muscle moments increased rapidly with loads at the feet. Additionally, the increased metabolic rate with the load carriage may be caused by increased ankle positive work during push-off [8]. Morrison et al. [9] also analyzed the motion entropy changes to the load carriage at a joint level and pointed out that the entropy of spine slide flexion increased while hip flexion entropy decreased. Kari et al. [11] pointed out the sex effect on the kinematics with loads: females used more hip and knee moments with loads compared to males during walking. Furthermore, Krajewski [12] studied the effect of load carriage magnitudes and different locomotion patterns (fast run and force marching) on knee moments.

Most studies investigating load carriages suggest a positive correlation exists between load mass and joint moments, as well as energetics. However, joint moments or joint work in one gait calculated by joint moments and angular displacement do not account for muscle activations during load carriage walking [13]. Researchers have made explorations into the muscle activation patterns during level walking with load carriages [4,5,14]. Karina et al. [4] found that the muscle activity changed differently with increased load masses to adjust to maintain balance and attenuate the loads placed on lower limbs. The muscle activations of the soleus, medial gastrocnemius (GA), lateral hamstrings (HA), and rectus femoris (RF) increased with load, and the muscle activation patterns were similar between men and women [5]. Kenneth et al. [14] studied the musculoskeletal stiffness during load carriages at different walking speeds and found the musculoskeletal stiffness increased as a function of both speed and load. Walsh et al. [15] investigated the effect of stable and unstable load carriages on muscles of older adults. They pointed out that unstable load carriages increased the activity of the RF and soleus, while stable load carriages increased the RF activity.

Subjects such as soldiers and hikers who habitually walk uphill with load carriages usually feel tired because of muscle fatigue. It is important to design assistive devices for soldiers and hikers according to the load carriage effects. A backpack load, for example, increases the dynamic forces on the human body. Huang et al. [16] and Yang et al. [17] designed suspended-load backpacks as an assistive device to reduce the dynamic forces.

Slope walking has been reported to lead to greater leg extensor muscle activities and joint moments. However, most of the studies investigated muscle activities [18–20] or joint moments [21–24] during slope walking without load carriages or only investigated the joint moment changes [9,10,12] and muscle activities [15,16,25] with load carriages during level walking. Whether the muscle activations such as the signal amplitude are influenced by the mixed factor of load mass and grade and whether the influence of the degrees of load mass and grade on different muscles are equal have not yet been investigated. It is important to know how the muscles are activated during one gait when slope walking with backpack loads for designing assistive devices, such as exoskeleton robots, to enhance people's movement abilities with backpack loads.

This study aimed at investigating the effects of load carriages on muscle activities during slope walking to provide suggestions for the design of assistive devices. We hypothesized that (1) hip, knee, and ankle extensor muscle signal amplitudes during one gait would increase during the slope walking compared to level walking, especially the hip extensor muscles, such as the gluteus maximus (GM) and HA; (2) the muscle signal amplitudes would increase pronouncedly with loads during slope walking; (3) the muscle signal amplitudes would increase at different degrees. The knee extensor muscles, such as the RF, would be activated more compared to the hip and ankle extensor muscles, such as GM, HA, and GA.

2. Methods

2.1. Subjects

Ten young male adults volunteered for this study (mean ± standard deviation; age: 24.10 ± 1.79 years, height: 175.30 ± 5.12 cm, and mass: 69.40 ± 8.15 kg). All subjects were familiar with treadmill walking and had no neuromuscular, cardiovascular, or orthopedic diseases. All subjects were provided with the informed consent form for the experiment, and the experiment was approved by the Ethics Committee of Beijing Sport University (No. 2019007H (2019.01–2021.01)).

2.2. Experimental Protocol

Subjects walked on a force treadmill (Bertec, Columbus, OH, USA), on which the walking grade and walking speed could be adjusted accordingly. Each subject was familiarized with walking on the treadmill for about 5 min with the walking speed set to 1.11 m/s and the walking grade set to 0°. The speed of 1.11 m/s (4 km/h) was selected according to the American College of Sports Medicine [22] and the literature on uphill and downhill walking [23]. Each subject was required to walk for 2 min on the treadmill with three mass backpack loads (10, 20, and 30 kg) during four grades (level (0°), 3, 5, and 10° grades). The level and slope walking on the treadmill without loads (0 kg) were also completed by each subject as a reference. Subjects were asked to perform all the load mass tests at one certain grade in order to shorten the experiment time. The load masses were in random order during one grade test, and the grade testes were also in random order. Subjects were asked to walk at one grade for 3 min with one load during one trial. Subjects rested for 3 min between different load mass trials and 30 min between different grade tests. The experimenters adjusted the load mass and the walking grade while the participants rested. The speed of the treadmill was set to 1.11 m/s in every trial. The temporal stride kinematics and surface electromyographic (EMG) during the final 30 s of each trial were recorded.

The temporal stride kinematics were calculated according to the ground force data recorded by the force platform in the treadmill. Two force platforms were embedded in the treadmill and recorded the ground interactive forces and moments between foot and ground. The software in the optical motion-capture system (Motion, Columbus, OH, USA) [26] calculated the center of force operation based on the forces and moments.

The EMG signals were collected by the wireless EMG system (Delsys Trigno™ Wireless EMG System (Natick, MA, USA)). The muscles selected included the GM, RF, HA, anterior tibialis (AT), and GA, which are the main activated muscles during human lower extremity movements [27]. The pre-amplified single differential electrodes (Trigno, Delsys, Natick, MA, USA) were placed on the muscle bellies after preparing the skin with alcohol (the schematic diagram of human lower limb muscles in this study is shown in Figure 1). The surface EMG (sEMG) signal sensors were fixed with double-sided tapes and bandages to prevent displacement between the sensors and muscles during walking.

This optical motion capture system (Motion, Columbus, OH, USA) can integrate the Delsys device and the Bertec force platforms by a data acquisition card (DAQ, National Instruments, Austin, TX, USA); thus, the sEMG signal and kinetic data can be collected simultaneously. The sampling frequency was selected as 1200 Hz.

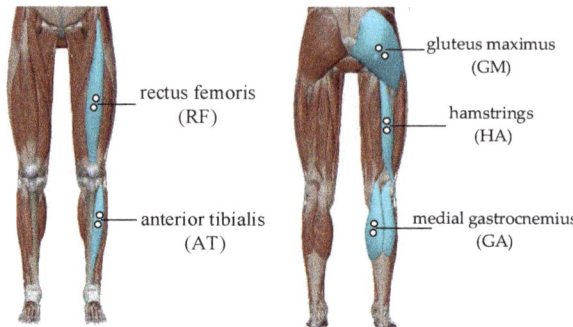

Figure 1. The schematic diagram of the human lower limb muscles in this study. The position of the two white points on one muscle represented the position of the electromyographic (EMG) electrodes attached.

2.3. Data Analysis

2.3.1. The Temporal Stride Parameters

The kinetic data were obtained by the output of the software provided by the optical motion-capture system (Cortex-64, Santa Rosa, CA, USA), which was linked with the force treadmill system (Bertec, Columbus, OH, USA). Raw kinetic data were smoothed using a 4th-order Butterworth filter with a cutoff frequency of 10 Hz [28]. We then used vertical ground reaction force data and a threshold of 20 N (on the basis of the standard deviation of the vertical ground reaction force signal during leg swing) [29] to determine the heel strike and toe-off for each leg and computed the temporal characteristics of each trial using custom software (MathWorks Inc., Natick, MA, USA). The step length was determined as the distance between the point where the left heel strike occurred and the point where the right heel strike occurred in the walking direction, and the step width was determined as the distance between the two heel strike points in the walking transverse distance [30].

2.3.2. The EMG Analysis

The raw EMG signals were filtered by a bidirectional Butterworth band-pass filter with cutoff values of 20 and 500 Hz [31,32] in a custom script written in MATLAB (MathWorks Inc., Natick, MA, USA). The signals were full-wave rectified and filtered by a low-pass filter at 10 Hz [33,34]. The filtered EMG signals were then used to calculate the root mean square (RMS EMG) with a window of 10 ms to describe the muscle activation during movement [33]. In addition, the filtered EMG signals were used to calculate the mean of the EMG (MEMG) to describe the work of one muscle during movement. Since the gait cycle was usually normalized to 0~100%, the sEMG data acquired synchronously should be also interpolated into 0~100% to describe how the muscles were activated during the gait [34,35]. Therefore, all the RMS EMGs were interpolated into 101 points corresponding to the gait cycle.

2.4. Statistical Analysis

We calculated the mean values of step length, step width, and RMS EMG, as well as MEMG, over ten consecutive strides. We then normalized the temporal stride parameters and determined the EMG parameters by calculating the ratio of the values during slope walking with loads to the values during level walking without loads. We used a two-factor (grade × load mass) analysis of variance for repeated measures to test the significant effects of the grade and load masses. When there was a significant effect ($p < 0.05$), Bonferroni corrected post hoc comparisons (adjusted $p < 0.0072$ (0.05/7, two dependent stride variables and five sEMG variables) [18,22–24,36] were carried out to evaluate the differences between the grades and load masses. All statistical analyses were conducted using SPSS software (IBM SPSS Statistics 22).

3. Results

3.1. Temporal Stride Kinematics

As the load mass and grade increased, subjects took a longer step length than level walking (Table 1). The changes in the normalized step widths were different between the load mass and grade groups. Both of the temporal stride kinematics were not significantly different from level walking without backpack loads (all $p > 0.05$).

Table 1. Normalized step lengths and step widths during different grades of walking with different load masses.

	Normalized Step Length				Normalized Step Width			
	0°	3°	5°	10°	0°	3°	5°	10°
0 kg	1.00	1.07 (0.06)	1.03 (0.06)	1.08 (0.07)	1.00	1.03 (0.05)	1.04 (0.07)	1.02 (0.05)
10 kg	1.06 (0.06)	1.10 (0.09)	1.06 (0.10)	1.05 (0.09)	0.98 (0.08)	0.98 (0.06)	1.04 (0.06)	1.02 (0.06)
20 kg	1.09 (0.05)	1.13 (0.09)	1.10 (0.08)	1.10 (0.08)	1.04 (0.06)	0.98 (0.09)	0.95 (0.06)	1.07 (0.01)
30 kg	1.10 (0.08)	1.08 (0.06)	1.06 (0.08)	1.02 (0.06)	1.09 (0.09)	1.00 (0.08)	0.97 (0.07)	1.03 (0.05)

All the step lengths and step widths were divided by the values during level walking without backpack loads. Therefore, the normalized step lengths and step widths were "1.00", and all the normalized step lengths and step widths were dimensionless in Table 1.

3.2. Muscle Activities

As expected, the mean muscle activities of the hip, knee, and ankle extensors generally increased with the increase of the load mass and grade (Figures 2–5 and Table S1). Both the grade and load mass had a significant effect on all muscles ($p < 0.05$), and none of the muscles showed significant grade-load-mass interactions ($p > 0.05$).

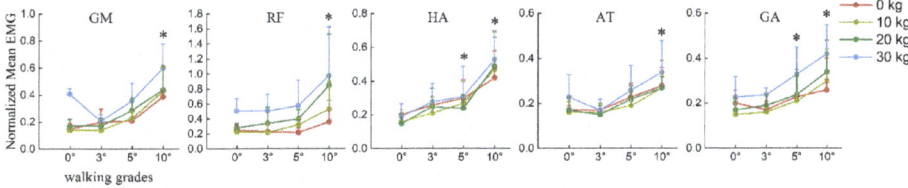

Figure 2. The mean EMG signals for muscles during different slope walking across all load masses in one gait from right heel strike to the next right heel strike, normalized to the mean activity during level walking without backpack loads. * Representing the mean EMG was significantly different from level walking across all the backpack loads, according to post hoc comparisons with a Bonferroni adjusted level of significance ($p < 0.0072$). The red line represented the normalized mean EMG of each muscle at different grades without backpack loads. The yellow one represented the normalized mean EMG of each muscle at different grades with 10-kg backpack loads. The green one represented the normalized mean EMG of each muscle at different grades with 20-kg backpack loads. The blue one represented the normalized mean EMG of each muscle at different grades with 30-kg backpack loads.

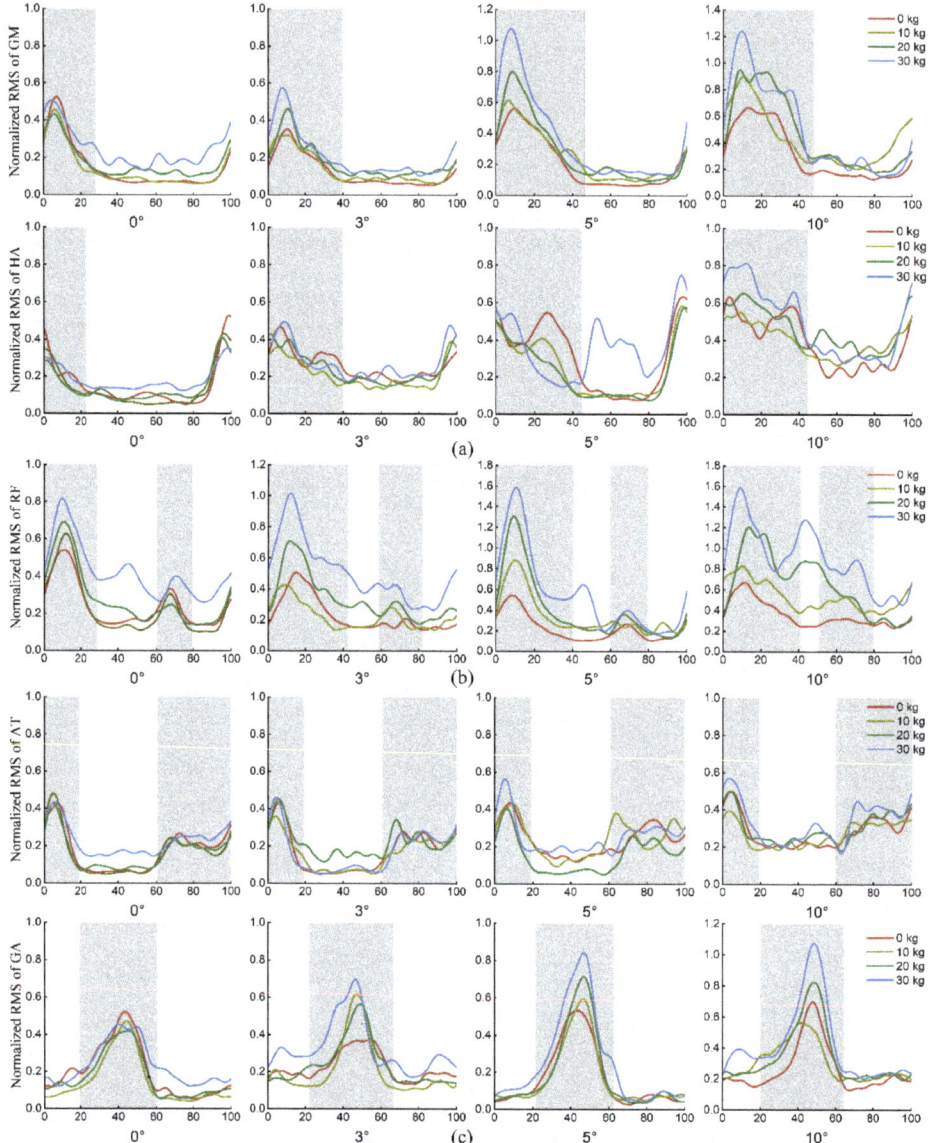

Figure 3. The muscle activity of leg muscles in one gait during different slope walking across all backpack loads, normalized to the mean activity during level walking without backpack loads: (**a**) The muscle activity of the hip extensor muscles. (**b**) The muscle activity of the knee extensor muscles. (**c**) The muscle activity of the ankle muscles. The different colors of the curves had the same representation as those colors in Figure 2. The gray area represented the higher muscle activation duration in one gait. RMS: root mean square.

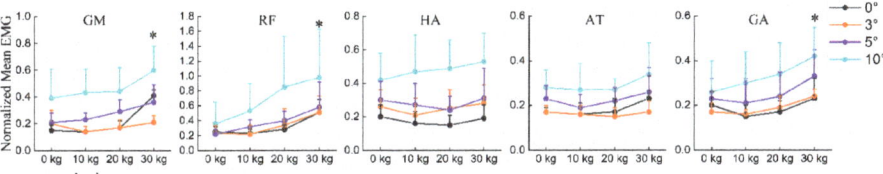

Figure 4. Mean EMG signals for muscles while walking across all grades with different backpack loads during one gait from right heel strike to the next right heel strike, normalized to the mean activity during level walking without backpack loads. * Representing the mean EMG was significantly different from walking without backpack loads across all the grades, according to post hoc comparisons with a Bonferroni adjusted level of significance ($p < 0.0072$). The line in dark gray represented the normalized mean EMG of each muscle with different load masses during level walking. The line in orange represented the normalized mean EMG of each muscle with different load masses during slope walking at grade 3°. The line in purple represented the normalized mean EMG of each muscle with different load masses during slope walking at grade 5°. The line in blue represented the normalized mean EMG of each muscle with different load masses during slope walking at grade 10°.

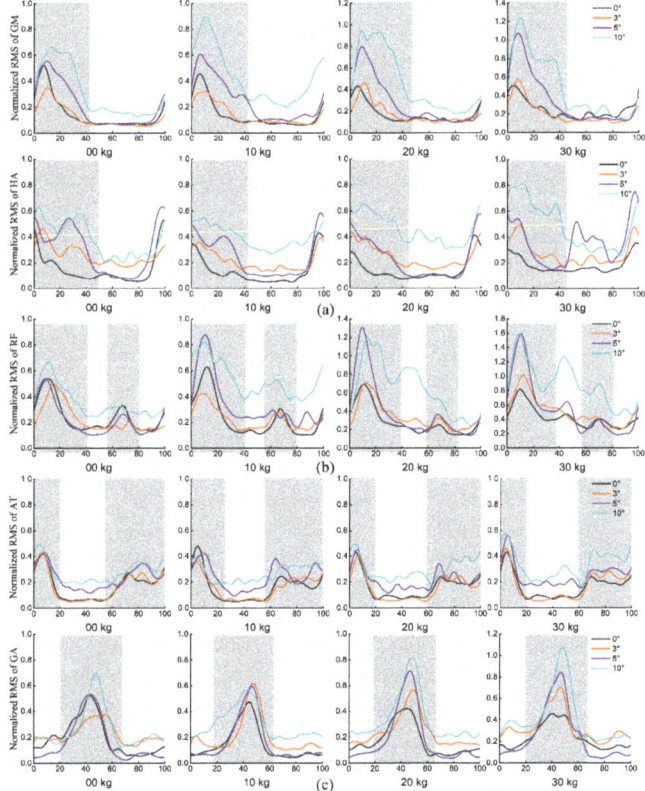

Figure 5. The muscle activity of leg muscles in one gait during walking with different backpack load masses across all grades, normalized to the mean activity during level walking without backpack loads: (**a**) The muscle activity of the hip extensor muscles. (**b**) The muscle activity of the knee extensor muscle. (**c**) The muscle activity of the ankle muscles. The different colors of the curves had the same representation as those colors in Figure 4. The gray area represented the higher muscle activation duration in one gait.

3.2.1. Grade Effects

The mean EMG signals of the hip, knee, and ankle extensor muscles increased generally during most of the slope walking, especially during the 10° slope walking (GM, $p = 1.32 \times 10^{-8}$; HA, $p = 2.33 \times 10^{-16}$; RF, $p = 0.2 \times 10^{-5}$; and GA, $p = 6.74 \times 10^{-9}$). Compared to the level walking, these increases were statistically significant for GM, RF, and AT at the 10° grade and for HA and GA at the 5° and 10° grades (Figure 2). Compared to the level walking with the same loads, the mean EMG of GM increased greatly during walking at the 10° grade by 46% to 207%, HA increased by 110% to 226%, RF increased by 44% to 203%, AT increased by 48% to 68%, and GA increased by 30% to 100% (shown in Table S2).

As the grade increased, the muscle activity of the hip extensor muscles (GM and HA, especially GM) increased both in the activation value and duration (Figure 3a). The maximum activation value of the GM changed from 0.52 to 1.24, and the activation duration increased from about 28% to 48% of one gait as the grade increased. The maximum activation value of the HA changed from 0.52 to 0.81, and the activation duration changed from 20% to about 45% of one gait as the grade increased.

The muscle activity of the knee extensor muscle (RF) increased most in the activation value, shown in Figure 3b. The maximum activation value of the RF increased from 0.82 to 1.60 during the early stance stage and from 0.4 to about 0.9 during the early swing stage.

As expected, the muscle activity of the ankle extensor (GA) increased considerably in the muscle activation value (Figure 3c). The maximum activation of the GA during the median and the late stances increased highly, from 0.52 to 1.07. Compared to the ankle extensor, the muscle activity of the ankle dorsiflexion (AT) increased slightly, from 0.48 to 0.57 during the early stance stage and swing stage.

3.2.2. Load Mass Effects

The mean EMG signals of the hip, knee, and ankle extensor muscles increased generally as the backpack load masses increased. Compared to walking without backpack loads, the increases were statistically significant for the GM and GA during walking with 30-kg loads (GM, $p = 0.000091$ and GA, $p = 0.00091$) and for the RF during walking with 30 kg ($p = 8.86 \times 10^{-7}$) (Figure 4). The increases in the HA and AT were not statistically significant ($p > 0.0072$). Compared to walking without loads at the same grade, the mean EMG of the GM increased by 5% to 173% with a 30-kg backpack load, the HA increased by −5% to 26%, the RF increased by 104% to 172%, the AT increased by 0% to 35%, and the GA increased by 15% to 61% (the data are shown in Table S3).

The muscle activity of the hip extensors (GM and HA) increased as the backpack load mass increased, as shown in Figure 5a. The maximum muscle activity of the GM increased greatly from 0.66 to 1.24 as the backpack load mass increased from 0 to 30 kg. The maximum muscle activity of the HA increased slightly from 0.63 to 0.81 as the load mass increased.

The knee extensor muscle RF increased greatly in muscle activation as the backpack load mass increased (Figure 5b). The maximum muscle activation of the RF increased greatly from 0.67 to 1.60 during the early stance stage as the load mass increased from 0 to 30 kg across all the slope walking.

The ankle extensor muscle GA increased greatly in muscle activation from 0.70 to 1.07 as the backpack load mass increased from 0 to 30 kg, and the dorsiflexion muscle AT increased slightly, from 0.50 to 0.58 (Figure 5c). The muscle activity demonstrated that the ankle extensor muscles were activated more than the flexor muscles during slope walking with backpack loads.

4. Discussion

This study quantified the hip, knee, and ankle muscle activations during level and slope walking with different backpack loads. Compared to level walking, the hip, knee, and ankle muscle activations increased generally during slope walking, especially the hip extensor muscle activations. The increased mean EMG of the leg muscles in this study were consistent with published findings [4,5,18–20]. Moreover, the increase became more pronounced with backpack loads, especially the hip and knee muscle activations. The hip extensor muscles increased the most with grades changing, and the knee extensor muscles increased the most with loads changing, which expanded our knowledge of muscle activation strategies during slope walking with backpack loads.

The results of this study supported our first hypothesis that the hip, knee, and ankle extensor muscle activations would increase during the slope walking, especially the hip extensor muscle activations, compared to level walking. In this study, all the leg extensor muscle activations increased during slope walking to raise the body's center of mass, which were consistent with prior studies [18–20]. In addition, the hip extensor muscle activations (GM and HA) increased remarkably more (the GM increased by 46% to 207% and the HA increased by 110% to 226%) than the ankle extensor muscle (GA increased by 30% to 100%) at steeper grades. The activation value and duration of the hip extensor muscles increased remarkably at the early stance stage during slope walking (shown in Figure 2). This demonstrates the pronounced role of hip extensor muscles during slope walking [18,23], which was also described by the greatest increase of the hip extension moment (increased from 1.01 to 1.37 when the treadmill gradient increased from 0% to 20% [22]) and the greatest increased power of the hip extensor muscles (increased by 85% at push-off and by 75% during mid-stance while walking on uneven terrain [21]). The hip extensors provided greater acceleration of the COM and generated more power for the trunk and ipsilateral leg during slope walking [19], which may also be the reason that the hip extensor muscles were more pronouncedly activated on slopes in our study.

The results of this study also supported our second hypothesis that muscle activations would increase pronouncedly with backloads during slope walking. The increases of the GM, RF, and GA became significant statistically when slope walking with a big backpack load (30 kg). Consistent with previous investigations [4,37,38], the mean amplitude of the RF and GA increased with loads in this study. The RF activation increased to provide more force and energy to extend the knee to attenuate the impact forces with heavy load carriage [38] and to maintain lower limb stability as the load mass increased [4]. The increase of the GA activations provided more power for walking by increasing the plantar flexing [38], which was thought to overcome the inertia associated with increasing backpack loads [39]. However, the mean EMG of the AT increased in this study, while the average amplitude of the AT remained unaffected [37,38]. This difference may be caused by different experimental designs in our study and theirs. The walking conditions in our study were slope walking with backpack loads, while their studies' conditions involved level walking. People elicited larger AT activity during slope walking to provide greater ankle dorsiflexion than level walking [19,22,28]. The slope grades may enlarge the influence of backpack loads on muscles.

The results of this study supported our third hypothesis that the muscle activations would increase at different degrees, and the knee extensor muscles would be activated more compared to the hip and ankle extensor muscles. Compared to walking without loads at the same grade across all slope walking, the mean EMG of the knee extensor muscle (RF) increased significantly by 104% to 172% with 30-kg backpack loads. The increase of the knee extensor muscle was much greater than that of the ankle extensor muscle (GA increased by 15% to 61% with 30-kg backpack loads relative to without loads across all grades). The knee extensor muscle increased most to provide greater force for body support during the early stance stage, which was consistent with other investigations [18,38,40]. Except for the knee extensor muscle activations, the hip extensor muscle GM activations also increased more pronouncedly than the ankle extensor muscle GA (GM increased by 5% to 173%). With the loads increasing, the energy and power for walking increased greatly [7,10]. The hip extensor muscle GM played an important role in the acceleration of the trunk [19]. Thus, the GM activations increased pronouncedly to provide more power for the acceleration of the trunk as the backpack loads increased. The results implied that the leg extensor muscles may have different contributions during walking with backpack loads. The knee extensor and hip extensor muscles may play a greater role during walking with heavy loads, which was also speculated by Harman [38].

In our present study, the EMG of the GM, HA, RF, AT, and GA were analyzed to investigate the muscle strategy during slope walking with backpack loads. However, one limitation of our study is that we did not acquire the kinematic data in the experiment that may give force to our work.

In addition, another limitation of our study is that the muscles analyzed were relatively few and most of them were focused on the leg extensor muscles. The muscles around the trunk, such as the external oblique muscles, were not analyzed in this study, which influenced pronouncedly during the inclined walking with backpack loads. The vastus medialis and vastus lateralis at the knee joint were influenced a lot during slope walking to provide more forces for lower limb stability [18,19], which were also not analyzed in this study. Thus, we should acquire the kinematics data and analyze more muscles by experiment or simulation [19,41] in the future to expand the insights into the muscle strategy during slope walking with backpack loads. Finally, considering the load intensity, only male participants were recruited in this study. Males and females may have different muscle-activation strategies during slope walking with backpack loads. Future studies may be needed to understand how muscle activations are influenced by the grade and loads using female subjects.

5. Conclusions

In this study, we explored the effects of backpack loads on leg muscle activations during slope walking. It was concluded that the hip, knee, and ankle extensor muscle activations increased during slope walking, and the hip muscle increased the most among the hip, knee, and ankle muscles. Moreover, muscle activations increased pronouncedly with loads during slope walking, and the knee extensor muscle activations increased more than the hip and ankle muscles. The results in our study imply that the hip and knee muscles play an important role during slope walking with loads. Our results are important for the design of assistant devices, such as exoskeleton robots, to enhance people's walking ability, especially for hikers and soldiers. The hip and knee extension movements during slope walking should be considerably assisted to lower the muscle activations. Future studies could explore the effects of loads and grades on more muscles and involve more participants, including female subjects, to expand the insights into the muscle strategy for providing more suggestions for the design of assistant devices.

Full postal address: Room A1043, Lee Shao Kee S&T Building, Department of Mechanical Engineering, Tsinghua University, Beijing 100084, China.

Supplementary Materials: The following are available online at http://www.mdpi.com/2076-3417/10/14/4890/s1: Table S1: Normalized mean (mean ± SD) EMG activities during inclined walking with a range of backpack loads, Table S2: The ratio of the EMG between inclined walking and level walking across all backpack loads, Table S3: The ratio of the EMG between walking with backpack loads and without backpack loads across all grades.

Author Contributions: Conceptualization, Y.L. and Q.S.; methodology, X.G.; software, Y.L. and M.Z.; validation, Y.L. and M.Z.; formal analysis, X.G.; investigation, Y.L. and L.Q.; resources, M.Z.; data curation, Y.L., L.Q., and M.Z.; writing—original draft preparation, Y.L.; writing—review and editing, Q.S. and X.G.; visualization, Y.L., L.Q., Q.S., and X.G.; supervision, X.G.; project administration, Y.L.; and funding acquisition, Q.S. All authors have read and agreed to the published version of the manuscript.

Funding: The study was funded by grants from the National Natural Science Foundation of China (Grant No. 51905035 and 51905291), the China Postdoctoral Science Foundation-funded project (Grant No. 2019M660478), and the Ministry of Science and Technology national key R&D program (Grant Number: 2017YFB1300500).

Acknowledgments: We thank Yue Zhou and Peidong Ma from Beijing Sports University for providing the lab experiments and giving suggestions for the analysis. We thank all the participants in this study.

Conflicts of Interest: The authors have no conflict of interest concerning this manuscript.

References

1. Nordb, I.; Prebensen, N.K. Hiking as mental and physical experience. In *Advances in Hospitality and Leisure*; Emerald Group Publishing Limited: Bingley, UK, 2015; pp. 169–186.
2. American College of Sports Medicine. *ACSM's Resource Manual for Guidelines for Exercise Testing and Prescription*; Lippincott Williams & Wilkins: Philadelphia, PA, USA, 2012.
3. Elliott, T.B.; Elliott, B.A.; Bixby, M.R. Risk factors associated with camp accidents. *Wilderness Environ. Med.* **2003**, *14*, 2–8. [CrossRef]

4. Simpson, K.M.; Munro, B.J.; Steele, J.R. Backpack load affects lower limb muscle activity patterns of female hikers during prolonged load carriage. *J. Electromyogr. Kinesiol.* **2011**, *21*, 782–788. [CrossRef] [PubMed]
5. Silder, A.; Delp, S.L.; Besier, T. Men and women adopt similar walking mechanics and muscle activation patterns during load carriage. *J. Biomech.* **2013**, *46*, 2522–2528. [CrossRef]
6. Keren, G.; Epstein, Y.; Magazanik, A.; Sohar, E. The energy cost of walking and running with and without a backpack load. *Eur. J. Appl. Physiol. Occup. Physiol.* **1981**, *46*, 317–324. [CrossRef]
7. Browning, R.C.; Modica, J.R.; Kram, R.; Goswami, A. The effects of adding mass to the legs on the energetics and biomechanics of walking. *Med. Sci. Sport Exerc.* **2007**, *39*, 515–525. [CrossRef]
8. Huang, T.W.; Kuo, A.D. Mechanics and energetics of load carriage during human walking. *J. Exp. Biol.* **2014**, *217*, 605–613. [CrossRef]
9. Morrison, A.; Hale, J.; Brown, S. Joint range of motion entropy changes in response to load carriage in military personnel. *Hum. Mov. Sci.* **2019**, *66*, 249–257. [CrossRef]
10. Liew, B.X.W.; Morris, S.; Netto, K. The effects of load carriage on joint work at different running velocities. *J. Biomech.* **2016**, *49*, 3275–3280. [CrossRef]
11. Loverro, K.L.; Hasselquist, L.; Lewis, C.L. Females and males use different hip and knee mechanics in response to symmetric military-relevant loads. *J. Biomech.* **2019**, *95*, 109280. [CrossRef]
12. Krajewski, K.T.; Dever, D.E.; Johnson, C.C.; Rawcliffe, A.J.; Ahamed, N.U.; Flanagan, S.D.; Mi, Q.; Anderst, W.J.; Connaboy, C. Load carriage magnitude and locomotion strategy alter knee total joint moment during bipedal ambulatory tasks in recruit-aged women. *J. Biomech.* **2020**, *105*, 109772. [CrossRef]
13. Lay, A.N.; Hass, C.J.; Gregor, R.J. The effects of sloped surfaces on locomotion: A kinematic and kinetic analysis. *J. Biomech.* **2006**, *39*, 1621–1628. [CrossRef] [PubMed]
14. Holt, K.G.; Wagenaar, R.C.; LaFiandra, M.E.; Kubo, M.; Obusek, J.P. Increased musculoskeletal stiffness during load carriage at increasing walking speeds maintains constant vertical excursion of the body center of mass. *J. Biomech.* **2003**, *36*, 465–471. [CrossRef]
15. Walsh, G.S.; Low, D.C.; Arkesteijn, M. Effect of stable and unstable load carriage on walking gait variability, dynamic stability and muscle activity of older adults. *J. Biomech.* **2018**, *73*, 18–23. [CrossRef] [PubMed]
16. Huang, L.; Yang, Z.; Wang, R.; Xie, L. Physiological and biomechanical effects on the human musculoskeletal system while carrying a suspended-load backpack. *J. Biomech.* **2020**, *108*, 109894. [CrossRef]
17. Yang, L.; Zhang, J.; Xu, Y.; Chen, K.; Fu, C. Energy Performance Analysis of a Suspended Backpack with an Optimally Controlled Variable Damper for Human Load Carriage. *Mech. Mach. Theory* **2020**, *146*, 103738. [CrossRef]
18. Franz, J.R.; Kram, R. The effects of grade and speed on leg muscle activations during walking. *Gait Posture* **2012**, *35*, 143–147. [CrossRef]
19. Pickle, N.T.; Grabowski, A.M.; Auyang, A.G.; Silverman, A.K. The functional roles of muscles during sloped walking. *J. Biomech.* **2016**, *49*, 3244–3251. [CrossRef]
20. Alexander, N.; Schwameder, H. Effect of sloped walking on lower limb muscle forces. *Gait Posture* **2016**, *47*, 62–67. [CrossRef]
21. Voloshina, A.S.; Kuo, A.D.; Daley, M.A.; Ferris, D.P. Biomechanics and energetics of walking on uneven terrain. *J. Exp. Biol.* **2013**, *216*, 3963–3970. [CrossRef]
22. Haggerty, M.; Dickin, D.C.; Popp, J.; Wang, H. The influence of incline walking on joint mechanics. *Gait Posture* **2014**, *39*, 1017–1021. [CrossRef]
23. Alexander, N.; Strutzenberger, G.; Ameshofer, L.M.; Schwameder, H. Lower limb joint work and joint work contribution during downhill and uphill walking at different inclinations. *J. Biomech.* **2017**, *61*, 75–80. [CrossRef]
24. Alexander, N.; Schwameder, H. Lower limb joint forces during walking on the level and slopes at different inclinations. *Gait Posture* **2016**, *45*, 137–142. [CrossRef] [PubMed]
25. Son, H. The Effect of Backpack Load on Muscle Activities of the Trunk and Lower Extremities and Plantar Foot Pressure in Flatfoot. *J. Phys. Ther. Sci.* **2013**, *25*, 1383–1386. [CrossRef]
26. Collins, S.H.; Adamczyk, P.G.; Ferris, D.P.; Kuo, A.D. A simple method for calibrating force plates and force treadmills using an instrumented pole. *Gait Posture* **2009**, *29*, 59–64. [CrossRef] [PubMed]
27. Behnke Robert, S. *Kinetic Anatomy*; Human Kinetics: Champaign, IL, USA, 2006.
28. Ehlen, K.A.; Reiser, R.F.; Browning, R.C. Energetics and biomechanics of inclined treadmill walking in obese adults. *Med. Sci. Sports Exerc.* **2011**, *43*, 1251–1259. [CrossRef] [PubMed]

29. Mills, P.M.; Barrett, R.S.; Morrison, S. Agreement between footswitch and ground reaction force techniques for identifying gait events: Inter-session repeatability and the effect of walking speed. *Gait Posture* **2007**, *26*, 1–326. [CrossRef] [PubMed]
30. Pirker, W.; Katzenschlager, R. Gait disorders in adults and the elderly. *Wien. Klin. Wochenschr.* **2017**, *129*, 81–95. [CrossRef]
31. Chen, S.-K.; Wu, M.-T.; Huang, C.-H.; Wu, J.-H.; Guo, L.-Y.; Wu, W.-L. The analysis of upper limb movement and EMG activation during the snatch under various loading conditions. *J. Mech. Med. Biol.* **2013**, *13*, 1350010. [CrossRef]
32. Liu, Y.; Hong, Y.; Ji, L. Dynamic Analysis of the Abnormal Isometric Strength Movement Pattern between Shoulder and Elbow Joint in Patients with Hemiplegia. *J. Healthc. Eng.* **2018**, *2018*. [CrossRef]
33. Konrad, P. The abc of emg. *Pract. Introd. Kinesiol. Electromyogr.* **2005**, *1*, 30–35.
34. Guan, X.; Liu, Y.; Gao, L.; Ji, L.; Wang, R.; Yang, M.; Ji, R. Trunk muscle activity patterns in a person with spinal cord injury walking with different un-powered exoskeletons: A case study. *J. Rehab. Med.* **2016**, *48*, 390–395. [CrossRef] [PubMed]
35. Guan, X.; Kuai, S.; Song, L.; Li, C.; Liu, W.; Liu, Y.; Ji, L.; Wang, R.; Zhang, Z. How Height and Weight of Patients with Spinal Cord Injury Affect the Spring Locations of Unpowered Energy-stored Exoskeleton. In Proceedings of the 41st Annual International Conference of the IEEE Engineering in Medicine and Biology Society (EMBC), Berlin, Germany, 23–27 July 2019.
36. Rupert, G., Jr. *Simultaneous Statistical Inference*; Springer Science & Business Media: Berlin/Heidelberg, Germany, 2012.
37. Harman, E. The effects on gait timing, kinetics and muscle activity of various loads carried on the back. *Med. Sci. Sports Exerc.* **1992**, *24*, S129. [CrossRef]
38. Harman, E.; Hoon, K.; Frykman, P.; Pandorf, C. *The Effects of Backpack Weight on the Biomechanics of Load Carriage*; Army Research Institute of Environmental Medicine: Natick, MA, USA, 2000.
39. Attwells, R.L.; Birrell, S.A.; Hooper, R.H.; Mansfield, N.J. Influence of carrying heavy loads on soldiers' posture, movements and gait. *Ergonomics* **2006**, *49*, 1527–1537. [CrossRef] [PubMed]
40. McGowan, C.P.; Neptune, R.R.; Clark, D.J.; Kautz, Z.A. Modular control of human walking: Adaptations to altered mechanical demands. *J. Biomech.* **2010**, *43*, 412–419. [CrossRef]
41. Dorn, T.W.; Wang, J.M.; Hicks, J.L.; Delp, S.L. Predictive Simulation Generates Human Adaptations during Loaded and Inclined Walking. *PLoS ONE* **2015**, *10*. [CrossRef] [PubMed]

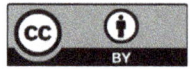

© 2020 by the authors. Licensee MDPI, Basel, Switzerland. This article is an open access article distributed under the terms and conditions of the Creative Commons Attribution (CC BY) license (http://creativecommons.org/licenses/by/4.0/).

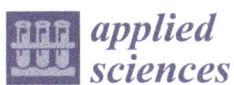 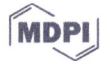

Article

Ankle Taping Effectiveness for the Decreasing Dorsiflexion Range of Motion in Elite Soccer and Basketball Players U18 in a Single Training Session: A Cross-Sectional Pilot Study

Carlos Romero-Morales [1], Carlos López-Nuevo [1], Carlos Fort-Novoa [1], Patricia Palomo-López [2], David Rodríguez-Sanz [3], Daniel López-López [4], César Calvo-Lobo [3] and Blanca De-la-Cruz-Torres [5],*

[1] Faculty of Sport Sciences, Universidad Europea, Villaviciosa de Odón, 28670 Madrid, Spain; carlos.romero@universidadeuropea.es (C.R.-M.); carlosenrique.lopez@universidadeuropea.es (C.L.-N.); carlosfortnovoa@gmail.com (C.F.-N.)
[2] University Center of Plasencia, Faculty of Podiatry, Universidad de Extremadura, 10600 Plasencia, Spain; patibiom@unex.es
[3] Facultad de Enfermería, Fisioterapia y Podología, Universidad Complutense de Madrid, 28040 Madrid, Spain; davidrodriguezsanz@ucm.es (D.R.-S.); cescalvo@ucm.es (C.C.-L.)
[4] Research, Health and Podiatry Group, Department of Health Sciences, Faculty of Nursing and Podiatry, Universidade da Coruña, 15403 Ferrol, Spain; daniellopez@udc.es
[5] Department of Physiotherapy, University of Seville, Avicena Street, 41009 Seville, Spain
* Correspondence: bcruz@us.es

Received: 21 April 2020; Accepted: 25 May 2020; Published: 28 May 2020

Abstract: Ankle sprains have been defined as the most common injury in sports. The aim of the present study was to investigate the ankle taping for the reduction of ankle dorsiflexion range of motion (ROM) and inter-limb in elite soccer and basketball players U18 in a single training session. Methods: A cross-sectional pilot study was performed on 38 male healthy elite athletes divided into two groups: a soccer group and a basketball group. Ankle dorsiflexion ROM and inter-limb asymmetries in a weight-bearing lunge position were assessed in three points: with no-tape, before the practice and immediately after the practice. Results: For the soccer group, significant differences ($p < 0.05$) were observed for the right ankle, but no differences for the asymmetry variable. The basketball group reported significant differences ($p < 0.05$) for the right ankle and symmetry. Conclusions: Ankle taping decreased the ankle dorsiflexion ROM in youth elite soccer and basketball players U18. These results could be useful as a prophylactic approach for ankle sprain injury prevention. However, the ankle ROM restriction between individuals without taping and individuals immediately assessed when the tape was removed after the training was very low.

Keywords: ankle sprain; taping; range of motion; soccer; basketball; prevention; musculoskeletal disorders; personalized treatment

1. Introduction

Ankle sprains have been defined as the most common injury in sports [1]. Worldwide, soccer and basketball are some of the most popular sports for both participation and viewing. These athletes reported the highest injury incidence ratios [2,3]. Elite soccer players experienced between 13 and 55 injuries per 1000 competitive hours. In addition, the lower limb is most commonly affected as foot, and ankle injuries were the most prevalent diagnoses in training or competition [4]. Regarding the basketball athletes, McKay et al. reported an ankle incidence rate of 3.85 per 1000 participations, landings being the most prevalent mechanism of injury [5]. Most cases of ankle sprain in basketball and soccer players occurred when the foot takes an over-plantar-flexed position during running or landing after a jump [6]. In addition, amateur and youth soccer players have a higher risk of suffering a lateral ankle sprain than professional players due to an increase of strength and training experience for the professional players [7].

Functional approaches, including prophylactic methods such as taping, bandaging, or bracing of the ankle to protect the ankle ligaments have been studied, with the aim of reducing the incidence rates of ankle sprain injuries since the 1990s [8].

In the past decade, several studies have been developed to assess the effectiveness of ankle taping for the protection of the ankle ligaments in maximal stress situations, such as an ankle sprain [9]. Ankle taping was associated with competition, rehabilitation, and prevention sport contexts over many years. Karlsson and Andreasson reported a restricted range of motion (ROM) for the ankle joint in individuals with ankle taping but with a decrease in the peroneus muscle reaction time assessed by electromyography [10]. Taping with or without pre-wrap has also been studied, i.e., Ricard et al. reported the effectiveness of the ankle taping to reduce the average inversion velocity, maximum inversion velocity, and time to maximum inversion velocity, but no differences between individuals with or without pre-wrap were observed [11]. Pederson et al. argued that ankle taping was effective in the reduction of inversion movement in a study carried out in rugby players. In addition, authors have also reported that there may be a functional restriction on inversion parameters after exercise with ankle taping [12]. Callaghan reported that the inversion-eversion ROM had been limited by up to 41% as ankle taping in a non-weight bearing position presented as a restriction of the frontal plane movements [13]. Kemler et al. reported in a systematic review that elastic bandages and ankle taping were effective for the ankle sprain episodes [14]. Kerkhoffs et al. conducted a systematic review regarding the different bandage approaches for ankle sprain situations, and they concluded that the taping method is effective to limit the ankle ROM. However, several complications have been observed, such as skin irritations and a longer time to return to work when compared with an elastic bandage [15]. Jeffries et al. reported that ankle taping should provide protection to the ankle joint without affecting the planned change-of-direction or reactive agility performance in basketball players [16].

Currently, research showed that ankle taping is often employed in elite sports in order to prevent the incidence and severity of lateral ankle sprains. Thus, the aim of the present study was to investigate in elite soccer and basketball players U18 the effectiveness of ankle taping in the reduction of ankle dorsiflexion ROM and inter-limb asymmetries throughout the training session. Thus, we assessed the ankle dorsiflexion ROM in a weight-bearing lunge position in three time-points: (1) with no-tape, (2) before the practice, and (3) immediately after the practice. Prior research concluded that the ankle taping would reduce the ankle joint dorsiflexion angle immediately after the taping. However, we hypothesized that the taping had lost the initial effectiveness for restricting the ankle dorsiflexion ROM at the end of the training session, as the last minutes of the training session were the period of time in which there was a high injury risk for the athletes.

2. Materials and Methods

2.1. Design

A cross-sectional observational study was performed in November 2019 following the Strengthening the Reporting of Observational Studies in Epidemiology (STROBE) recommendations.

2.2. Participants

A total sample of 38 healthy male individuals aged between 15 and 17 years was recruited from two elite sports and divided into two groups following their sports discipline: A group composed of elite soccer players (n = 18) and B group composed of elite basketball players (n = 20). All the players were taped in both ankle joints, usually for training and competitions with a prescription of the medical doctors from their clubs. Elite U18 individuals followed a training schedule of 3 hours-per-day, 5 days-per-week and played 1 to 2 matches in a week [17]. In addition, both groups were composed of individuals who have played at least 1 time with the national team [18]. Subjects were excluded if: they underwent a physical therapy treatment, suffered any musculoskeletal injury the last 6 weeks, had skins allergy and any history of lower limb surgery, did not complete all the training sessions, and had other foot orthoses.

2.3. Ethical Considerations

The Research and Ethics Committee from the Universidad Europea de Madrid has been approved this research (Villaviciosa de Odón, Madrid, Spain. Record code: 10-04-2019. CIPI/19/157). Before participating in the study, the players and parents were fully informed about the protocol and written informed consent was obtained by the parents of the players. The Declaration of Helsinki was fully respected throughout the study.

2.4. Taping: Procedure and Materials

Ankle taping was performed by two physiotherapists—one for the soccer team and one for the basketball team—both with more than 5 years of experience in taping methods in accordance with Williams et al. [19] procedures and the Sports Medicine Australia [20] guidelines protocol. Before the taping, all of the ankles were covered with a pre-wrap (Rehabmedic, Barcelona, Spain) by the physiotherapist in order to prevent skin alterations for daily use [21]. For the ankle taping, two anchor strips were applied around the leg 10 cm above the malleoli with a 38-mm self-adhesive tape (Leukotape, BSN Medical, Stockholm, Sweden). Secondly, with the foot maintained in a neutral position, two strips were placed from the medial side of the anchor tape and fixing to the lateral side. [19] The "figure sixes" for the subtalar joint were initially placed onto the medial anchor through the plantar surface of the foot to attach back onto the medial anchor. Finally, all the free endings and spaces without tape were covered to complete the ankle taping [19].

2.5. Training Sessions

The training session, in which subjects were evaluated in both groups, consisted of a 90-min technical session and was structured in 3 phases: warm-up (15-min), tactical skills (15-min), and scrimmage (60-min). This session did not comprise of a pre-game or post-game session.

2.6. Outcome Measurements

Ankle ROM assessment was developed by the *Dorsiflex* app (v.2.0, Balsalobre-Fernández, 2017, Madrid, Spain) installed on an iPhone 8 (iOS 12.1, Apple Inc., Cupertino, CA, USA). To measure dorsiflexion ROM, the iPhone 8 was placed at the tibial tuberosity to assess the angle between the tibia and the ground in a weight-bearing lunge position. This procedure was repeated with both legs, and the *Dorsiflex* app reported the dorsiflexion angle for each leg and the percent of asymmetry between the legs. In addition, the *Dorsiflex* app was considered as a valid, reliable, rapid, and easy-to-use tool to assess the ankle ROM and asymmetries in a weight-bearing lunge position [22]. Measurements were made in 3 time periods: (1) baseline, before the practice without bandage; (2) pre-training, immediately after the baseline measurement and before the training session; post-training, immediately after the end of the training session.

2.7. Statistical Analysis

SPSS v.23.0 for macOS (IBM SPSS Statistics for macOS, NY: IBM Corp) was used for statistical analysis. The Shapiro-Wilk test was used to check the normality data distribution. For each group separately, one-way analysis of variance (ANOVA) and Bonferroni's correction were developed to assess significant differences between the three-time points (basal, pre-training and post-training) and check the multiple comparisons, respectively. The effect size was calculated with the Eta^2 coefficient.

In order to observe the difference between groups, the Student's t-test—parametric data—and U Mann-Whitney test—no parametric data—were applied to test sociodemographic data between groups. To assess the effects of intra-subjects (time) and inter-subject (treatment groups) values on the dependent variables, a two-way ANOVA for repeated measures was performed (considering the significance of the Greenhouse–Geisser correction when the Mauchly test rejected the sphericity). The Bonferroni post-hoc test was employed for multiple comparisons. Furthermore, the effect size was calculated by the Eta^2 coefficient. The level of significance was set at $p < 0.05$ with an α error of 0.05 (95% confidence interval) and the desired power of 80% (β error of 0.2).

3. Results

Regarding Table 1, the height and weight showed significant differences ($p < 0.05$) between groups. For the soccer group, significant differences were observed for the right ankle [F (2,32) = 7.558; $p = 0.002$ (0.321)] and left ankle [F (2,32) = 9.813; $p = 0.001$ (0.380)], but no differences for the asymmetry variable. The basketball group reported significant differences for the right ankle [F (2,36) = 17.687; $p = 0.001$ (0.496)], the left ankle [F (2,36) = 35.204; $p = 0.001$ (0.662)] and the symmetry [F (2, 36); $p = 0.001$ (0.247)]. (Table 2) The Bonferroni corrections showed significant differences ($p < 0.05$) in the soccer group's right and left ankle between the baseline and pre-training and between the baseline and post-training moments for the right ankle whereas for the basketball group significant differences ($p < 0.05$) were shown for the right and left ankle between baseline and pre-training and in the right and left ankle between pre-training and post-training (Table 3).

The statistical analysis to assess the comparison of the ankle taping between soccer and basketball players reported significant differences in all variables for the time: right ankle [F (2, 68) = 19.022; $p = 0.001$ (0.359)]; left ankle [F (2, 68) = 34.339; $p = 0.001$ (0.503)] and asymmetry [F (2,68) = 7.842; $p = 0.001$ (0.187)].

In addition, the interaction time x group showed significant differences for the asymmetry [F (2, 68) = 0.415; $p = 0.002$ (0.012)]. (Figures 1–3) The Bonferroni corrections for the interaction between groups reported significant differences ($p < 0.05$) for the right ankle, the left ankle and the asymmetry variables between baseline and pre-training moments and the left ankle as well as the asymmetry between pre-training and post-training moments (Table 4).

Table 1. Sociodemographic data of the sample.

Data	Soccer Group (n = 17)	Basketball Group (n = 19)	Total Sample (n = 38)	p Value
Age, years	16.00 ± 1.0 †	15.00 ± 1.00 †	16.00 ± 2.00 †	0.005 ††
Height, m	1.73 ± 0.1 *	1.92 ± 0.12 †	1.83 ± 0.12 *	0.001 ††
Weight, kg	68.45 ± 6.75 *	82.04 ± 11.06 *	75.62 ± 11.45 *	0.001 **
BMI (kg/m^2)	22.61 ± 1.63 *	21.93 ± 2.53 †	22.29 ± 1.83 †	0.332 ††

Abbreviations: BMI, body mass index. * Mean ± standard deviation (SD) was applied. ** The Student T-test was performed for independent samples. † Median ± interquartile range (IR) was used. †† The Mann-Whitney U-test was performed.

Table 2. One-way ANOVA for the ankle ROM and asymmetry variables.

Group	Baseline	Pre-Training	Post-Training	Time F (Df); p (Eta^2)
Soccer				
Right ankle	39.71 ± 5.33	36.00 ± 6.55	36.88 ± 5.32	$F(2,32) = 7.558; p = 0.002 (0.321)$
Left ankle	38.82 ± 4.87	34.58 ± 5.86	37.49 ± 5.10	$F(2,32) = 9.813; p = 0.001 (0.380)$
Asymmetry	6.44 ± 3.44	10.40 ± 6.90	6.25 ± 5.68	$F(2,32) = 3.213; p = 0.057 (0.167)$
Basketball				
Right ankle	41.00 ± 6.6	37.67 ± 6.4	40.58 ± 5.6	$F(2,36) = 17.687; p = 0.001 (0.496)$
Left ankle	39.56 ± 6.7	34.9 ± 5.3	38.70 ± 5.7	$F(2,36) = 35.204; p = 0.001 (0.662)$
Asymmetry	4.56 ± 3.9	8.7 ± 5.1	5.95 ± 4.5	$F(2,36) = 5.913; p = 0.001 (0.247)$

Abbreviations: ANOVA, analysis of variance; ROM, range of motion. Values are mean ± SD unless otherwise indicated.

Table 3. Bonferroni correction values for the intra-subject (time) effects.

Measure	Right Ankle p Value	Left Ankle p Value	Asymmetry p Value
Soccer			
Baseline			
Pre-training	0.007	0.001	0.116
Post-training	0.021	0.611	1.000
Pre-training			
Post-training	1.000	0.054	0.184
Basketball			
Baseline			
Pre-training	0.001	0.001	0.007
Post-training	1.000	0.575	0.361
Pre-training			
Post-training	0.001	0.001	0.286

Table 4. Two-way ANOVA and Bonferroni correction values for the intra-subject effects of the total sample.

	Two-Way ANOVA Values	
	Time F (Df): p (Eta^2)	Time x Group F (Df); p (Eta^2)
Right ankle	$F(2,68) = 19.022; p = 0.001 (0.359)$	$F(2,68) = 2.585; p = 0.083 (0.071)$
Left ankle	$F(2,68) = 34.393; p = 0.001 (0.503)$	$F(2,68) = 0.316; p = 0.730 (0.009)$
Asymmetry	$F(2,68) = 7.842; p = 0.001 (0.187)$	$F(2,68) = 0.415; p = 0.002 (0.012)$

	Bonferroni correction values		
Measure	Right ankle p value	Left ankle p value	Asymmetry p value
Baseline			
Pre-training	0.001	0.001	0.001
Post-training	0.009	0.206	1.000
Pre-training			
Post-training	0.009	0.001	0.032

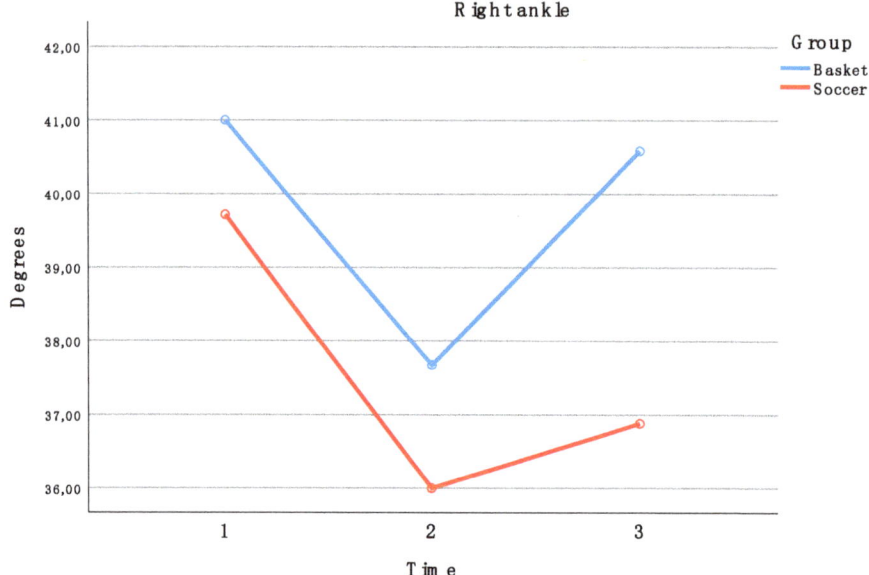

Figure 1. Right ankle ROM values for each group in three measurement times.

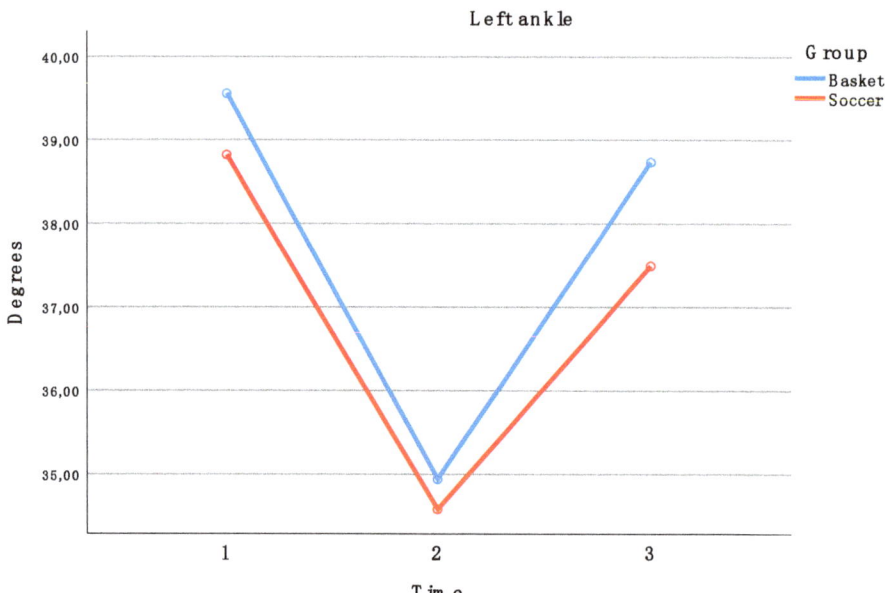

Figure 2. Left ankle ROM values for each group in three measurement times.

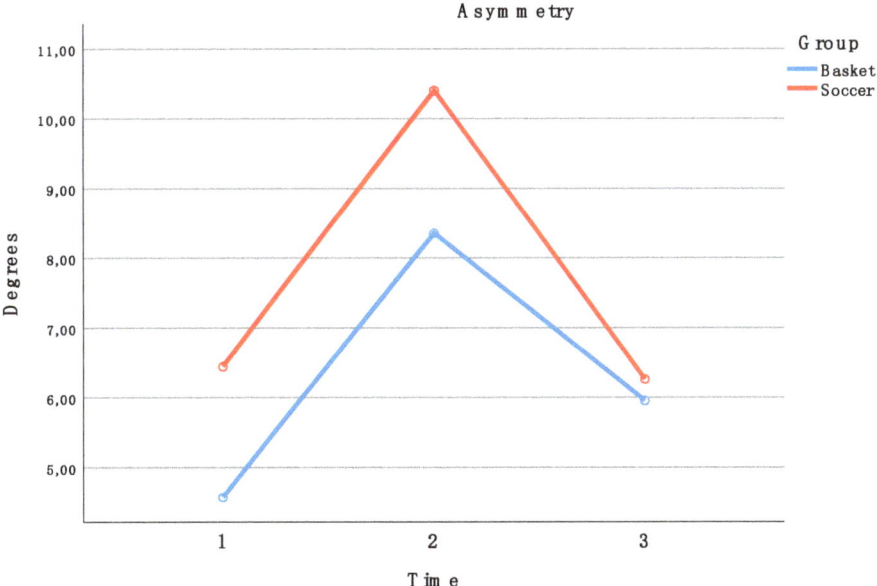

Figure 3. Asymmetry values for each group in three measurement times.

4. Discussion

This research compared the ankle taping on ankle mobility during three specific moments on a daily basis in youth elite soccer and basketball players. The results of the present study suggest that a prophylactic approach, such as ankle taping, is effective for the ROM restriction of the ankle joint immediately after the taping application in soccer and basketball players without differences between groups. However, in the final minutes of the session, where the intensity and the fatigue levels were at its highest peak [23], the ROM values were similar to the baseline values.

According to the findings of the present study, several authors reported the effectiveness of the ankle taping for the ankle ROM restriction [10,12]. For example, Quackenbush et al. argued that the ankle taping was an effective prophylactic method without decreasing jump performance in athletes. [24] Willeford et al. performed a study in collegiate football players and reported that with a bandage of the ankle joint —self-adherent and lace-up ankle brace —a ROM restriction was produced without affecting the dynamic balance [25]. According to the results of the present study, an ankle dorsiflexion ROM increase was observed immediately post-match in soccer players and basketball players—without a bandage [26,27]. However, in both groups, a decrease of ankle dorsiflexion ROM was observed 48 h post-match. Therefore, prevention and recovery strategies in order to minimize the ankle dorsiflexion restriction should be performed in soccer and basketball players. Regarding muscle fatigue and biomechanics, chronic ankle instability and fatigue were related to postural control by disturbances detected on sagittal-plane joints adjacent to the ankle, which may have influence in the ankle dorsiflexion ROM values after training sessions [28].

In addition to the above, landing mechanisms have been defined as a risk factor for ankle sprains in sports populations, De Ridder et al. argued that taping is able to stabilize the ankle joint prior to touch down, placing the ankle joint in a safe position before the landing phase [29]. In addition, Chinn et al. reported that the changes in the foot positioning in individuals with ankle taping could be a protective effect for the prevention of the lateral ankle sprains [30]. In addition, ankle taping increases the confident sense in dynamic-balance activities [31].

Regarding the ankle dorsiflexion asymmetry concept, Rabin et al. determined that weight-bearing ankle ROM should not be assumed to be bilaterally symmetrical [32]. However, the results of the present study reported an asymmetry increase when the taping was applied. Currently, research about the normative values for weight-bearing ankle ROM symmetries reported a dorsiflexion ROM increase of 23% in male military subjects for the dominant side with respect no-dominant side [32]. In the context of the ankle dorsiflexion asymmetry in professional soccer players, Moreno-Pérez et al. reported that ankle dorsiflexion ROM increased after a match in the dominant ankle but decreased 48 h post-match when the post-match assessments in both ankles—dominant and non-dominant—were compared [26]. In this line, a recent study reported that the ankle dorsiflexion ROM was increased post-match from pre-match in both dominant and non-dominant limbs and decreased 48 h post-game in semi-professional players [27]. An asymmetry increase immediately after the ankle tape application could be explained by the restriction of the musculoskeletal structures which surround the ankle joint or alterations of the sensitive proprioception mechanisms due to the taping application [33].

Other useful taping alternatives for ankle sprain prevention could be the kinesiology tape, [7] kinesiotape, [34], or distal fibular taping [35].

4.1. Clinical Considerations

Based on the prior literature and the findings of the present study, it could be supported that ankle taping was an effective and prophylactic method to reduce the ankle dorsiflexion ROM and, consequently, for the prevention of ankle sprain in sports populations. However, the fact that no differences were observed for the soccer left ankle, both basketball ankles from baseline to post-training values could be defined as the ankle taping having "dynamic effectiveness". Therefore, further research is needed in order to develop new strategies to maintain the initial effectiveness throughout the training session and games. For example, the addition of active stripes or to intensify the ankle taping in the training pauses and games half-times.

4.2. Limitations and Future Lines

Some limitations should be acknowledged in the present study. Although the physical therapist had more than 5 years of experience in taping strategies and functional assessments, the fact that both teams had not been taped and assessed by the same therapist may be a limitation as a human bias for the ankle dorsiflexion ROM and asymmetry were variables. Another limitation could be the fact that just one session was evaluated for each group. Weight, height, and BMI variables were descriptive variables and were found obvious differences between groups. It would be interesting to take them into account for the comparison between groups. In addition, the differences between these two sports in training skills in the footwork and training sessions specific exercises could also be a limitation.

Further research is needed in order to evaluate dynamic balance, landing situations, and lower limb stability with a pressure platform. In addition, electromyography or ultrasound imaging assessments for the muscular activation and the muscle architecture of the muscles related to the ankle joint could be useful to explore the effects of the ankle taping in a deep manner. Several authors reported the effectiveness of ankle taping also in psychological aspects such as better perceptions of confidence and reassurance; thus, it would be interesting to study these variables in soccer and basketball populations.

5. Conclusions

Ankle taping decreased the ankle dorsiflexion ROM in youth elite soccer and basketball players U18. These results could be useful as a prophylactic approach for ankle sprain injury prevention. However, the ankle ROM restriction between individuals without taping, and individuals immediately assessed when the tape was removed after the training was very low. Thus, further research is needed in order to develop new strategies to maintain the initial effectiveness throughout the training session and games.

Author Contributions: Conceptualization, B.D.-L.-C.-T. and C.R.-M.; data curation, D.R.-S., C.L.-N. and C.F.-N.; methodology, P.P.-L., D.R.-S. and D.L.-L.; formal analysis, C.R.-M., D.L.-L. and C.C.-L.; investigation, P.P.-L., C.L.-N. and C.F.-N.; supervision, C.R.-M. and B.D.-L.-C.-T.; writing—original draft preparation, B.D.-L.-C.-T., C.R.-M., D.R.-S. and C.C.-L.; writing—review and editing, B.D.-L.-C.-T., C.R.-M., D.L.-L. and C.C.-L. All authors have read and agreed to the published version of the manuscript.

Funding: This research received no external funding.

Acknowledgments: The authors thank all of the dancers, doctors and physiotherapists that participated in this project and acknowledge their valuable and essential contribution to the study.

Conflicts of Interest: The authors declare no conflict of interest.

References

1. Cordova, M.L.; Ingersoll, C.D.; LeBlanc, M.J. Influence of ankle support on joint range of motion before and after exercise: A meta-analysis. *J. Orthop. Sports Phys. Ther.* **2000**, *30*, 170–182. [CrossRef] [PubMed]
2. Newman, J.S.; Newberg, A.H. Basketball injuries. *Radiol. Clin. N. Am.* **2010**, *48*, 1095–1111. [CrossRef] [PubMed]
3. McLeod, T.V.; Israel, M.; Christino, M.A.; Chung, J.S.; McKay, S.D.; Lang, P.J.; Bell, D.R.; PRiSM Sports Specialization Research Interest Group; Chan, C.M.; Crepeau, A.; et al. Sport Participation and Specialization Characteristics Among Pediatric Soccer Athletes. *Orthop. J. Sport Med.* **2019**, *7*, 2325967119832399. [CrossRef] [PubMed]
4. Walls, R.J.; Ross, K.A.; Fraser, E.J.; Hodgkins, C.W.; Smyth, N.A.; Egan, C.J.; Calder, J.; Kennedy, J.G. Football injuries of the ankle: A review of injury mechanisms, diagnosis and management. *World J. Orthop.* **2016**, *7*, 8–19. [CrossRef] [PubMed]
5. McKay, G.D.; Goldie, P.A.; Payne, W.R.; Oakes, B.W. Ankle injuries in basketball: Injury rate and risk factors. *Br. J. Sports Med.* **2001**, *35*, 103–108. [CrossRef] [PubMed]
6. Kobayashi, T.; Gamada, K. Lateral Ankle Sprain and Chronic Ankle Instability: A Critical Review. *Foot Spec.* **2014**, *7*, 298–326. [CrossRef]
7. Kim, M.K.; Shin, Y.J. Immediate Effects of Ankle Balance Taping with Kinesiology Tape for Amateur Soccer Players with Lateral Ankle Sprain: A Randomized Cross-Over Design. *Med. Sci. Monit.* **2017**, *23*, 5534–5541. [CrossRef]
8. Kemler, E.; van de Port, I.; Schmikli, S.; Huisstede, B.; Hoes, A.; Backx, F. Effects of soft bracing or taping on a lateral ankle sprain: A non-randomised controlled trial evaluating recurrence rates and residual symptoms at one year. *J. Foot Ankle Res.* **2015**, *8*, 13. [CrossRef]
9. Wilkerson, G.B.; Kovaleski, J.E.; Meyer, M.; Stawiz, C. Effects of the subtalar sling ankle taping technique on combined talocrural-subtalar joint motions. *Foot Ankle Int.* **2005**, *26*, 239–246. [CrossRef]
10. Karlsson, J.; Andreasson, G.O. The effect of external ankle support in chronic lateral ankle joint instability. An electromyographic study. *Am. J. Sports Med.* **1992**, *20*, 257–261. [CrossRef]
11. Ricard, M.D.; Sherwood, S.M.; Schulthies, S.S.; Knight, K.L. Effects of tape and exercise on dynamic ankle inversion. *J. Athl. Train.* **2000**, *35*, 31–37. [PubMed]
12. Pederson, T.S.; Ricard, M.D.; Merrill, G.; Schulthies, S.S.; Allsen, P.E. The effects of spatting and ankle taping on inversion before and after exercise. *J. Athl. Train.* **1997**, *32*, 29–33. [PubMed]
13. Callaghan, M.J. Role of ankle taping and bracing in the athlete. *Br. J. Sports Med.* **1997**, *31*, 102–108. [CrossRef] [PubMed]
14. Kemler, E.; van de Port, I.; Backx, F.; van Dijk, C.N. A systematic review on the treatment of acute ankle sprain: Brace versus other functional treatment types. *Sports Med.* **2011**, *41*, 185–197. [CrossRef]
15. Kerkhoffs, G.M.M.J.; Struijs, P.A.A.; Marti, R.K.; Assendelft, W.J.J.; Blankevoort, L.; van Dijk, C.N. Different functional treatment strategies for acute lateral ankle ligament injuries in adults. *Cochrane Database Syst. Rev.* **2002**, CD002938. [CrossRef]
16. Jeffriess, M.D.; Schultz, A.B.; McGann, T.S.; Callaghan, S.J.; Lockie, R.G. Effects of Preventative Ankle Taping on Planned Change-of-Direction and Reactive Agility Performance and Ankle Muscle Activity in Basketballers. *J. Sports Sci. Med.* **2015**, *14*, 864–876.

17. Morales, C.R.; Polo, J.A.; Sanz, D.R.; Lopez, D.L.; Gonzalez, S.V.; Buria, J.L.A.; Lobo, C.C. Ultrasonography features of abdominal perimuscular connective tissue in elite and amateur basketball players: An observational study. *Rev. Assoc. Med. Bras.* **2018**, *64*, 936–941. [CrossRef]
18. Romero-Morales, C.; Almazán-Polo, J.; Rodríguez-Sanz, D.; Palomo-López, P.; López-López, D.; Vázquez-González, S.; Calvo-Lobo, C. Rehabilitative Ultrasound Imaging Features of the Abdominal Wall Muscles in Elite and Amateur Basketball Players. *Appl. Sci.* **2018**, *8*, 809. [CrossRef]
19. Williams, S.A.; Ng, L.; Stephens, N.; Klem, N.; Wild, C. Effect of prophylactic ankle taping on ankle and knee biomechanics during basketball-specific tasks in females. *Phys. Ther. Sport* **2018**, *32*, 200–206. [CrossRef]
20. Chatswood, N.S. *Sports Medicine Austraila. Sports Medicine for Sports Trainers*, 10th ed.; Chatswood, N.S., Ed.; Mosby Inc: St. Louis, MO, USA, 2013.
21. Cordova, M.L.; Takahashi, Y.; Kress, G.M.; Brucker, J.B.; Finch, A.E. Influence of external ankle support on lower extremity joint mechanics during drop landings. *J. Sport Rehabil.* **2010**, *19*, 136–148. [CrossRef]
22. Balsalobre-Fernández, C.; Romero-Franco, N.; Jiménez-Reyes, P. Concurrent validity and reliability of an iPhone app for the measurement of ankle dorsiflexion and inter-limb asymmetries. *J. Sports Sci.* **2019**, *37*, 249–253. [CrossRef] [PubMed]
23. Clemente, F.M.; Mendes, B.; da Bredt, S.G.T.; Praça, G.M.; Silvério, A.; Carriço, S.; Duarte, E. Perceived Training Load, Muscle Soreness, Stress, Fatigue, and Sleep Quality in Professional Basketball: A Full Season Study. *J. Hum. Kinet.* **2019**, *67*, 199–207. [CrossRef] [PubMed]
24. Quackenbush, K.E.; Barker, P.R.J.; Stone Fury, S.M.; Behm, D.G. The effects of two adhesive ankle-taping methods on strength, power, and range of motion in female athletes. *N. Am. J. Sports Phys. Ther.* **2008**, *3*, 25–32. [PubMed]
25. Willeford, K.; Stanek, J.M.; McLoda, T.A. Collegiate Football Players' Ankle Range of Motion and Dynamic Balance in Braced and Self-Adherent-Taped Conditions. *J. Athl. Train.* **2018**, *53*, 66–71. [CrossRef]
26. Moreno-Pérez, V.; Soler, A.; Ansa, A.; López-Samanes, Á.; Madruga-Parera, M.; Beato, M.; Romero-Rodríguez, D. Acute and chronic effects of competition on ankle dorsiflexion ROM in professional football players. *Eur. J. Sport Sci.* **2020**, *20*, 51–60. [CrossRef]
27. Moreno-Pérez, V.; Del Coso, J.; Raya-González, J.; Nakamura, F.Y.; Castillo, D. Effects of basketball match-play on ankle dorsiflexion range of motion and vertical jump performance in semi-professional players. *J Sports Med. Phys. Fitness* **2020**, *60*, 110–118. [CrossRef]
28. Gribble, P.A.; Hertel, J.; Denegar, C.R.; Buckley, W.E. The Effects of Fatigue and Chronic Ankle Instability on Dynamic Postural Control. *J. Athl. Train.* **2004**, *39*, 321–329.
29. De Ridder, R.; Willems, T.; Vanrenterghem, J.; Verrelst, R.; De Blaiser, C.; Roosen, P. Taping Benefits Ankle Joint Landing Kinematics in Individuals With Chronic Ankle Instability. *J. Sport Rehabil.* **2018**, *1*, 1–16.
30. Chinn, L.; Dicharry, J.; Hart, J.M.; Saliba, S.; Wilder, R.; Hertel, J. Gait kinematics after taping in participants with chronic ankle instability. *J. Athl. Train.* **2014**, *49*, 322–330. [CrossRef]
31. Simon, J.; Donahue, M. Effect of ankle taping or bracing on creating an increased sense of confidence, stability, and reassurance when performing a dynamic-balance task. *J. Sport Rehabil.* **2013**, *22*, 229–233. [CrossRef]
32. Rabin, A.; Kozol, Z.; Spitzer, E.; Finestone, A.S. Weight-bearing ankle dorsiflexion range of motion-can side-to-side symmetry be assumed? *J. Athl. Train.* **2015**, *50*, 30–35. [CrossRef] [PubMed]
33. Han, J.; Anson, J.; Waddington, G.; Adams, R.; Liu, Y. The Role of Ankle Proprioception for Balance Control in relation to Sports Performance and Injury. *BioMed Res. Int.* **2015**, *2015*, 842804. [CrossRef] [PubMed]
34. Wang, Y.; Gu, Y.; Chen, J.; Luo, W.; He, W.; Han, Z.; Tian, J. Kinesio taping is superior to other taping methods in ankle functional performance improvement: A systematic review and meta-analysis. *Clin. Rehabil.* **2018**, *32*, 1472–1481. [CrossRef] [PubMed]
35. Simsek, S.; Yagci, N. Acute effects of distal fibular taping technique on pain, balance and forward lunge activities in Chronic Ankle Instability. *J. Back Musculoskelet Rehabil.* **2019**, *32*, 15–20. [CrossRef] [PubMed]

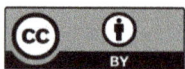

© 2020 by the authors. Licensee MDPI, Basel, Switzerland. This article is an open access article distributed under the terms and conditions of the Creative Commons Attribution (CC BY) license (http://creativecommons.org/licenses/by/4.0/).

 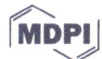

Article

Effects of Upper-Limb, Lower-Limb, and Full-Body Compression Garments on Full Body Kinematics and Free-Throw Accuracy in Basketball Players

Duo Wai-Chi Wong [1,2], Wing-Kai Lam [3,4,5,*], Tony Lin-Wei Chen [1], Qitao Tan [1], Yan Wang [1,2] and Ming Zhang [1,2,*]

1. Department of Biomedical Engineering, Faculty of Engineering, The Hong Kong Polytechnic University, Hong Kong 999077, China; duo.wong@polyu.edu.hk (D.W.-C.W.); tony.l.chen@connect.polyu.hk (T.L.-W.C.); matthew.tan@connect.polyu.hk (Q.T.); annie.y.wang@polyu.edu.hk (Y.W.)
2. The Hong Kong Polytechnic University Shenzhen Research Institute, Shenzhen 518057, China
3. Guangdong Provincial Engineering Technology Research Center for Sports Assistive Devices, Guangzhou Sport University, Guangzhou 510000, China
4. Department of Kinesiology, Shenyang Sport University, Shenyang 110102, China
5. Li Ning Sports Science Research Center, Li Ning (China) Sports Goods Company, Beijing 101111, China
* Correspondence: gilbertlam@li-ning.com.cn (W.-K.L.); ming.zhang@polyu.edu.hk (M.Z.); Tel.: +86-010-80801108 (W.-K.L.); +852-2766-4939 (M.Z.)

Received: 1 April 2020; Accepted: 6 May 2020; Published: 19 May 2020

Abstract: Compression garments can enhance performance and promote recovery in athletes. Different body coverage with compression garments may impose distinct effects on kinematic movement mechanics and thus basketball free-throw accuracy. The objective of this study was to examine basketball free-throw shooting accuracy, consistency and the range of motion of body joints while wearing upper-, lower- and full-body compression garments. Twenty male basketball players performed five blocks of 20 basketball free-throw shooting trials in each of the following five compression garment conditions: control-pre, top, bottom, full (top + bottom) and control-post. All conditions were randomized except pre- and post-control (the first and last conditions). Range of motion of was acquired by multiple inertial measurement units. Free-throw accuracy and the coefficient of variation were also analyzed. Players wearing upper-body or full-body compression garments had significantly improved accuracy by 4.2% and 5.9%, respectively ($p < 0.05$), but this difference was not observed with shooting consistency. Smaller range of motion of head flexion and trunk lateral bending ($p < 0.05$) was found in the upper- and full-body conditions compared to the control-pre condition. These findings suggest that an improvement in shooting accuracy could be achieved by constraining the range of motion through the use of upper-body and full-body compression garments.

Keywords: range of motion; basketball shooting; proprioception

1. Introduction

Basketball is one of the most popular sports; at least 450 million people play basketball worldwide, ranging from registered elite players to amateurs [1]. Basketball skills can be categorized into offensive skills, including shooting, passing and dribbling and defensive skills, including blocking and stealing [2]. While shooting is the mean to score in the game, free-throws (or foul shots) are considered as one of the easiest movements, yet they can significantly influence the outcome of a game [3,4]. Movement mechanics and coordination are key to free-throwing performance [5,6] and may be regulated by wearing compression garments [7].

Compression garment can enhance performance and recovery in various sports [7,8]. Specifically, compression garments improve joint awareness, reduce muscle soreness and encourage blood circulation and thus, promote recovery [9]. Conversely, some studies have argued that upper-body compression garment may impose negative effects in hot environments and the claimed benefits may only be confined to perception of comfort [10,11]. Different movement tasks, selection of indicators, and the physical status of the athletes may also contribute to the variability and effectiveness of using compression garments during exercise, whereas garment design, such as type, coverage and tightness, may affect the functions of the garment [9]. The tightness of the compression garment has been hypothesized to change the interfacial pressure of the body [12]; however, there is a lack of studies exploring the influence of body coverage with different compression garments.

The benefits of compression garments could be attributed to the enhancement of proprioception to improve movement mechanics [13]. Hooper et al. [14] demonstrated the relationship between throwing velocity and accuracy, and improved proprioceptive signals in upper-body compression garments for baseball athletes. The compression on the cutaneous receptors or muscle spindle receptors not only enhanced the sensory information, but also filtered irrelevant mechanoreceptor information [15]. Depending on the task, the nervous system integrated these signals or information at multiple levels to mediate cutaneous and muscle afferent feedback, which is imperative for smooth coordination of movements [15–17].

There is insufficient evidence to support the use of compression garments (upper-body or lower-body) to enhance basketball performance. Atkins et al. [7] showed that wearing lower-body compression garments overnight produced negligible effects on the countermovement jump, repeated sprint and agility test performances, despite improvements in perceived fatigue and muscle soreness. Other evidence indicated that lower-leg compression garments were found to significantly reduce the range of abduction motion of the hip joint during a drop vertical jump, but produced minimal effects on the kinematics/kinetics of other lower extremity joints [13].

Furthermore, lower-body compression was shown to improve lower limb balance and stability in active females during a single-leg balance task [18]. Poor stability results in higher motion variability and may potentially weaken shooting accuracy [6,19,20]. How these findings affect other functional performances (e.g., basketball shooting) requires further investigation. Since compression garments produce mechanical restraints on body segments and joints, range of motion (ROM) has been one of the key parameters for the evaluation of kinematic effects during exercise in previous basketball studies [13,21].

Considering the relationship between compression garment coverage (upper-body, lower-body and combined) on the kinematics and shooting performance of basketball specific maneuvers is currently questionable, coaches and athletes are eager to understand what type of compression garment coverage could help them improve performance and consistency of performance. The objective of this study was to examine the effect of upper- and lower-body compression garment coverage (top, bottom and full) on the full body range of motion (ROM) and shooting accuracy of basketball free-throws. It was hypothesized that a certain compression garment condition would improve free-throw performance and consistency compared to the no-compression garment control group.

2. Materials and Methods

2.1. Participants

Twenty ($n = 20$) male basketball players were recruited from local universities. Their average age, height and body mass were 22.6 ± 1.1 years, 179.4 ± 3.4 cm and 72.7 ± 8.2 kg, respectively. All participants had at least 4 years of experiences in playing basketball and were right hand dominant single-handed shooters. The average basketball training experience and training time were 8.5 ± 2.4 years and 5.2 ± 1.6 h per week, respectively. All participants were physically fit and healthy and reported no injuries over the previous 6 months. Ethical approval (IRB-2017-BM-006) was granted from the institutional ethics committee. Written informed consent was obtained from all participants.

2.2. Experimental Conditions and Procedure

All free-throw shooting conditions were performed in our biomechanical laboratory. The free-throw distance and the height of the basketball rim were set according to the International Basketball Federation standards [19]. The participants performed single-handed free-throws under five different garment conditions, control-pre: no garment pre-control, Top: upper-body compression garment (Li Ning, Powershell, AULM043-I, Beijing, China), Bottom: lower-body compression garment bottom (Li Ning, Powershell, AUDL101-1, Beijing, China), full: both upper-body and lower-body compression garment and control-post: no garment post-control, as shown in Figure 1. Control-pre and control-post were the first and the last test conditions. The remaining three compression garment conditions (top, bottom and full) were randomly assigned as the second to the fourth conditions across participants. As the experimental protocol compared the first and last conditions, we were able to evaluate the fatigue effect [22]. For each free-throw condition, 20 free-throw shooting trials were performed. Testing of the next condition started immediately after the participant changed their garments.

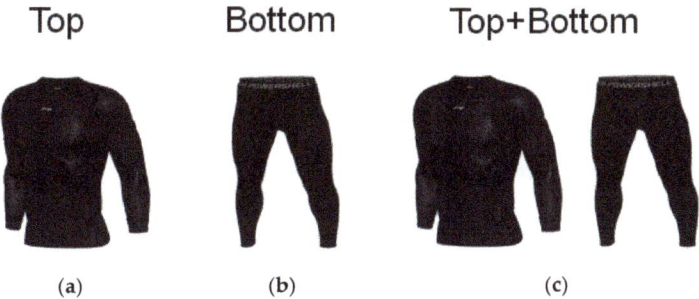

Figure 1. Compression garment conditions: (**a**) top; (**b**) bottom; (**c**) full (top + bottom).

The control conditions (control-pre and control-post) were self-selected comfortable sportswear that were not compression garments. The experimenters measured the height, waist and chest circumference of the participants to determine the appropriate garment [23]. The appropriate compression garment size was pre-determined by the manufacturer's sizing guidelines and was based on the body height and mass of each participant. Next, we assigned participants compression garments one size smaller than the pre-determined appropriate size in order to increase the interfacial pressure, as recommended by the experimental protocol detailed by Williams and colleagues [12].

A motion capturing system with multiple inertial measurement units (MyoMOTION, Noraxon, Inc., Scottsdale, AZ, USA) was used to measure full-body kinematics during the free-throw shooting trials. The inertial measurement units (IMU) were attached and strapped to each body segment according to the instrument guidelines. During each free-throw trial, the participants performed shooting from the same position behind the free-throw line. The sampling frequency of the IMU was 200 Hz. The kinematic data during the free-throw motion were post-processed using Matlab software (MathWorks, Inc., Natick, MA, USA) using a 6 Hz cutoff 4th order Butterworth low-pass filter.

2.3. Outcome Measures

Outcome measures including performance score (accuracy) and joint ROM variables were investigated. The performance score was gauged using an ordinal six-point (0 to 5 point) scoring system. Five, four and three points denoted a clean score, that the ball hit the rim and went in, and that the ball hit the backboard and went in, respectively. Two, one and zero points denoted that the ball hit the rim and missed, hit the backboard and missed and missed complete, respectively, as illustrated in Table 1 [19,24]. The consistency of the score was also assessed by the coefficient of variation (i.e., the ratio of the standard deviation to the mean of the trials).

Table 1. The six-point basketball shooting performance score system.

Performance	Scored			Missed		
	Clean (Swish)	Rim & In	Backboard & In	Rim & Out	Backboard & Out	Complete Miss
Score	5	4	3	2	1	0

ROM of the head, trunk, elbow, shoulder, wrist, hip, knee and ankle joints in the sagittal, coronal and frontal planes were calculated. Data were averaged across trials for each participant in each condition which served as the targeted average profile for subsequent statistical analysis [25]. We did not view the within-participant effect (trial) of ROM as an independent observation or random factor to be analyzed.

2.4. Data Analysis

All statistical analysis was performed in SPSS 21 (IBM, New York, NY, USA). Prior to statistical analysis, the Shapiro–Wilk test was performed to check for the normality of the kinematic data, and it was satisfied. The Wilcoxon signed-rank test was performed to compare free-throw performance scores between the control-pre- and control-post-control conditions to ensure that there was no learning or fatigue effect (i.e., Control pre- and post-control were not significantly different). Furthermore, one-way repeated measures analysis of variance (ANOVA) was performed to examine any significant difference for joint ROM variables between the control-pre, top, bottom and full conditions, followed by the post hoc pairwise comparison of Least Significant Difference (LSD) if a significant main effect was found. We chose the LSD approach as our research hypothesis was more focused on planned comparisons. As such, we regarded the ANOVA as an additional constraint [26]. Similarly, the comparison for the performance score and the coefficient of variation was performed using a nonparametric test (Friedman test), with the post hoc pairwise Wilcoxon signed-rank test, as the performance score was gauged in an ordinal scale. Level of significance was set at $p = 0.05$. The indices of effect size for the ANOVA and post hoc pairwise comparison were partial η^2 and Cohen's d, respectively.

3. Results

3.1. Control-Pre and Control-Post Conditions

There was no significant difference in performance score between the control-pre (Median = 2.975) and control-post (Median = 3.075) conditions (Z = −1.430, $p = 0.153$). Similarly, there was no significant difference in the coefficient of variation of performance score between the control-pre and control-post conditions (Z = −1.382, $p = 0.167$). We assumed that there was no pronounced carry-over or fatigue effect that significantly affected performance over the course of the experiment.

3.2. Free-Throw Accuracy

There were no significant differences in free-throw performance score ($\chi^2(4) = 6.510$, $p = 0.089$) or the coefficient of variation of the performance score ($\chi^2(4) = 5.629$, $p = 0.131$) between the conditions (control-pre, top, bottom or full). However, post hoc pairwise comparison showed that the free-throw performance scores of the top (Median = 3.1, Z = −2.357, $p = 0.018$) and full (Median = 3.15, Z = −2.112, $p = 0.035$) conditions were significantly larger than that of the control-pre condition (Median = 2.975), as shown in Tables 2 and 3.

Table 2. Descriptive statistics of the averaged and coefficient of variation of the free-throw performance score.

Condition	Performance Score		Coefficient of Variation (%)
	Median	Mean (Standard Deviation)	Mean (Standard Deviation)
Control-Pre	2.975	2.975 (0.419)	38.04 (6.67)
Top	3.100 *	3.168 (0.382)	36.78 (7.05)
Bottom	3.050	3.035 (0.411)	37.06 (7.07)
Full	3.150 *	3.175 (0.385)	36.19 (7.58)
Control-Post	3.075	3.123 (0.476)	35.88 (8.61)

* significant difference ($p < 0.05$) compared to the control-pre condition by post hoc Wilcoxon signed-rank test.

Table 3. Probability values (p-value) of the average (upper right triangle) and coefficient of variation (lower left triangle) of the free-throw performance score.

Coefficient of Variation	Performance Score			
	Control-Pre	Top	Bottom	Full
Control-Pre		0.018 *	0.230	0.035 *
Top	0.296		0.152	0.888
Bottom	0.227	0.654		0.159
Full	0.107	0.794	0.344	

* significant difference ($p < 0.05$) by post hoc Wilcoxon signed-rank test.

3.3. Full-Body Joint Range of Motion (RoM)

One-way ANOVA repeated measures showed that the variation in compression garments imposed significant effects on the ROM of head flexion ($p = 0.014$, partial $\eta^2 = 0.169$), trunk lateral bending ($p = 0.024$, partial $\eta^2 = 0.152$), left shoulder flexion ($p = 0.041$, partial $\eta^2 = 0.152$), right shoulder rotation ($p = 0.048$, partial $\eta^2 = 0.128$) and left knee flexion ($p = 0.003$, partial $\eta^2 = 0.212$). Post hoc pairwise comparison showed that the top condition significantly reduced the head flexion ($p = 0.037$; d = 0.503; 1.346, 95% CI 0.376 to 2.315) and trunk lateral bending ($p = 0.042$; d = 0.487; 1.039, 95% CI 0.041 to 2.036) ROM compared with the control-pre condition (Table 4). Similarly, the full condition significantly reduced head flexion ($p = 0.009$; d = 0.650; 1.346, 95% CI 0.376 to 2.315) and trunk lateral bending ($p = 0.028$; d = 0.532; 1.446, 95% CI 0.173 to 2.718) ROM compared to the control-pre condition.

Table 4. Descriptive statistics and one-way ANOVA repeated measures outcome of the range of motion of head and trunk in different compression garment conditions.

	Range of Motion, Mean (Standard Deviation)				ANOVA Repeated Measure	
	Control-Pre	Top	Bottom	Full	Effect Size	p-Value
Head FL/EX	10.57 (3.81)	9.53 (3.1) [a]	9.75 (3.37)	9.22 (3.07) [A]	0.169	0.014 *
Head lateral bending	6.14 (2.83)	5.80 (2.69)	6.05 (2.99)	5.87 (2.62)	0.019 [g]	0.694
Head axial rotation	13.17 (8.04)	17.11 (12.74)	15.02 (10.49)	14.42 (8.63)	0.053	0.368
Trunk FL/EX	19.20 (6.24)	17.15 (5.96)	18.43 (5.85)	18.15 (6.42)	0.11	0.082
Trunk lateral bending	10.21 (4.24)	9.17 (4.38) [a]	9.88 (3.63)	8.77 (4.01) [a]	0.152	0.024 *
Trunk axial rotation	11.05 (4.56)	11.46 (5.04)	10.99 (4.36)	11.39 (4.37)	0.018 [g]	0.687

FL/EX: flexion/extension; * significant difference ($p < 0.05$) using one-way ANOVA repeated measures; [g] Greenhouse–Geisser correction to adjust the lack of sphericity; [a] and [A] denote $p < 0.05$ and $p < 0.0125$ than the control-pre condition.

Compared to that of the bottom condition, both the top ($p = 0.01$; d = 0.642; 3.422, 95% CI 0.929 to 5.915) and full ($p = 0.003$; d = 0.778; 3.530, 95% CI 1.405 to 5.655) conditions significantly reduced the ROM of the left shoulder flexion, while the top condition had significantly larger right shoulder rotation compared with the control-pre ($p = 0.013$; d = 0.611; 38.316, 95% CI −8.98 to 67.65) and bottom ($p = 0.041$; d = 0.491; 23.028, 95% CI 1.08 to 44.976) conditions (Table 5). The control-pre condition had significantly larger left knee flexion ROM than the bottom ($p = 0.026$; d = 0.539; 2.605, 95% CI 0.345 to 4.864) and full ($p = 0.002$; d = 0.804; 2.908, 95% CI 1.214 to 4.602) conditions. Similarly, the top condition had a significantly larger left knee flexion ROM than the bottom ($p = 0.044$; d = 0.482; 2.047, 95% CI 0.059 to 4.035) and full ($p = 0.018$; d = 0.585; 2.351, 95% CI, 0.469 to 4.232) conditions (Table 6).

Table 5. Descriptive statistics and one-way ANOVA repeated measures outcome of the range of motion of the upper limb in different compression garment conditions.

	Range of Motion, Mean (Standard Deviation)				ANOVA Repeated Measure	
	Control-Pre	Top	Bottom	Full	Effect Size	p-Value
L elbow FL/EX	49.35 (23.12)	51.38 (23.28)	50.95 (22.82)	51.24 (24.05)	0.048	0.417
R elbow FL/EX	93.30 (13.27)	89.43 (12.46)	89.14 (13.79)	89.82 (14.38)	0.098	0.116
L shoulder FL/EX	30.06 (12.77)	26.98 (11.58)	30.40 (12.66) [B]	26.87 (10.48) [C]	0.152 [g]	0.041 *
R shoulder FL/EX	44.11 (18.88)	40.48 (16.96)	44.01 (19.11)	41.47 (17.2)	0.148 [g]	0.148
L shoulder AB/AD	124.84 (113.81)	125.37 (132.49)	133.85 (120.05)	132.36 (124.17)	0.022 [g]	0.66
R shoulder AB/AD	72.93 (51)	75.01 (55.07)	76.05 (48.47)	78.02 (71.69)	0.012 [g]	0.821
L shoulder rotation	50.50 (40.81)	58.41 (51.4)	67.74 (83.18)	59.95 (61.04)	0.089 [g]	0.176
R shoulder rotation	90.38 (45.46)	128.70 (81.71) [a]	105.67 (67.28) [b]	118.07 (73.94)	0.128	0.048 *
L wrist RA/UL	35.80 (26.08)	34.93 (27)	35.12 (28.48)	38.26 (32.93)	0.036	0.552
R wrist RA/UL	70.79 (27.55)	79.36 (29.02)	71.34 (33.37)	77.37 (31.8)	0.071 [g]	0.249
L wrist FL/EX	39.21 (33.56)	39.37 (41.11)	42.20 (43.93)	42.90 (45.34)	0.011 [g]	0.885
R wrist FL/EX	105.39 (34.39)	109.35 (36.59)	110.83 (35.36)	106.85 (35.66)	0.026	0.675
L palm rotation	49.54 (47.21)	51.35 (48.84)	60.70 (72.13)	52.23 (55.49)	0.067 [g]	0.269
R palm rotation	93.97 (46)	126.74 (77.75)	113.01 (81.54)	110.93 (66.53)	0.117	0.066

FL/EX: flexion/extension; AB/AD: abduction/adduction; RA/UL: Radial/Ulnar deviation; * significant difference ($p < 0.05$) using one-way ANOVA repeated measures; [g] Greenhouse–Geisser correction to adjust the lack of sphericity; [a] denotes $p < 0.05$ than the control-pre condition; [b] and [B] denote $p < 0.05$ and $p < 0.0125$ than the top condition; [C] denotes $p < 0.0125$ than the bottom condition.

Table 6. Descriptive statistics and one-way ANOVA repeated measures outcome of the range of motion of the lower limb in different compression garment conditions.

	Range of Motion, Mean (Standard Deviation)				ANOVA Repeated Measure	
	Control-Pre	Top	Bottom	Full	Effect Size	p-Value
L hip FL/EX	23.56 (6.8)	22.58 (6.65)	22.34 (7.8)	21.81 (7.19)	0.076 [g]	0.22
R hip FL/EX	26.47 (4.49)	25.14 (6.02)	26.19 (6.26)	25.93 (5.85)	0.065	0.274
L hip AB/AD	5.69 (1.73)	6.46 (2.38)	5.57 (1.64)	6.28 (2.36)	0.069	0.251
R hip AB/AD	6.95 (2.6)	7.22 (2.72)	6.31 (2.42)	6.97 (2.62)	0.069	0.248
L hip rotation	9.99 (3.57)	10.03 (3.52)	9.31 (3.04)	9.45 (2.53)	0.043 [g]	0.445
R hip rotation	12.62 (3.89)	12.83 (4.19)	12.43 (4.17)	12.30 (4.61)	0.013	0.861
L knee FL/EX	51.86 (8.63)	51.30 (8.15)	49.25 (10.08) [a, b]	48.95 (9.37) [A, b]	0.212	0.003 *
R knee FL/EX	53.77 (7.33)	52.90 (7.88)	53.61 (6.61)	52.94 (6.67)	0.036	0.549
L knee rotation	10.64 (4.39)	11.35 (5.59)	10.26 (3.99)	10.35 (4.21)	0.051 [g]	0.37
R knee rotation	14.96 (4.52)	14.72 (6.12)	15.68 (5.86)	15.43 (5.01)	0.031	0.61
L knee AB/AD	7.15 (4.52)	7.92 (4.46)	6.81 (2.89)	7.00 (3.28)	0.029 [g]	0.587
R knee AB/AD	8.32 (3.72)	7.67 (3.84)	9.10 (4.32)	8.48 (3.58)	0.048	0.418
L ankle PL/DO	61.22 (16.82)	64.36 (8.64)	61.71 (8.01)	61.83 (9.08)	0.049 [g]	0.362
R ankle PL/DO	60.93 (11.16)	61.97 (6.1)	60.76 (7.49)	61.82 (8.21)	0.019 [g]	0.682
L ankle EV/IV	25.31 (14.66)	22.84 (13.08)	24.29 (11.37)	23.38 (12.54)	0.041	0.49
R ankle EV/IV	26.49 (13.19)	23.04 (11.28)	22.95 (8.38)	21.27 (10.34)	0.123	0.056
L ankle AB/AD	15.28 (4.08)	15.47 (4.5)	15.52 (4.76)	16.12 (5.18)	0.016 [g]	0.732
R ankle AB/AD	13.98 (3.73)	14.69 (4.46)	15.17 (4.9)	14.43 (4.14)	0.077	0.204

FL/EX: flexion/extension; AB/AD: abduction/adduction; EV/IV: eversion/inversion; PL/DO: plantarflexion/dorsiflexion; * significant difference ($p < 0.05$) using one-way ANOVA repeated measures; [g] Greenhouse–Geisser correction to adjust the lack of sphericity; [a] and [A] denote $p < 0.05$ and $p < 0.0125$ than the control-pre condition; [b] denotes $p < 0.05$ than the top condition.

4. Discussion

This study examined the effect of upper and lower-body compression garments on the body kinematics and shooting accuracy of basketball free-throws. Our study found that upper-body (top) or full-body (top + bottom) compression garments significantly improved the performance of basketball free-throws; however, there was no significant improvement in the consistency of performance. Overall, mechanically, compression garments had a significant influence on the ROM of the head flexion, trunk lateral bending, left (non-dominant side) shoulder flexion, right (dominant side) shoulder rotation and left knee flexion as indicated by the ANOVA findings. Post hoc comparisons showed that wearing either upper- or full-body garments constrained the ROM of head flexion and trunk lateral bending which could be associated with improved trunk stability and thus, improved performance [27]. The relationship between the condition of the head movement and stability and free-throw accuracy was advocated previously, but not well understood [28]. On the other hand, garment coverage of the lower body (bottom or full-body gear) significantly reduced the ROM of the left (non-dominant) side knee joint in the sagittal plane, but not the right (dominant) side, because experienced players tended to adjust the knee joint of the dominant side to greater extent for better performance [29]. Theoretically, compression of the knee joint enhanced proprioception and thus performance [30,31] notwithstanding that our study did not demonstrate an improved shooting score for lower-body (bottom) garments. In addition, the reduced head flexion and trunk lateral bending ROM could implicate successful shooting performance.

Elbow and wrist movements are determinants of free-throw performance and player skill levels [20]. Skilled players coordinate the shooting arm by constantly compromising between elbow and wrist movements to adapt to subtle changes in release parameters of the ball (e.g., release height, angle of ball projection, velocity at ball release) [20]. In addition, more highly skilled players tend to maximize the ROM of the wrist joint [20]. top compression garments help to constrain the ROM of the elbow, and thus players can focus on optimizing distal joint (wrist) motion only [20]. In our study, although there were no significant main effects on the ROM of the elbow and wrist joints, pairwise comparisons showed that upper-body (top) garments significantly reduced the ROM of the right (dominant) side elbow, but increased that of the wrist radial/ulnar deviation and palmar rotation compared to that of the control-pre condition. This was likely due to the fact that the uncovered wrist joint compensated the reduced motion of the elbow [20]. In fact, some statisticians argued that conducting and interpreting post hoc analyses could still be valid even though the main effect was not significant [32,33].

The enhanced proprioception by compression garments may also facilitate the organization of compensatory behavior between joints for better performance. This was supported by existing studies that the proprioception (joint position sense) of the elbow and wrist joints was correlated with the success rate of the free-throw tasks [34]. More highly skilled players managed to optimize their performance based on the perceptual consequence of their actions [35].

A previous study suggested that the shoulder joint plays an important role in the action of basketball free-throws. Kaya et al. [36] found that free-throw performance was significantly correlated with the peak torque of the shoulder joint muscles and the shoulder joint position sense at 160° in the dominant side. While we anticipated that compression garments would amplify the proprioception [30], enhance stability and reduce the ROM of the shooting limb (right side), our study found that the ROM of the upper-body was significantly smaller when wearing top compression garments than when wearing bottom garments. Although there were no significant differences compared to that of the control-pre condition, we believe that the increased trend of the joint ROM may indicate that wearing lower-body (bottom) garments alone had a negative effect on the shoulder joint. From the kinetic chain perspective, intervention at the lower limb level may alter energy generation which can be transferred to the upper limbs and thus considerably influences upper limb movement tasks (e.g., racket and ball speed in racket sports) [19,37]. The influence of lower limb garments on the upper limbs may also be the reason that the full-body garments did not have an effect on the elbow and wrist joints, despite upper-body garments having an effect.

There were some limitations in this study. First, although we demonstrated no carry-over effect as revealed by the fact that there was no significant difference between the performance score of the control-pre and control-post conditions, there was an improvement trend on both the performance score and consistency. We believed that the randomized order assigned on the garment condition could minimize the carry-over effect. Second, our short adaptation time for each compression garment condition may not be adequate enough, despite that there is no consensus on the duration of adaptation in the past studies. Future studies may consider tests with longer adaptation in different days or weeks or considering the variation of kinematic variables [38]. Third, we presented only joint ROM in this study. More comprehensive analysis with discrete variables (peak angle, angular velocity), joint power, muscle force, proprioception as well as stability should be considered to evaluate their influence and underlying mechanism on the free-throw shooting performance. Asymmetry sport activity (e.g., single-handed shooting) may produce unique sequential coordination of the upper and lower limb with coherent patterns of muscle activation [39]. Forth, our study confined to non-professional basketball players. Playing level and sex effects may contribute to variations in movement strategy, skeletal alignment and muscle strength and could also be investigated. Lastly, the compression garments may impose different levels of pressure on the participants depending on their body built. Future study shall consider measuring the compression level in each condition.

5. Conclusions

Players wearing upper-body or full-body compression garment significantly improved basketball free-throw accuracy by 4.2% and 5.9%, respectively, but not on the intertrial consistency. full body kinematics data suggested that the improved performance could be attributed to the reduced ROM of head flexion and lateral bending of the trunk. Future studies investigating the relationship between shooting performance in basketball, reduced ROM and enhanced proprioception or stability are required.

Author Contributions: Conceptualization, D.W.-C.W. and W.-K.L.; data curation, D.W.-C.W. and T.L.-W.C.; formal analysis, D.W.-C.W. and T.L.-W.C.; funding acquisition, M.Z.; investigation, T.L.-W.C., Q.T. and Y.W.; methodology, D.W.-C.W., T.L.-W.C. and Q.T.; supervision, W.-K.L. and M.Z.; writing—original draft, D.W.-C.W.; writing—review & editing, W.-K.L. All authors have read and agreed to the published version of the manuscript.

Funding: This research was funded by the Key R&D Program granted by the Ministry of Science and Technology of China, Grant Number 2018YFB1107000; the National Natural Science Foundation of China, Key Program Grant Number 11732015 and General Program Grant Number 11972315; and the General Research Fund granted by the Hong Kong Research Grant Council, Grant Number PolyU152065/17E and PolyU152002/15E.

Conflicts of Interest: W.-K.L. is an employee of Li Ning Sports Goods Company Limited which supplied the compression garments and footwear in the experiments. Other authors declared no potential conflict of interest.

References

1. Drinkwater, E.J.; Pyne, D.B.; McKenna, M.J. Design and interpretation of anthropometric and fitness testing of basketball players. *Sports Med.* **2008**, *38*, 565–578. [CrossRef] [PubMed]
2. Krause, J.V.; Nelson, C. *Basketball Skills & Drills*; Human Kinetics: Champaign, IL, USA, 2018.
3. Sampaio, J.; Janeira, M. Statistical analyses of basketball team performance: Understanding teams' wins and losses according to a different index of ball possessions. *Int. J. Perform. Anal. Sport* **2003**, *3*, 40–49. [CrossRef]
4. Csataljay, G.; O'Donoghue, P.; Hughes, M.; Dancs, H. Performance indicators that distinguish winning and losing teams in basketball. *Int. J. Perform. Anal. Sport* **2009**, *9*, 60–66. [CrossRef]
5. Okazaki, V.H.; Rodacki, A.L.; Satern, M.N. A review on the basketball jump shot. *Sports Biomech.* **2015**, *14*, 190–205. [CrossRef] [PubMed]
6. Verhoeven, F.M.; Newell, K.M. Coordination and control of posture and ball release in basketball free-throw shooting. *Hum. Mov. Sci.* **2016**, *49*, 216–224. [CrossRef] [PubMed]
7. Atkins, R.; Lam, W.-K.; Scanlan, A.T.; Beaven, C.M.; Driller, M. Lower-body compression garments worn following exercise improves perceived recovery but not subsequent performance in basketball athletes. *J. Sports Sci.* **2020**, *38*, 1–9. [CrossRef]
8. Marqués-Jiménez, D.; Calleja-González, J.; Arratibel, I.; Delextrat, A.; Terrados, N. Are compression garments effective for the recovery of exercise-induced muscle damage? A systematic review with meta-analysis. *Physiol. Behav.* **2016**, *153*, 133–148. [CrossRef]
9. MacRae, B.A.; Cotter, J.D.; Laing, R.M. Compression garments and exercise: Garment considerations, physiology and performance. *Sports Med.* **2011**, *41*, 815–843. [CrossRef]

10. Leoz-Abaurrea, I.; Aguado-Jiménez, R. Upper Body Compression Garment: Physiological Effects While Cycling in a Hot Environment. *Wilderness Environ. Med.* **2017**, *28*, 94–100. [CrossRef]
11. Ali, A.; Creasy, R.H.; Edge, J.A. Physiological effects of wearing graduated compression stockings during running. *Eur. J. Appl. Physiol.* **2010**, *109*, 1017–1025. [CrossRef]
12. Brophy-Williams, N.; Driller, M.W.; Shing, C.M.; Fell, J.W.; Halson, S.L. Confounding compression: The effects of posture, sizing and garment type on measured interface pressure in sports compression clothing. *J. Sports Sci.* **2015**, *33*, 1403–1410. [CrossRef] [PubMed]
13. Zamporri, J.; Aguinaldo, A. The Effects of a Compression Garment on Lower Body Kinematics and Kinetics During a Drop Vertical Jump in Female Collegiate Athletes. *Orthop. J. Sports Med.* **2018**, *6*, 2325967118789955. [CrossRef] [PubMed]
14. Hooper, D.R.; Dulkis, L.L.; Secola, P.J.; Holtzum, G.; Harper, S.P.; Kalkowski, R.J.; Comstock, B.A.; Szivak, T.K.; Flanagan, S.D.; Looney, D.P. Roles of an upper-body compression garment on athletic performances. *J. Strength Cond. Res.* **2015**, *29*, 2655–2660. [CrossRef] [PubMed]
15. Barss, T.S.; Pearcey, G.E.; Munro, B.; Bishop, J.L.; Zehr, E.P. Effects of a compression garment on sensory feedback transmission in the human upper limb. *J. Neurophysiol.* **2018**, *120*, 186–195. [CrossRef]
16. Zehr, P.E.; Collins, D.F.; Chua, R. Human interlimb reflexes evoked by electrical stimulation of cutaneous nerves innervating the hand and foot. *Exp. Brain Res.* **2001**, *140*, 495–504. [CrossRef]
17. Zehr, E.P.; Collins, D.F.; Frigon, A.; Hoogenboom, N. Neural control of rhythmic human arm movement: Phase dependence and task modulation of Hoffmann reflexes in forearm muscles. *J. Neurophysiol.* **2003**, *89*, 12–21. [CrossRef]
18. Michael, J.S.; Dogramaci, S.N.; Steel, K.A.; Graham, K.S. What is the effect of compression garments on a balance task in female athletes? *Gait Posture* **2014**, *39*, 804–809. [CrossRef]
19. Lam, W.-K.; Lee, W.C.-C.; Ng, S.-O.; Zheng, Y. Effects of foot orthoses on dynamic balance and basketball free-throw accuracy before and after physical fatigue. *J. Biomech.* **2019**, *96*, 109338. [CrossRef]
20. Button, C.; Macleod, M.; Sanders, R.; Coleman, S. Examining movement variability in the basketball free-throw action at different skill levels. *Res. Q. Exerc. Sport* **2003**, *74*, 257–269. [CrossRef]
21. Montgomery, P.G.; Pyne, D.B.; Hopkins, W.G.; Dorman, J.C.; Cook, K.; Minahan, C.L. The effect of recovery strategies on physical performance and cumulative fatigue in competitive basketball. *J. Sports Sci.* **2008**, *26*, 1135–1145. [CrossRef]
22. Thomas, J.R.; Nelson, J.K.; Silverman, S.J. *Research Methods in Physical Activity*; Human Kinetics: Champaign, IL, USA, 2015.
23. Watkins, W.B. Compression garment sizing: Challenges, issues, and a solution. *Plast. Surg. Nurs.* **2010**, *30*, 85–87. [CrossRef] [PubMed]
24. Martin, L. *Sports Performance Measurement and Analytics: The Science of Assessing Performance, Predicting Future Outcomes, Interpreting Statistical Models, and Evaluating the Market Value of Athletes*; FT Press: Upper Saddle River, NJ, USA, 2016.
25. Newell, J.; Aitchison, T.; Grant, S. *Statistics for Sports and Exercise Science: A Practical Approach*; Routledge: Abingdon, UK, 2014.
26. Holm, S. A simple sequentially rejective multiple test procedure. *Scand. J. Stat.* **1979**, *6*, 65–70.
27. Doan, B.; Kwon, Y.-H.; Newton, R.; Shim, J.; Popper, E.; Rogers, R.; Bolt, L.; Robertson, M.; Kraemer, W. Evaluation of a lower-body compression garment. *J. Sports Sci.* **2003**, *21*, 601–610. [CrossRef] [PubMed]
28. Humphries, K.M.; Ward, J.; Coats, J.; Nobert, J.; Amonette, W.; Dyess, S. Immediate effects of lower cervical spine manipulation on handgrip strength and free-throw accuracy of asymptomatic basketball players: A pilot study. *J. Chiropr. Med.* **2013**, *12*, 153–159. [CrossRef]
29. Ammar, A.; Chtourou, H.; Abdelkarim, O.; Parish, A.; Hoekelmann, A. Free throw shot in basketball: Kinematic analysis of scored and missed shots during the learning process. *Sport Sci. Health* **2016**, *12*, 27–33. [CrossRef]
30. Ghai, S.; Driller, M.; Ghai, I. Effects of joint stabilizers on proprioception and stability: A systematic review and meta-analysis. *Phys. Ther. Sport* **2017**, *25*, 65–75. [CrossRef]
31. Ghai, S.; Driller, M.W.; Masters, R.S.J.G. The influence of below-knee compression garments on knee-joint proprioception. *Gait Posture* **2018**, *60*, 258–261. [CrossRef]
32. Hsu, J. *Multiple Comparisons: Theory and Methods*; CRC Press: Boca Raton, FL, USA, 1996.

33. Maxwell, S.E.; Delaney, H.D.; Kelley, K. *Designing Experiments and Analyzing Data: A Model Comparison Perspective*; Routledge: Abingdon, UK, 2017.
34. Sevrez, V.; Bourdin, C. On the role of proprioception in making free throws in basketball. *Res. Q. Exerc. Sport* **2015**, *86*, 274–280. [CrossRef]
35. Handford, C.; Davids, K.; Bennett, S.; Button, C. Skill acquisition in sport: Some applications of an evolving practice ecology. *J. Sports Sci.* **1997**, *15*, 621–640. [CrossRef]
36. Kaya, D.; Callaghan, M.J.; Donmez, G.; Doral, M.N. Shoulder joint position sense is negatively correlated with free-throw percentage in professional basketball players. *Isokinet. Exerc. Sci.* **2012**, *20*, 189–196. [CrossRef]
37. Reid, M.; Elliott, B.; Alderson, J. Lower-limb coordination and shoulder joint mechanics in the tennis serve. *Med. Sci. Sports Exerc.* **2008**, *40*, 308. [CrossRef] [PubMed]
38. Lam, W.; Maxwell, J.; Masters, R. Analogy versus explicit learning of a modified basketball shooting task: Performance and kinematic outcomes. *J. Sports Sci.* **2009**, *27*, 179–191. [CrossRef] [PubMed]
39. Chen, T.L.-W.; Wong, D.W.-C.; Wang, Y.; Ren, S.; Yan, F.; Zhang, M. Biomechanics of fencing sport: A scoping review. *PLoS ONE* **2017**, *12*, e0171578. [CrossRef] [PubMed]

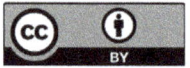

© 2020 by the authors. Licensee MDPI, Basel, Switzerland. This article is an open access article distributed under the terms and conditions of the Creative Commons Attribution (CC BY) license (http://creativecommons.org/licenses/by/4.0/).

Article

Effect of Football Shoe Collar Type on Ankle Biomechanics and Dynamic Stability during Anterior and Lateral Single-Leg Jump Landings

Yunqi Tang [1,2], Zhikang Wang [2], Yifan Zhang [2], Shuqi Zhang [3], Shutao Wei [4], Jiahao Pan [4] and Yu Liu [1,*]

1. Key Laboratory of Exercise and Health Sciences of the Ministry of Education, Shanghai University of Sport, Shanghai 200438, China; tangyunqi@sust.edu.cn
2. College of Art & Design, Shaanxi University of Science & Technology, Xi'an 710021, China; 1710073@sust.edu.cn (Z.W.); 1710035@sust.edu.cn (Y.Z.)
3. Department of Kinesiology & Center for Orthopaedic & Biomechanics Research, Boise State University, Boise, ID 83725, USA; shuqizhang@boisestate.edu
4. 361° (CHINA) CO., LTD., Xiamen 361009, China; st.wei@361sport.com (S.W.); toby881012@gmail.com (J.P.)
* Correspondence: yuliu@sus.edu.cn; Tel.: +86-21-65507860

Received: 13 March 2020; Accepted: 5 May 2020; Published: 13 May 2020

Abstract: In this study, we investigated the effects of football shoes with different collar heights on ankle biomechanics and dynamic postural stability. Fifteen healthy college football players performed anterior and lateral single-leg jump landings when wearing high collar, elastic collar, or low collar football shoes. The kinematics of lower limbs and ground reaction forces were collected by simultaneously using a stereo-photogrammetric system with markers (Vicon) and a force plate (Kistler). During the anterior single-leg jump landing, a high collar shoe resulted in a significantly smaller ankle dorsiflexion range of motion (ROM), compared to both elastic ($p = 0.031$, dz = 0.511) and low collar ($p = 0.043$, dz = 0.446) types, while also presenting lower total ankle sagittal ROM, compared to the low collar type ($p = 0.023$, dz = 0.756). Ankle joint stiffness was significantly greater for the high collar, compared to the elastic collar ($p = 0.003$, dz = 0.629) and low collar ($p = 0.030$, dz = 1.040). Medial-lateral stability was significantly improved with the high collar, compared to the low collar ($p = 0.001$, dz = 1.232). During the lateral single-leg jump landing, ankle inversion ROM ($p = 0.028$, dz = 0.615) and total ankle frontal ROM ($p = 0.019$, dz = 0.873) were significantly smaller for the high collar, compared to the elastic collar. The high collar also resulted in a significantly smaller total ankle sagittal ROM, compared to the low collar ($p = 0.001$, dz = 0.634). Therefore, the high collar shoe should be effective in decreasing the amount of ROM and increasing the dynamic stability, leading to high ankle joint stiffness due to differences in design and material characteristics of the collar types.

Keywords: collar height; kinematics; kinetics; dynamic stability; ankle injury

1. Introduction

Football is the most popular sport in the world, has the largest number of participants, and is associated with a high risk of injury at the professional, amateur, and youth levels during practices and matches [1–5]. It is estimated that somewhere between 13 and 35 players get injured every 1000 competitive hours. The most common incidence of injuries occurs in the lower limbs, mostly ankle sprains [1,5,6]. Dvorak et al. studied injury incidences in the 2010 International Federation of Association Football World Cup. They found that ankle sprains were the most prevalent injury in practices or matches [6]. The impacts of ankle sprains can be severe and include considerable medical expenses, decreased fitness or endurance levels, and missed matches. Furthermore, a common complication of ankle sprains is chronic ankle instability, which results in episodes of the ankle giving way, recurrent sprains, and persistent symptoms such as pain, swelling, limited motion, weakness, and diminished self-reported function. This includes functional and mechanical impairments in isolation, or both [7].

In order to lower football injury risk, shoe manufacturers have attempted to design different cleat configurations that can handle a variety of field conditions, such as turf or grass. In an early study, researchers reported that decreasing the number of cleats and their size may reduce the risk of knee injury [8]. Queen et al. determined that turf cleats could decrease the pressure and force beneath the forefoot, compared to other types of cleats that might minimize metatarsal injury risk on grass [9]. However, Torg et al. examined the mechanical properties of rotational torsion resistance to explain the relation between turf shoes and surface conditions at five temperatures, suggesting that only flat turf football shoes could lower the sprain risk incidence under all conditions [10]. Adjusting cleat configurations could potentially minimize the risk of injuries such as knee sprains and stress fractures on specific field conditions. However, at present, no clear experimental evidence exists to determine the positive effect of cleat configurations on improved ankle stability or decreased ankle sprains.

Increased ankle stability and the prevention of ankle sprains by increasing the shoe collar height have been examined for basketball shoes [11–15]. High collar basketball shoes exhibit a smaller ankle inversion range of motion (ROM), smaller ankle inversion and external rotation at initial contact, and smaller peak inversion velocity, compared to low collar shoes, but no significant difference in kinetic parameters during side-step cutting are observed [11,12]. During jumping tasks, research has revealed that ankle joints show a smaller peak plantarflexion moment and power when wearing basketball shoes with high collars, compared to low collars [13]. According to other research, high collar basketball shoes result in delayed pre-activation timing and decreased amplitude of muscle activity [14]. Therefore, high collar basketball shoes are one factor used to reduce injury potential [16].

Based on the experience with basketball shoes, similar footwear technology has been implemented in football shoes in an attempt to mitigate injury risk. Researchers have observed the ankle inversion between high and low collar football shoes using an inversion platform, which can be rotated 35° to induce a sudden ankle inversion [17]. This research has indicated that high collar shoes significantly reduce the amount and rate of inversion. Additionally, using an arthrometer foot plate, researchers have found that high collar shoes are more effective in decreasing inversion ROM and velocity [18]. However, the research method employed in these previous studies does not accurately portray real-world practices and matches when only the ankle inversion is available. Additionally, although the peak ankle plantarflexion moment and power are significantly smaller in high collar, compared to low collar basketball shoes during landing jumps [13], knowledge of the effects of football shoe collar types on ankle dorsiflexion/plantar flexion movement is currently limited. Furthermore, according to previous studies, around 31% to 46% of football injuries, especially for the knee and ankle, are induced by losing balance or inducing a sprain after landing [19,20]. Hence, for football shoes, questions remain regarding how ankle kinematics and kinetics behave in both dorsiflexion-plantarflexion and inversion-eversion dynamic movements when performing jumping and landing maneuvers.

It should be noted that postural stability has been used to examine the risk of ankle sprain [21,22], and a deficiency in postural stability could play a significant role in increasing ankle sprain risk [20]. A study has found that high collar boots have smaller postural sway, compared to low collar boots, and thereby collar height might have a positive effect on postural control [23]. In a recent study, however, a high collar football shoe did not enhance static postural stability, compared to a low collar shoe [18]. Thus, limited research is available regarding the effects of shoe collars on postural stability. Evidence from a psychological study shows that elastic ankle taping or stiff ankle bracing provides beneficial effects by increasing the feeling of confidence and stability during dynamic-balance tasks [24]. However, direct evidence is conflicting on the beneficial impact on dynamic balance [25–28]. The lack of consistent findings may be due to a lack of measuring more sensitive parameters. The dynamic postural stability index (DPSI) measures three directional components of the ground reaction force during single-leg jump landings. Furthermore, DPSI and its directional components can detect differences in dynamic stability in different football collar types [29]. Therefore, DPSI provides a measure of dynamic stability that has high precision and reliability [30].

Determining the effect of high collar football shoes on ankle biomechanics and DPSI during single-leg jump landings might provide further insight into the biomechanics and dynamic stability of playing football. The purpose of the study aims to determine differences in shoe collar types (i.e., low collar, elastic collar, and high collar) on ankle biomechanics and DPSI during anterior and lateral single-leg jump landings. Our first hypothesis was that smaller ankle ROM, moment, and joint stiffness would result from the high collar football shoe, compared to the elastic or low collar shoes, in both tasks. Our second hypothesis was that dynamic stability would improve when wearing a high collar football shoe, compared to an elastic or low collar shoe, in both tasks.

2. Materials and Methods

2.1. Participants

Fifteen healthy male college football players (age: 21.2 ± 2.0 years; height: 172.4 ± 5.3 cm; body mass: 66.5 ± 9.7 kg) were recruited in this study. The inclusion criteria were (1) at least three years football training experience; (2) foot length of U.S. size 8 for heel-to-toe length; (3) right leg dominant (preferred for kicking); (4) not having sustained a lower limb injury within the past 12 months, including ankle sprain, fractures, or surgeries; and (5) no history of neural or vestibular diseases. The University Ethics Board approved this study, and all participants gave written informed consent before they participated in this study.

2.2. Equipment

Three commercially available football shoes (U.S. size 8, Vapor Untouchable 3; Nike, Portland, OR, USA), which are very popular for football players, were tested in the current study. All shoes were built on the same shoe platform and had identical lightweight upper sections, carbon fiber, thermoplastic polyurethane plates, and cleats, but different shoe collar types: high collar (mass: 300 g; collar height: 70 mm; material: high intensity knitted fabric), elastic collar (mass: 310 g; collar height: 35 mm; material: low intensity knitted fabric), and low collar (mass: 300 g; collar height: 0 mm, material: nil) (Figure 1).

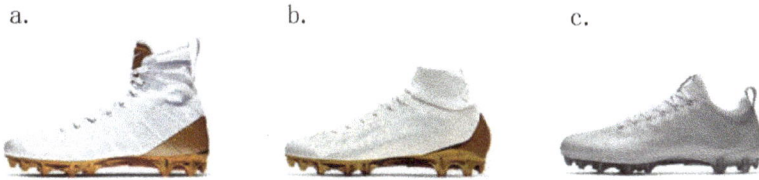

Figure 1. Football shoes used in the current study. (**a**) high collar shoe, (**b**) elastic collar shoe, (**c**) low collar shoe.

The testing environment was an indoor artificial turf-top football ground. The three-dimensional kinematics were measured using a ten-camera Vicon Vantage motion capture system (Vantage 8; Vicon, Oxford, UK), which was arranged around the artificial turf football ground, at a sampling rate of 200 Hz. These cameras are widely used to capture motion trajectory in sports science and biomechanics to optimize human movement [31,32]. The ground reaction force, which was measured for the dominant lower limb, was collected simultaneously using a 600 × 900 mm force plate (9287C; Kistler, Winterthur, Switzerland), which was recessed in the middle of the artificial turf football ground, at a sampling rate of 1000 Hz. The force plate was also used to record the forces exerted by the foot when standing, walking, or running [31,32]. A 900 × 600 × 10 mm artificial turf cover was fixed on the surface of the force plate through screws at each corner (Figure 2). The kinematics and kinetic data were collected and synchronized using a Nexus Lock (Lock +; Vicon, Oxford, UK) with Nexus software (Nexus 2.6.1; Oxford, UK). The Nexus Lock is Vicon's control box for connecting, integrating, and synchronizing third-party devices with the Vicon motion capture system.

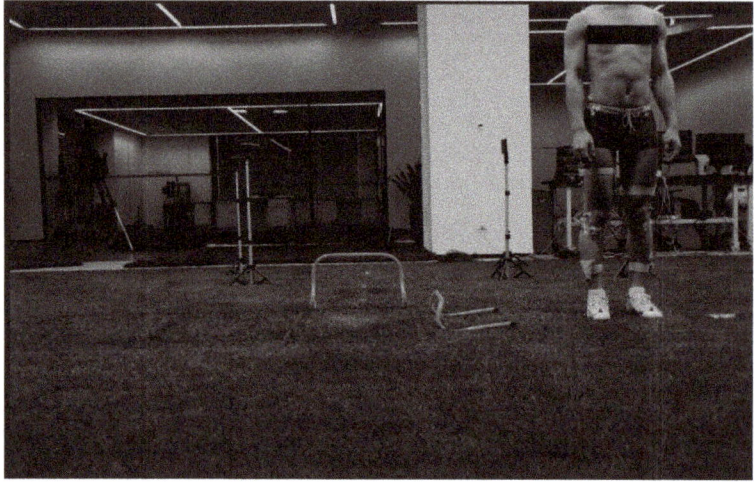

Figure 2. Experimental setup.

Thirty-six retroreflective markers (diameter: 14 mm) were attached to the lower limbs using bio-adhesive tapes. The reflective markers were placed on both the right and left limbs of the iliac crest; anterior superior iliac spine; posterior superior iliac spine; lateral/medial prominence of the lateral femora epicondyle; proximal tip of the head of the fibula; anterior border of the tibial tuberosity; lateral/medial prominence of the lateral malleolus; dorsal margin of the first, second, and fifth metatarsal head; and four four-marker rigid clusters were attached bilaterally onto the thigh and shank.

2.3. Protocol

Each participant performed two tasks, anterior and lateral single-leg jump landings, in one day. Therefore, participants were asked to implement either the anterior single-leg jump landing or the lateral single-leg jump landing, while wearing either low, elastic, or high collar football shoes. All of the tasks were first randomized, and then the shoe order was randomized. Prior to data collection, anatomical and tracking reflective markers were placed on the lower limbs, according to the Istituto Ortopedico Rizzoli (IOR) lower limb model [31]. Meanwhile, the shoelaces were tied by an experimenter and the same type of sport socks were worn, in order to avoid the effects of various shoelaces and socks on the results. Participants were provided five practice trials for each task, to become familiar with the reflective markers and tasks. The anterior and lateral single-leg jump landings were normalized by jump distance according to body height, which was 40% and 33% of body height, respectively [33,34]. Additionally, 30 cm and 15 cm hurdles were placed at 10 cm from the edge of the force plate in anterior and lateral single-leg jump landings, respectively. During data collection, participants were positioned at a normalized distance, then they jumped onto the center of the force plate and landed on their dominant leg after receiving the "start" signal from the researcher. For each condition, each participant was required to stabilize as quickly as possible, place their hands on their waist during landing, and remain motionless on the landing leg for 10 s. Trials were discarded and repeated for the following reasons: (1) moving the foot before jumping, (2) touching or collapsing the hurdle during jumping, or (3) losing balance or removing hands from the waist during landing. To prevent fatigue, 2 min and 5 min breaks were provided between trials and tasks. Trials of each condition were collected for three successful jump landings tasks.

2.4. Data Analysis

Visual3D software (C-motion, Inc.; Germantown, MD, USA) was used to analyze the marker positions and force plate data, which were filtered with a low-pass Butterworth filter with cut-off frequencies of 14 Hz and 50 Hz, respectively. The ankle joint angle was defined using the segment coordinate system for the virtual foot segment, which set the ankle joint angle to zero degrees in the static standing, to be aligned with the segment coordinate system for the shank. The ankle joint moment was calculated using Newton–Euler inverse dynamics with the proximal segment of the shank as the reference segment, which was normalized to each participant's body mass. Ankle joint stiffness was calculated as the change in ankle joint moment divided by the change in ankle joint angle from initial contact to peak dorsiflexion [35].

The DPSI is the composite of the vertical (VSI), anteroposterior (APSI), and medial-lateral (MLSI) components, and was computed following the method of Wikstrom et al. [30] using the customized Visual3D software. The square root of the mean square deviation of force, which was the fluctuation from the baseline along each axis of the force plate, was calculated. The APSI and MLSI were assessed using the fluctuations from 0, and the VSI was calculated using the fluctuation from the subject's body weight. The square root of the sum of the squares of APSI, MLSI, and VSI constituted total DPSI.

These variables were calculated using the first 3 s following initial contact, identified as the force threshold exceeding 10 N. The time interval of 3 s is recommended by Wikstrom et al. for studies of sports performance [36]. For anterior single-leg jump landings, the variables of interest included: (1) ankle dorsiflexion ROM, which refers to the total ankle dorsiflexion excursion; (2) ankle eversion ROM, which refers to the total ankle eversion excursion; (3) total ankle ROM in the sagittal and frontal planes, which refers to the total angle changes in the ankle joint in both planes; (4) peak ankle plantarflexion moment, which refers to the maximum plantarflexion moment; (5) peak ankle inversion moment, which refers to the maximum inversion moment; (6) ankle joint stiffness; and (7) APSI, MLSI, VSI, and DPSI, which refer to the assessments of dynamic postural stability. For lateral single-leg jump landings, the variables of interest were similar to the anterior single-leg jump landing, but with two extra variables: (1) ankle inversion ROM, which is the total ankle inversion excursion; and (2) peak eversion moment, which is the maximum eversion moment. The variables of interest are listed in Tables 1 and 2.

Table 1. Mean (standard deviation) of biomechanical variables and pairwise post hoc *p*-value (Cohen's dz) in ankle joint during tasks in the high-, elastic-, and low collar shoe conditions.

Variables	Shoe Collar Condition			Pairwise Post Hoc		
	High	Elastic	Low	H vs. E	H vs. L	E vs. L
Anterior single-leg jump landing						
Dorsiflexion ROM (°) *	10.40 (5.19)	12.83 (4.28)	12.50 (4.16)	0.031 (0.511)	0.043 (0.446)	0.718 (0.078)
Eversion ROM (°)	10.47 (3.48)	11.72 (3.43)	10.09 (2.76)	0.286 (0.362)	0.691 (0.121)	0.030 (0.524)
Peak plantarflexion moment (Nm/kg)	2.38 (0.38)	2.21 (0.36)	2.24 (0.35)	0.095 (0.459)	0.789 (0.383)	1.000 (0.084)
Peak inversion moment (Nm/kg)	0.48 (0.24)	0.58 (0.43)	0.51 (0.31)	0.442 (0.287)	0.696 (0.108)	0.437 (0.187)
Lateral single-leg jump landing						
Dorsiflexion ROM (°)	18.11 (5.13)	20.50 (3.50)	20.62 (2.39)	0.058 (0.544)	0.059 (0.627)	0.907 (0.040)
Eversion ROM (°)	8.85 (3.13)	11.04 (4.29)	9.20 (4.74)	0.005 (0.583)	0.752 (0.087)	0.116 (0.407)
Inversion ROM (°) *	12.10 (3.15)	15.00 (5.88)	12.97 (4.25)	0.028 (0.615)	0.323 (0.233)	0.054 (0.396)
Peak plantarflexion moment (Nm/kg)	2.42 (0.36)	2.39 (0.49)	2.51 (0.48)	1.000 (0.070)	1.000 (0.212)	0.785 (0.247)
Peak inversion moment (Nm/kg)	0.29 (0.21)	0.37 (0.32)	0.31 (0.21)	0.402 (0.296)	0.704 (0.095)	0.496 (0.222)
Peak eversion moment (Nm/kg)	0.35 (0.30)	0.41 (0.26)	0.38 (0.26)	0.471 (0.214)	0.689 (0.107)	0.743 (0.115)

Note. * represents a significant difference within a subject factor. High (H), Elastic (E), and Low (L) represent three football shoe conditions: high collar, elastic collar, and low collar, respectively.

Table 2. Mean (standard deviation) of dynamic postural stability index and pairwise post hoc *p*-value (Cohen's dz) during tasks in the high-, elastic-, and low collar shoe conditions.

Variables	Shoe Collar Condition			Pairwise Post Hoc		
	High	Elastic	Low	H vs. E	H vs. L	E vs. L
	Anterior single-leg jump landing					
APSI	0.17 (0.014)	0.17 (0.022)	0.17 (0.024)	1.000 (0.101)	1.000 (0.131)	0.714 (0.194)
MLSI *	0.039 (0.004)	0.040 (0.007)	0.045 (0.006)	1.000 (0.204)	0.001 (1.232)	0.051 (0.116)
VSI	0.42 (0.049)	0.42 (0.050)	0.43 (0.059)	1.000 (0.035)	0.387 (0.234)	0.312 (0.263)
DPSI	0.45 (0.045)	0.45 (0.050)	0.46 (0.058)	1.000 (0.016)	0.569 (0.220)	0.526 (0.225)
	Lateral single-leg jump landing					
APSI	0.064 (0.007)	0.063 (0.007)	0.063 (0.010)	1.000 (0.116)	1.000 (0.087)	1.000 (0.007)
MLSI *	0.14 (0.009)	0.14 (0.009)	0.14 (0.012)	0.982 (0.203)	0.359 (0.411)	0.060 (0.588)
VSI	0.39 (0.038)	0.38 (0.049)	0.38 (0.048)	1.000 (0.078)	1.000 (0.159)	1.000 (0.071)
DPSI	0.42 (0.038)	0.41 (0.047)	0.40 (0.060)	1.000 (0.058)	0.547 (0.340)	0.614 (0.270)

Note. * represents a significant difference within a subject factor. High (H), Elastic (E), and Low (L) represent three football shoe conditions: high collar, elastic collar, and low collar, respectively.

2.5. Statistical Analyses

The residual of each dependent variable was assessed for normality using a one-sample Kolmogorov–Smirnov test (α = 0.05). Differences between shoe conditions were examined using two (for anterior and lateral single-leg jump landings) one-way within-subject analyses of variance (ANOVA). Pairwise post hoc analyses were conducted to assess significant differences in the main effects. Wilks's Λ and effect size (ηp^2) were calculated, and Cohen's dz effect sizes were used to interpret the effect of pairwise comparisons. An alpha level of 0.05 was used for statistical analysis. SPSS (19.0, IBM Inc.; Chicago, IL, USA) was used to conduct all statistical analyses.

3. Results

All the variables of interest were normally distributed. Mean (standard deviation) values of each ankle biomechanical variable and the stability index for each collar type, which were estimated intra-subject first and then inter-subject, are shown in Tables 1 and 2, respectively.

3.1. Anterior Single-Leg Jump Landing

The result of the ANOVA indicated a significant shoe effect on dorsiflexion ROM ($F_{2,28}$ = 3.829, p = 0.035, Wilks's Λ = 0.675, ηp^2 = 0.639), total ROM in the sagittal plane ($F_{2,28}$ = 7.554, p = 0.006, Wilks's Λ = 0.590, ηp^2 = 0.854), ankle joint stiffness ($F_{2,28}$ = 7.431, p = 0.009, Wilks's Λ = 0.445, ηp^2 = 0.810), and MLSI ($F_{2,28}$ = 7.418, p = 0.004, Wilks's Λ = 0.382, ηp^2 = 0.884). Post hoc pairwise tests indicated that the high collar resulted in a significantly smaller dorsiflexion ROM, compared to the elastic collar (p = 0.031, dz = 0.511) and low collar (p = 0.043, dz = 0.446) (Table 1), while a significantly smaller total ROM was observed for the high collar, compared to the low collar (p = 0.023, dz = 0.756) in the sagittal plane (Figure 3). The ankle joint stiffness was significantly larger for the high collar, compared to the low collar (p = 0.030, dz = 1.040) and elastic collar (p = 0.003, dz = 0.629) (Figure 4). MLSI was significantly smaller for the shoe with the high collar, compared to the low collar (p = 0.004, dz = 1.232) (Table 2). No other main effects of shoe conditions were detected (Tables 1 and 2).

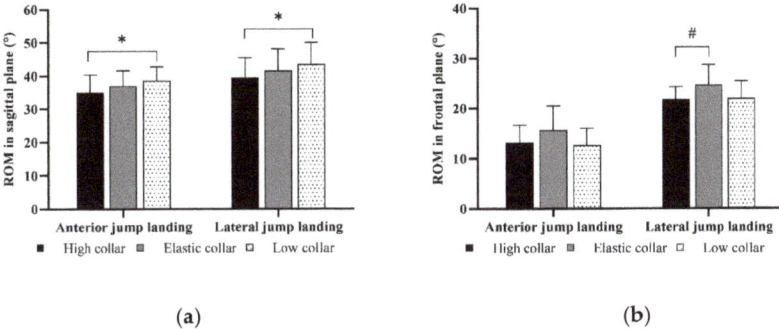

Figure 3. Range of motion (ROM) in the sagittal (**a**) and frontal (**b**) planes for both anterior and lateral jump landings in three shoe conditions: high collar, elastic collar, and low collar. * indicates a significant pairwise difference between the high collar and low collar; # indicates a significant pairwise difference between the high collar and elastic collar.

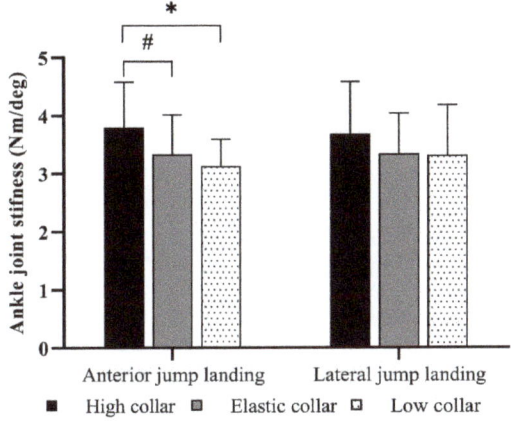

Figure 4. Ankle joint stiffness for both anterior and lateral jump landings in three shoe conditions: high collar, elastic collar, and low collar. * indicates a significant pairwise difference between the high collar and low collar; # indicates a significant pairwise difference between the high collar and elastic collar.

3.2. Lateral Single-Leg Jump Landing

There were significant differences in inversion ROM ($F_{2,28}$ = 4.344, p = 0.029, Wilks's Λ = 0.690, ηp^2 = 0.658), total ROM in both sagittal ($F_{2,28}$ = 6.404, p = 0.009, Wilks's Λ = 0.373, ηp^2 = 0.813) and frontal ($F_{2,28}$ = 6.655, p = 0.006, Wilks's Λ = 0.571, ηp^2 = 0.846) planes, ankle joint stiffness ($F_{2,28}$ = 3.783, p = 0.040, Wilks's Λ = 0.703, ηp^2 = 0.610), and MLSI ($F_{2,28}$ = 7.554, p = 0.041, Wilks's Λ = 0.664, ηp^2 = 0.601) between shoe conditions. Post hoc pairwise tests indicated that inversion ROM was significantly smaller for the high collar, compared to the elastic collar (p = 0.028, dz = 0.615) shoe (Table 1). The high collar resulted in a significantly smaller total ROM, compared to the low collar (p = 0.001, dz = 0.634) in the sagittal plane (Figure 3), while the elastic collar resulted in a significantly larger ROM, compared to the high collar (p = 0.019, dz = 0.873) in the frontal plane (Figure 3). No other pairwise differences were observed for ankle joint stiffness and MLSI (Tables 1 and 2).

4. Discussion

In the present study, we determined the effects of football shoes with different collar conditions on dynamic stability and ankle biomechanical characteristics during anterior and lateral single-leg jump landings. Our results indicate that the high collar football shoe resulted in smaller dorsiflexion ROM and total ROM in the sagittal plane during the anterior single-leg jump landing, while it also decreased inversion ROM and total ROM in the sagittal and frontal planes during the lateral single-leg jump landing. We also found that ankle joint stiffness was significantly larger for the high collar football shoe during anterior and lateral single-leg jump landings, which contradicted our original hypothesis. For dynamic stability, only MLSI showed significant differences during both landing tasks, which was greater when wearing the high collar football shoe and lesser in other conditions; this is partly consistent with our original hypothesis.

The ankle ROM during the anterior single-leg jump landing suggested that the high collar significantly constrained ankle movement, compared to the elastic and low collars. These findings are consistent with Yang et al. and Rowson et al., who reported that peak ankle dorsiflexion or total ankle ROM during a sagittal maneuver was reduced as collar height increases [13,37]. They suggested that collar height and material play an important role in influencing the flexibility and deformation of the whole shoe [13,37]. Additionally, the high collar basketball shoes with strips of plastic that are positioned at the collar's anterior and posterior to the medial and lateral malleoli showed a more restricted ROM of the ankle joint in the sagittal and frontal planes, compared to no plastic condition [16]. It is noteworthy that the elastic collar could not constrain the ankle movement, which might have been due to the low rigidity or high elasticity of the collar material. However, there was no significant change in the frontal plane's ROM. One possible reason is that our healthy participants might have had few inversion-eversion movements during the anterior single-leg jump landings, because our results detected significant differences in inversion and total ankle ROM in the frontal plane between the high and elastic collar, but not between the high and low collar during lateral single-leg jump landings. The elastic collar, similar to ankle taping, likely provides a feeling of confidence and stability [18,24]. This result, in our perspective, is in disagreement with a recent report that indicated that high collar basketball shoes do not restrict the peak inversion angle (29.3° vs. 28.3°) and ROM (17.4° vs. 15.2°) in a self-initiated drop landing on an inversion platform [14]. However, our findings are supported by Richard et al., who found that a high collar football shoe effectively reduces the amount of inversion by 4.5° (38.1° vs. 42.6°) after an inversion platform drop [17]. It is possible that a self-initiated drop landing on an inversion platform does not reach the limitation boundary of the inversion for a high collar basketball shoe. During side-step cutting, Liu et al. and Lam et al. found that the ankle inversion angle, peak inversion velocity, and total inversion ROM are reduced as collar height increases [11,12]. Therefore, there is a restricted angle for an inverted ankle joint position, which might effectively increase ankle joint stability and reduce the risk of ankle sprain injury [11,12]. In our study, the dorsiflexion and total sagittal ROM showed moderate-to-large effect sizes with the high collar, compared to the other collars. Therefore, the football shoe's higher collar height used in this study could constrain ankle dorsiflexion and the inversion angle during both longitude and widthwise tasks, potentially reducing the risk of ankle sprain injury.

Several prior studies have examined the effect of collar conditions on ankle kinetics. Lam et al. detected no difference from collar conditions on the ankle inversion moment during side-step cutting [12]. In addition, Yang et al. reported that high collar basketball shoes could reduce the plantarflexion moment during lay-up jumps, but not drop jumps [13]. The authors suggested that these differential findings were caused by different upper limb positions, movement patterns, and force requirements, as well as the coordination of active and antagonist muscles [13]. These findings are in agreement with our results showing either no significant change or a small effect size in the ankle inversion moment for both tasks; however, different jump maneuvers that are high-frequency and risky during practices or matches still need to be tested. Interestingly, ankle joint stiffness was significantly increased when wearing the high collar football shoe, compared to the other shoes. Theoretically, ankle joint stiffness is calculated using the change in joint moment divided by the change in joint angle [35]. Although the change in ankle moment was not measured in our study, it is possible that the enhanced ankle joint stiffness from the high collar football shoe may be due to a decrease in total ankle

ROM in the sagittal plane. Given the primary role that joint stiffness plays in lower limb injuries [38], overuse injuries at the ankle joint might increase as collar height increases.

Our findings also suggest that MLSI is improved as the height of the football shoe collar increases. A couple of studies have examined the effect of collar height on static or dynamic postural stability [18,39]. However, according to previous research, adequate dorsiflexion ROM is essential for dissipating the ground reaction force [40] and has a positive influence on DPSI [30]; these findings conflict with the results of our study. However, evidence from ankle taping and bracing indicate an increased sense of confidence and stability [24]. Inconsistent findings across studies regarding the dynamic stability of ankle taping or bracing might be due to subjects with or without injury [25–28]. Furthermore, although the current study showed a significant difference in MLSI between shoe conditions during lateral single-leg jump landings, post hoc analysis indicated no pairwise difference, and small effect size. Therefore, this phenomenon still needs to be confirmed, and additional quantitative studies on DPSI are warranted.

There are some limitations to the present study. First, only healthy male college football players were recruited as subjects. Players with functional ankle instability may have different responses to shoe collar conditions, especially for DPSI. Second, it should be noted that our current findings were limited to anterior and lateral single-leg jump landings. Future studies should investigate other typical movements that have high injury risk, such as side-step cutting. Third, different types of shoes may have different mass, which could affect biomechanical responses. A better-controlled experiment is to match the shoe mass across conditions. Fourth, the long-term effect of shoe collar conditions on the incidence of lower limb injuries has yet to be examined. Long-term prospective studies are needed. Finally, the current study only focused on the biomechanical changes at the ankle joint, while knee and hip joint kinematics and kinetics and muscle activity data were not collected.

5. Conclusions

In the current study, the association between the collar condition of football shoes and ankle biomechanics and dynamic postural stability was analyzed. Ankle joint ROM and MLSI during a single-leg jump landing were reduced and improved as the height of the collar increased, respectively. In addition, higher ankle joint stiffness was found for the high collar, compared to the low collar football shoe. Ankle biomechanics and MLSI information from different collar types may be useful in designing football footwear and implementing training. Future prospective investigations are warranted to determine the influence of different shoe collar heights, ankle kinematics/kinetics, and DPSI on lower extremity risks.

Author Contributions: This paper is a result of the collaboration of all authors. All authors have previous experience in sport biomechanics that was shared in order to reach the results discussed in this paper. Conceptualization: Y.T. and Z.W.; data curation: Z.W. and Y.Z.; formal analysis: Y.T. and J.P.; funding acquisition: Y.L.; investigation: Y.Z.; methodology: Y.Z. and S.W.; project administration: Y.L. and J.P.; resources: Y.T. and Y.L.; software: Z.W. and J.P.; supervision: Y.L.; validation: S.Z., S.W., and Y.L.; visualization: Z.W.; writing—original draft: Y.T.; writing—review and editing: S.Z., Y.L., and J.P. All authors have read and agreed to the published version of the manuscript.

Funding: This research was funded by the National Natural Science Foundation of China (No. 11932013) and the National Key Research and Development Program of China (2018YFF0300501).

Acknowledgments: The authors thank all participants for their contributions.

Conflicts of Interest: The authors declare no conflicts of interest.

References

1. Walls, R.J.; Ross, K.A.; Fraser, E.J.; Hodgkins, C.W.; Smyth, N.A.; Egan, C.J.; Calder, J.; Kennedy, J.G. Football injuries of the ankle: A review of injury mechanisms, diagnosis and management. *World J. Orthop.* **2016**, *7*, 8–19. [CrossRef] [PubMed]
2. Ekstrand, J. Epidemiology of football injuries. *Lancet* **2008**, *23*, 73–77. [CrossRef]

3. Pfirrmann, D.; Herbst, M.; Ingelfinger, P.; Simon, P.; Tug, S. Analysis of injury incidences in male professional adult and elite youth soccer players: A systematic review. *J. Athl. Train.* **2016**, *51*, 410–424. [CrossRef] [PubMed]
4. Wong, P.; Hong, Y. Soccer injury in the lower extremities. *Br. J. Sports Med.* **2005**, *39*, 473–482. [CrossRef]
5. Hwang-Bo, K.; Joo, C.H. Analysis of injury incidences in the Korea national men's soccer teams. *J. Exerc. Rehabilit.* **2019**, *15*, 861–866. [CrossRef]
6. Dvorak, J.; Junge, A.; Derman, W.; Schwellnus, M. Injuries and illnesses of football players during the 2010 FIFA World Cup. *Br. J. Sports Med.* **2011**, *45*, 626–630. [CrossRef]
7. Hertel, J.; Corbett, R.O. An updated model of chronic ankle instability. *J. Athl. Train.* **2019**, *54*, 572. [CrossRef]
8. Torg, J.S.; Quedenfeld, T. Effect of shoe type and cleat length on incidence and severity of knee injuries among high school football players. *Res. Q.* **1971**, *42*, 203–211.
9. Queen, R.M.; Charnock, B.L.; Garrett, W.E.; Hardaker, W.M.; Sims, E.L.; Moorman, C.T. A comparison of cleat types during two football-specific tasks on FieldTurf. *Br. J. Sports Med.* **2008**, *42*, 278–284. [CrossRef]
10. Torg, J.S.; Stilwell, G.; Rogers, K. The effect of ambient temperature on the shoe-surface interface release coefficient. *Am. J. Sports Med.* **1996**, *24*, 79–82. [CrossRef]
11. Liu, H.; Wu, Z.; Lam, W.K. Collar height and heel counter-stiffness for ankle stability and athletic performance in basketball. *Res. Sports Med.* **2017**, *25*, 209–218. [CrossRef] [PubMed]
12. Lam, G.W.; Park, E.J.; Lee, K.K.; Cheung, J.T. Shoe collar height effect on athletic performance, ankle joint kinematics and kinetics during unanticipated maximum-effort side-cutting performance. *J. Sports Sci.* **2015**, *33*, 1738–1749. [CrossRef] [PubMed]
13. Yang, Y.; Fang, Y.; Zhang, X.; He, J.; Fu, W. Does shoe collar height influence ankle joint kinematics and kinetics in sagittal plane maneuvers? *J. Sports Sci. Med.* **2017**, *16*, 543–550. [PubMed]
14. Fu, W.; Fang, Y.; Liu, Y.; Hou, J. The effect of high-top and low-top shoes on ankle inversion kinematics and muscle activation in landing on a tilted surface. *J. Foot Ankle Res.* **2014**, *7*, 14. [CrossRef]
15. Brizuela, G.; Llana, S.; Ferrandis, R.; Garcia-Belenguer, A.C. The influence of basketball shoes with increased ankle support on shock attenuation and performance in running and jumping. *J. Sports Sci.* **1997**, *15*, 505–515. [CrossRef]
16. Thacker, S.B.; Stroup, D.F.; Branche, C.M.; Gilchrist, J.; Weitman, E.A. The prevention of ankle sprains in sports. a systematic review of the literature. *Am. J. Sports Med.* **1999**, *27*, 753–760. [CrossRef]
17. Sherman, N.W.; Daniel, M. Effects of high-top and low-top shoes on ankle inversion. *J. Phys. Educ. Recreat. Dance* **2002**, *73*, 6. [CrossRef]
18. Pizac, D.A.; Swanik, C.B.; Glutting, J.J.; Kaminski, T.W. Evaluating postural control and ankle laxity between taping and high-top cleats in high school football players. *J. Sport Rehabilit.* **2016**, *27*, 1–26. [CrossRef]
19. Grimmer, K.; Williams, J. Injury in junior Australian Rules footballers. *J. Sci. Med. Sport* **2003**, *6*, 328–338. [CrossRef]
20. Jones, D.; Louw, Q.; Grimmer, K. Recreational and sporting injury to the adolescent knee and ankle: Prevalence and causes. *Aust. J. Physiother.* **2000**, *46*, 179–188. [CrossRef]
21. McGuine, T.A.; Greene, J.J.; Best, T.; Leverson, G. Balance as a predictor of ankle injuries in high school basketball players. *Clin. J. Sport Med.* **2000**, *10*, 239–244. [CrossRef] [PubMed]
22. Willems, T.M.; Witvrouw, E.; Delbaere, K.; Mahieu, N.; De Bourdeaudhuij, I.; De Clercq, D. Intrinsic risk factors for inversion ankle sprains in male subjects: A prospective study. *Am. J. Sports Med.* **2005**, *33*, 415–423. [CrossRef] [PubMed]
23. Lord, S.R.; Bashford, G.M.; Howland, A.; Munroe, B.J. Effects of shoe collar height and sole hardness on balance in older women. *J. Am. Geriatr. Soc.* **1999**, *47*, 681–684. [CrossRef] [PubMed]
24. Simon, J.; Donahue, M. Effect of ankle taping or bracing on creating an increased sense of confidence, stability, and reassurance when performing a dynamic-balance task. *J. Sport Rehabilit.* **2013**, *22*, 229–233. [CrossRef] [PubMed]
25. Fayson, S.D.; Needle, A.R.; Kaminski, T.W. The effects of ankle Kinesio taping on ankle stiffness and dynamic balance. *Res. Sports Med.* **2013**, *21*, 204–216. [CrossRef] [PubMed]
26. Lee, B.G.; Lee, J.H. Immediate effects of ankle balance taping with kinesiology tape on the dynamic balance of young players with functional ankle instability. *Technol. Health Care* **2015**, *23*, 333–341. [CrossRef]

27. Papadopoulos, E.S.; Nikolopoulos, C.S.; Athanasopoulos, S. The effect of different skin–ankle brace application pressures with and without shoes on single-limb balance, electromyographic activation onset and peroneal reaction time of lower limb muscles. *Foot* **2008**, *18*, 228–236. [CrossRef]
28. Persson, U.M.; Arthurs, C. Dynamic postural stability in gaelic football players during a single leg drop-landing, a comparison of ankle tape and lace-up brace. *Br. J. Sport Med.* **2011**, *45*, 362. [CrossRef]
29. Bowser, B.J.; Rose, W.C.; McGrath, R.; Salerno, J.; Wallace, J.; Davis, I.S. Effect of footwear on dynamic stability during single-leg jump landings. *Int. J. Sports Med.* **2017**, *38*, 481–486. [CrossRef]
30. Wikstrom, E.A.; Tillman, M.D.; Smith, A.N.; Borsa, P.A. A new force-plate technology measure of dynamic postural stability: The dynamic postural stability index. *J. Athl. Train* **2005**, *40*, 305–309.
31. Zhang, S.; Pan, J.; Li, L. Non-linear changes of lower extremity kinetics prior to gait transition. *J. Biomech.* **2018**, *77*, 48–54. [CrossRef] [PubMed]
32. Pan, J.; Liu, C.; Zhang, S.; Li, L. Tai chi can improve postural stability as measured by resistance to perturbation related to upper limb movement among healthy older adults. *Evid. Based Complement. Altern.* **2016**, *2016*, 9710941. [CrossRef] [PubMed]
33. Sell, T.C. An examination, correlation, and comparison of static and dynamic measures of postural stability in healthy, physically active adults. *Phys. Ther. Sport* **2012**, *13*, 80–86. [CrossRef] [PubMed]
34. Williams, V.J.; Nagai, T.; Sell, T.C.; Abt, J.P.; Rowe, R.S.; McGrail, M.A.; Lephart, S.M. Prediction of dynamic postural stability during single-leg jump landings by ankle and knee flexibility and strength. *J. Sport Rehabilit.* **2016**, *25*, 266–272. [CrossRef] [PubMed]
35. Farley, C.T.; Houdijk, H.H.P.; Ciska, V.S.; Ciska, V.S.; Micky, L. Mechanism of leg stiffness adjustment for hopping on surfaces of different stiffnesses. *J. Appl. Physiol.* **1998**, *85*, 1044–1055. [CrossRef]
36. Wikstrom, E.A.; Tillman, M.D.; Borsa, P.A. Detection of dynamic stability deficits in subjects with functional ankle instability. *Med. Sci. Sports Exerc.* **2005**, *37*, 169–175. [CrossRef]
37. Rowson, S.; McNally, C.; Duma, S.M. Can footwear affect achilles tendon loading? *Clin. J. Sport Med.* **2010**, *20*, 344–349. [CrossRef]
38. Hamill, J.; Moses, M.; Seay, J. Lower extremity joint stiffness in runners with low back pain. *Res. Sports Med.* **2007**, *17*, 260–273. [CrossRef]
39. Fong, C.M.; Blackburn, J.T.; Norcross, M.F.; McGrath, M.; Padua, D.A. Ankle-dorsiflexion range of motion and landing biomechanics. *J. Athl. Train.* **2011**, *46*, 5–10. [CrossRef]
40. Debusk, H.; Hill, C.M.; Chander, H.; Knight, A.C.; Babski-Reeves, K. Influence of military workload and footwear on static and dynamic balance performance. *Int. J. Ind. Ergonom.* **2018**, *64*, 51–58. [CrossRef]

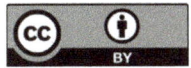

© 2020 by the authors. Licensee MDPI, Basel, Switzerland. This article is an open access article distributed under the terms and conditions of the Creative Commons Attribution (CC BY) license (http://creativecommons.org/licenses/by/4.0/).

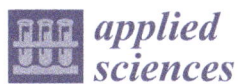 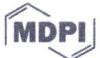

Article

Concurrent Validity and Reliability of My Jump 2 App for Measuring Vertical Jump Height in Recreationally Active Adults

Špela Bogataj [1,2], Maja Pajek [2], Slobodan Andrašić [3,*] and Nebojša Trajković [4]

1. Department of Nephrology, University Medical Centre, 1000 Ljubljana, Slovenia; spela.bogataj@kclj.si
2. Faculty of Sport, University of Ljubljana, 1000 Ljubljana, Slovenia; maja.pajek@fsp.uni-lj.si
3. Faculty of Economics, University of Novi Sad, 24000 Subotica, Serbia
4. Faculty of Sport and Physical Education, University of Novi Sad, 21000 Novi Sad, Serbia; nele_trajce@yahoo.com
* Correspondence: slobodan.andrasic@ef.uns.ac.rs; Tel.: +381-63-517-329

Received: 28 April 2020; Accepted: 27 May 2020; Published: 30 May 2020

Featured Application: My Jump 2 app is a valid and reliable tool for the assessment of vertical jump in recreationally active participants. It is relatively easy to use, affordable, and portable. My Jump 2 can be used in different fields as an alternative to laboratory testing.

Abstract: This study aimed to examine the reliability, validity, and usefulness of the smartphone-based application, My Jump 2, against Optojump in recreationally active adults. Participants (18 women, 28.9 ± 5.6 years, and 26 men, 30.1 ± 10.6 years) completed squat jumps (SJ), counter-movement jumps (CMJ), and CMJ with arm swing (CMJAS) on Optojump and were simultaneously recorded using My Jump 2. To evaluate concurrent validity, jump height, calculated from flight time attained from each device, was compared for each jump type. Test-retest reliability was determined by replicating data analysis of My Jump 2 recordings on two occasions separated by two weeks. High test-retest reliability (Intraclass correlation coefficient (ICC) > 0.93) was observed for all measures in both male and female athletes. Very large correlations were observed between the My Jump 2 app and Optojump for SJ ($r = 0.95$, $p = 0.001$), CMJ ($r = 0.98$, $p = 0.001$), and CMJAS ($r = 0.98$, $p = 0.001$) in male athletes. Similar results were obtained for female recreational athletes for all jumps ($r > 0.94$, $p = 0.001$). The study results suggest that My Jump 2 is a valid, reliable, and useful tool for measuring vertical jump in recreationally active adults. Therefore, due to its simplicity and practicality, it can be used by practitioners, coaches, and recreationally-active adults to measure vertical jump performance with a simple test as SJ, CMJ, and CMJAS.

Keywords: measurement; healthy athletes; jump performance; smartphones; My Jump 2; reliability; validity

1. Introduction

Physical fitness is important for older adults to maintain their independence and enhance wellbeing [1]. Therefore, it is of great importance to measure physical fitness in adults regularly. Vertical jump tests were recognized as the most common means for assessing physical fitness in various populations [2–4]. Moreover, a fundamental step in jump training studies is a vertical jump test. It is also a common method for assessing lower limb power in a physical education class, gym, or other sports programs [5]. Furthermore, it serves as an indicator of athletes fatigue during in-season [6]. Due to its simplicity and important outcome information, vertical jump tests are broadly used by coaches, strength and conditioning professionals, and professionals in health care. The most frequently used vertical jumps are squat jump (SJ), counter-movement jump (CMJ), and drop jump (DJ).

The most commonly used instruments for measuring the vertical jump characteristics have been photoelectric cell systems, force platforms, linear position transducers, infrared cells, contact mats, and video recording [7–12]. The great majority of mentioned instruments presents good validity and reliability in measuring different jumps with the force plate considered as the "gold standard". However, most of the above-mentioned instruments are not cheap and not widely accessible for different populations. Accordingly, due to the fact that these tools are expensive and not easy for transport, practical value for measuring vertical jumps in recreationally active adults is questionable.

Technology improvements led to the integration of high-speed cameras in mobile phones. The mobile application My Jump 2 takes advantage of these cameras to record slow-motion videos of different jump tasks. It gives us information about jump height by selecting the take-off and landing frame. Its validity and reliability were previously reported in male sport science students for drop jumps [8], elderly people [13], and in professional cerebral palsy football players for SJ and CMJ [14]. To the authors' knowledge, there is only one study [15] that analyzed the concurrent validity and reliability of a My Jump app for measuring vertical jump in recreationally active adults. However, the participants were younger men (22 years), and only CMJ was evaluated. There is evidence that the reliability of jumping explosiveness in physical performance tests might vary between men and women [16]. Therefore, it is necessary to check the validity and reliability of the My Jump app with recreational male and female adults. Moreover, in the study mentioned above, My Jump has recorded videos with iPhone 5 s app at 120 fps. As mentioned earlier, the key limiting factor to the accuracy of the app is the frame rate [8]. Therefore, the 240 fps camera on iPhone X was expected to make a significant improvement in the app's performance regarding reliability and validity.

Due to smartphone apps popularity, portability, affordability, and advanced technology, it is important to check the accuracy of these apps for measuring variables related to physical performance and health. Therefore, the present study aimed to investigate the reliability, validity, and usefulness of the My Jump 2 app in comparison to reliable and validated Optojump photoelectric cells system in measuring SJ, CMJ, and CMJ with arm swing (CMJAS) in recreationally active adults. The current research covered a heterogeneous sample with a bigger age range as contrasting to the homogeneous sample in most studies. Our goal was to reassess the app validity in a more heterogeneous sample that has diverse jumping capabilities in order to overcome possible errors in measurements.

2. Materials and Methods

2.1. Participants

A total of 44 participants volunteered to partake in the research. The sample consisted of 18 women (age—28.9 ± 5.6 years; height—169.6 ± 6.2 cm; weight—60.5 ± 8.7 kg) and 26 men (age—30.1 ± 10.6 years; height—178.2 ± 16.2 cm; weight—85.9 ± 23.8 kg) who were recreationally active and had membership in the local gym in Subotica, Serbia where the testing was performed. Participants completed general health and demographic survey and were excluded if they had a history of diseases, injuries in the past six months, or physical condition that may affect testing. All participants were asked if they regularly participated in vigorous physical activity and about the type of activity. Additionally, data were collected regarding the training background and training frequency during one week. On the day of testing, they were healthy, without any heart or pulmonary disease, and injury-free. Before the testing, they were not involved in any strength, jumping, or high-intensity training for 48 h. They were informed about the testing procedures, and before the start, they signed written informed consent. The research adhered to the Declaration of Helsinki and was approved by the local ethics committee (ref. 12/1041).

2.2. Procedures

All participants were familiarized with SJ, CMJ, and CMJAS techniques one day before testing at the same place where the testing was conducted. Assistants also have introduced the participants with the proper technique before testing by video and live demonstration and the explanation of the correct technique.

Before testing, they carried out a standardized 10 min warm-up that consisted of lower-body dynamic stretches, jogging, skipping, and vertical jumps based on similar jump warm-up protocols used in previous studies [15,17]. Their body mass was measured to the nearest 0.1 kg with electronic scale TANITA BC 540 (TANITA Corp., Arlington Heights, IL, USA) and body height with a stadiometer (SECA Instruments Ltd., Hamburg, Germany) to the nearest 1 cm. The leg length and height with bended knees at about 90° were measured using a measuring tape to the nearest 1 cm. Leg length was measured from the anterior iliac spine to the tiptoe in the laying position. Height at 90° was measured vertically from the anterior iliac spine to the ground in an optimal jump performance position (the angle at approximately 90°). Then, each participant performed three SJs, three CMJs, and three CMJs free arms with the instruction to jump as high as possible. For all jumps, it was recommended that the participants leave the floor at take-off with the knees and ankles extended and land in a similarly extended position [18]. Between the trials, there was a two-minute passive rest. The highest jump of each technique was taken into analysis. The jumps were recorded with the Optojump photoelectric cell system (Optojump photocell system; Microgate, Bolzano, Italy) and with an iPhone X (Apple Inc., Cupertino, CA, USA) through My Jump 2 app at the same time. The participants repeated the testing procedure after two weeks with the same conditions and in the same order as during the first testing.

Squat jump performance [19]

Participants were instructed to start the jump in the position of 90° knee flexion with the feet shoulder-width apart and with their hands on their waist. They were asked to jump for maximum height and maintain their hand on the waist. Counter-movement was discouraged, and in case of any mistake, the jump was repeated.

Counter-movement jump performance [20]

The CMJ starting position was a standing position with a straight torso and knees fully extended with the feet shoulder-width apart. Participants were asked to keep their hands on their waist throughout the whole jump. They were instructed to perform a quick downward movement (approximately 90° of knee flexion), and afterward a fast upward movement to jump as high as possible.

Counter-movement jump free arms performance

The CMJAS technique is similar to CMJ with the exception of arm movement. Participants were instructed to swing back with their arms during downward movement and forward during upward movement.

Optojump photoelectric cell system

The Optojump system consists of two parallel bars placed approximately 1 m apart and parallel to each other (see Figure 1). The bars are equipped with 33 optical light-emitting diodes (LEDs) with continuous communication of the transmitting and the receiving bar. The LEDs are positioned 0.3 cm from the ground level and at a 3.125 cm interval. The height of the jump is calculated as follows: $h = 0.5g \times t^2$, where h is the height of the jump, g is the acceleration of gravity, t is half of the flight time. The Optojump achieved strong concurrent validity for jump height in comparison with the force platform (ICC = 0.99; 95% CI (confidence interval) = 0.97; 0.99; $p < 0.001$) and was recognised as an reliable instrument for field-based vertical jump assessments [18].

My Jump 2 app

The app My Jump 2 for iPhone X was used to calculate the jump height by manually selecting the take-off frame and landing frame (Figure 1) of the video. The app determines the jump height using the equation h = t^2 × 1.22625 described by Bosco et al. [21] where h stands for the jump height (in meters) and t for flight time (in seconds). All collections were made with the same phone and by the same evaluator with no professional experience in video analysis. The evaluator was always recording from the same position (approximately 1 m height) and with the same distance from the participants (approximately 1.5 m), enabling the clear view of participants lower limbs. We used the sagittal plane because it showed that identification of the exact take-off and landing frames was more easily viewed, compared to a frontal plane view [22].

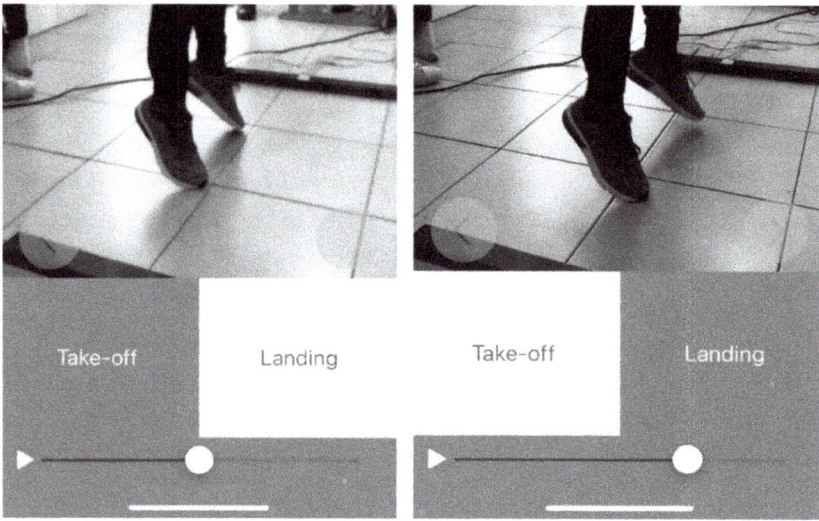

Figure 1. Take-off and landing phase frames on My Jump 2 app.

2.3. Statistical Analysis

Descriptive statistics were presented using means and standard deviations. Shapiro–Wilk test was used to check the data normality. Systematic bias between sessions and tools was evaluated using the paired samples t-test [18]. Standardized differences in mean (with 95% confidence intervals; CI) were calculated to determine the magnitude of the change across and between tests. According to Hopkins et al. [16], Cohen d effect size (ES) magnitudes of change were classified as trivial (>0.2), small (0.2–0.5), moderate (0.5–0.8), large (0.8–1.60), and very large (>1.60). Reliability between test-retest was analyzed using intraclass correlation coefficient (ICC), typical error (TE) expressed as coefficient of variation (CV%), and smallest worthwhile change (SWC) according to Excel spreadsheet provided by Hopkins (2007) [23]. Regarding the ICC analysis, a single measure, two-way mixed, absolute-agreement parameter was used [24]. The highest jump from each subject on both testing sessions, retrieved from the My Jump 2, was used. ICC was interpreted as <0.1 = low, <0.3 = moderate, <0.5 = high, <0.7 = very high, <0.9 = nearly perfect, and <1.0 = perfect. A good reliability was considered if following criteria was fulfilled: CV < 5% and ICC > 0.69 [25]. Test usefulness was determined based on the comparison of SWC (0.2 multiplied by the between-subject SD, based on Cohen's ES) to TE [26]. The following criteria were used to establish the usefulness of tests: "Marginal" (TE > SWC), "OK" (TE = SWC), and "Good" (TE < SWC).

The concurrent validity of the app was tested with Pearson's product-moment correlation coefficient (r). Additionally, the agreement between Optojump and My Jump 2 data was then examined graphically using Bland and Altman's plots in which the difference between both devices was plotted against the mean of the two devices [27].

3. Results

Participants' descriptive characteristics are presented in Table 1.

Table 1. Descriptive characteristics.

	Male (n = 26)	Female (n = 18)
Age (years)	30.1 ± 10.6	28.9 ± 5.6
Height (cm)	178.2 ± 16.2	169.6 ± 6.2
Weight (kg)	85.9 ± 23.8	60.5 ± 8.7
Leg length (cm)	108.1 ± 4.7	106.1 ± 4.5
Years of training	10.5 ± 7.6	9.8 ± 6.6
Training hours per week	6.2 ± 2.1	3.9 ± 1.1

Note: Values are expressed as mean ± SD.

3.1. Reliability

Similar SJ (test = 29.6 ± 6.0 cm; retest = 30.8 ± 6.6 cm), CMJ (test = 31.9 ± 6.6; retest = 34.2 ± 6.9 cm) and CMJAS (test = 39.4 ± 9.7 cm; retest = 39.7 ± 10.0 cm) values were observed between testing sessions in male recreationally active adults. Non-significant differences ($p > 0.05$) were observed between testing sessions for SJ (ES = trivial; CI 95% (0.4; 2.1)), CMJ (ES = small; CI 95% (1.6; 2.9)), and CMJAS (ES = trivial; CI 95% (−0.5; 1.1)) as observed in Table 2. High test-retest reliability (ICC > 0.93; TE < 5% for CMJ and CMJAS, respectively) was observed for all measures.

Table 2. Test-retest reliability and usefulness of My Jump 2 in male recreationally active adults.

	SJ	CMJ	CMJAS
Test (cm)	29.6 ± 6.0	31.9 ± 6.6	39.4 ± 9.7
Retest (cm)	30.8 ± 6.6	34.2 ± 6.9	39.7 ± 10.0
ES	0.19 (trivial)	0.34 (small)	0.03 (trivial)
Diff (95% CI)	1.2 (0.4; 2.1)	2.3 (1.6; 2.9)	0.3 (−0.5;1.1)
ICC (95% CI)	0.93 (0.86;0.96)	0.96 (0.93; 0.97)	0.97 (0.95; 0.99)
TE (95% CI)	1.8 (1.5;2.3)	1.3 (1.1;1.7)	2.0 (1.6;2.6)
CV% (95% CI)	5.8 (4.7; 7.6)	4.1 (3.4; 5.5)	5.0 (4.0; 6.6)
SWC%	1.2 (4.3%)	1.3 (4.0%)	2.0 (5.3%)
Rating	marginal	OK	OK

Abbreviations: SJ, squat jump; CMJ, countermovement jump; ES, effect size; Diff, difference; CI, confidence interval; ICC, intraclass correlation coefficient; TE, typical error; CV, coefficient of variation; SWC, smallest worthwhile change.

Table 3 shows the test retest results for SJ (test = 23.9 ± 6.0 cm; retest = 25.8 ± 6.8 cm), CMJ (test = 26.8 ± 6.3; retest = 27.3 ± 6.2 cm), and CMJAS (test = 29.3 ± 6.0 cm; retest = 30.2 ± 6.4 cm) in female recreationally active adults. There were no significant differences ($p > 0.05$) between testing sessions for SJ (ES = small; CI 95% (1.0; 2.8)), CMJ (ES = trivial; CI 95% (−0.1; 1.1)), and CMJAS (ES = trivial; CI 95% (0.2; 1.6)). High test-retest reliability (ICC > 0.94; TE < 5% for CMJ and CMJAS, respectively) was observed for all measures.

3.2. Test Usefulness

The TE for SJ for both male and female participants was greater than the presumed SWC; consequently, these measures were rated as "marginal." In contrast, TE for CMJ and CMJAS for both genders were similar or lower than SWC and was rated as "OK" and "good".

Table 3. Test-retest reliability and usefulness of My Jump 2 in female recreationally active adults.

	SJ	CMJ	CMJAS
Test (cm)	23.9 ± 6.0	26.8 ± 6.3	29.3 ± 6.0
Retest (cm)	25.8 ± 6.8	27.3 ± 6.2	30.2 ± 6.4
ES	0.30 (small)	0.08 (trivial)	0.15 (trivial)
Diff (95% CI)	1.90 (1; 2.8)	0.5 (−0.1; 1.1)	0.9 (0.2; 1.6)
ICC (95% CI)	0.94 (0.86; 0.97)	0.97 (0.93; 0.98)	0.97 (0.92; 0.98)
TE (95% CI)	1.6 (1.3; 2.3)	1.1 (0,8; 1.5)	1.2 (0.9; 1.6)
CV% (95% CI)	7.2 (5.6; 10.3)	4.3 (3.4; 6.1)	4.3 (3.3; 6.0)
SWC%	1.3 (5.1%)	1.2 (4.5%)	1.2 (4.2%)
Rating	marginal	good	OK

3.3. The Validity of the Test

There were no significant differences ($p > 0.05$) between the My Jump 2 app and Optojump for all jumps in male participants with trivial effects size (from −0.03 to −0.09) (Table 4). Very large correlations were observed between the My Jump 2 app and Optojump for SJ ($r = 0.95$, $p = 0.001$), CMJ ($r = 0.98$, $p = 0.001$), and CMJAS ($r = 0.98$, $p = 0.001$).

Table 4. Descriptive statistics and validity analysis in male recreationally active adults based on Pearson's r.

	My Jump 2	Optojump	Diff. (95% CI)	ES	r (95% CI)	Rating
SJ	29.6 ± 6.0	30.0 ± 6.3	0.40 (−3.26; 2.46)	−0.07	0.95 (0.91; 0.97)	Very large
CMJ	31.9 ± 6.6	32.5 ± 7.1	0.60 (−3.79; 2.59)	−0.09	0.98 (0.95;0.99)	Very large
CMJAS	39.4 ± 9.7	39.7 ± 9.5	0.30 (−4.76; 4.16)	−0.03	0.98 (0.97;0.99)	Very large

Abbreviations: r, Pearson's correlation coefficient.

Similar results were obtained for female recreationally active adults (Table 5). No significant differences ($p > 0.05$) were observed between the My Jump 2 app and Optojump for all jumps in female recreational athletes with trivial effects size (from −0.09 to −0.19). Very large correlations were observed between the My Jump 2 app and Optojump for all jumps ($r > 0.94$, $p = 0.001$).

Table 5. Descriptive statistics and validity analysis in female recreationally active adults based on Pearson's r.

	My Jump 2	Optojump	Diff. (95% CI)	ES	r (95% CI)	Rating
SJ	23.9 ± 6.0	24.5 ± 7.5	0.6 (−3.79; 2.59)	−0.09	0.97 (0.93; 0.99)	Very large
CMJ	26.8 ± 6.3	27.7 ± 7.8	0.9 (−4.90; 3.10)	−0.13	0.96 (0.91;0.98)	Very large
CMJAS	29.3 ± 6.0	30.7 ± 8.4	1.4 (−5.51; 2.71)	−0.19	0.94 (0.87;0.98)	Very large

Figures 2–4 show the level of agreement for all jumps. Bland and Altman's plot depicting limits of agreement for SJ height between the Optojump and My Jump 2 show that the majority of data points are within the 95% CI's (Figure 2).

Further analysis of the Bland–Altman plots in male athletes revealed very low R^2 values ($R^2 \leq 0.10$), meaning outcomes estimated from My Jump 2 had no predisposition to overestimate or underestimate jump performance. On the contrary, in female participants, the plot shows bias related to the magnitude of jump height ($R^2 = 0.74$), such that, at lower jump heights, values derived from Optojump data tended to be higher than those from My Jump 2, resulting in positive difference scores. Moreover, the mean bias between the two methods for all jumps was 0.51 cm.

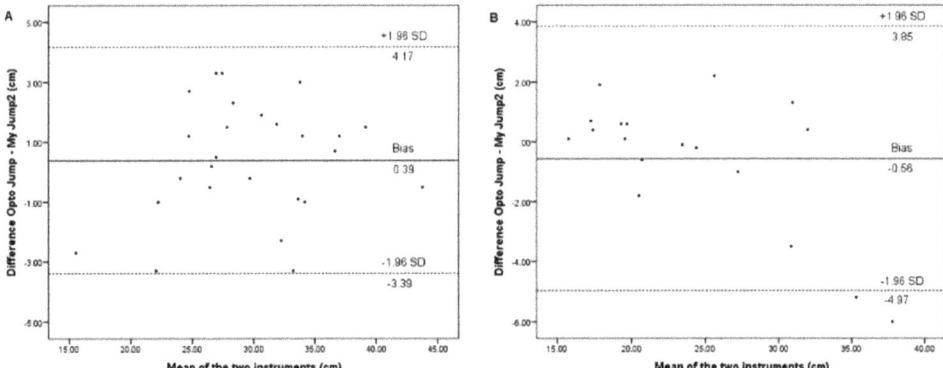

Figure 2. Level of agreement (Bland–Altman) with 95% limits of agreement (dashed lines) and the mean difference (solid line) between My Jump 2 and the Optojump for SJ in (**A**) male and (**B**) female participants.

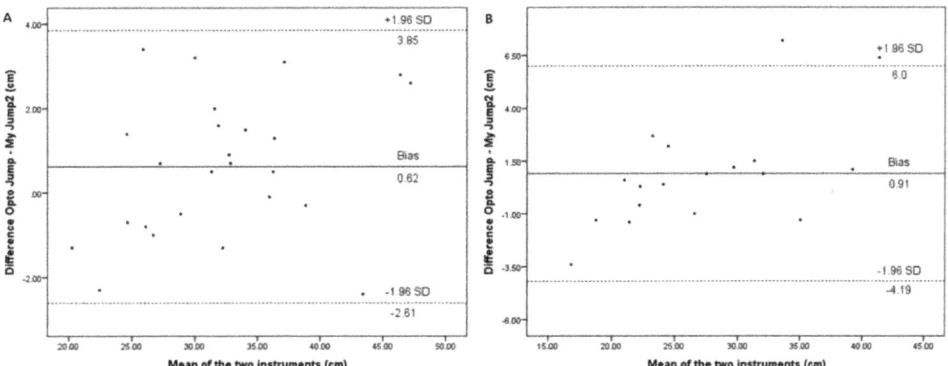

Figure 3. Level of agreement (Bland–Altman) with 95% limits of agreement (dashed lines) and the mean difference (solid line) between My Jump 2 and the Optojump for CMJ in (**A**) male and (**B**) female participants.

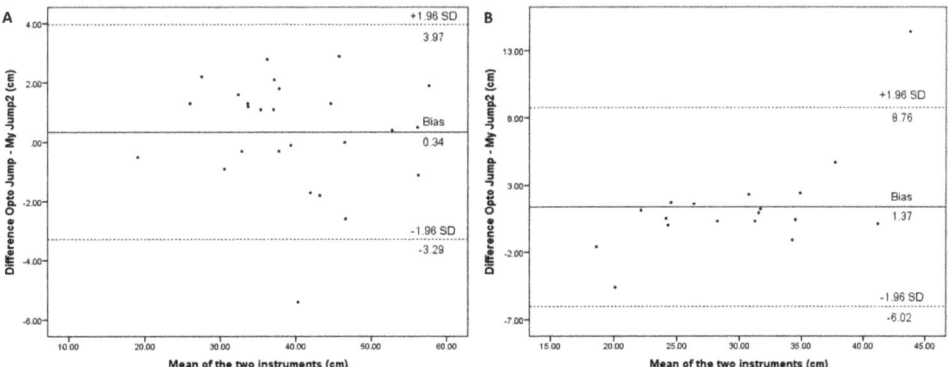

Figure 4. Level of agreement (Bland–Altman) with 95% limits of agreement (dashed lines) and the mean difference (solid line) between My Jump 2 and the Optojump for CMJAS in (**A**) male and (**B**) female participants.

4. Discussion

The CMJ and SJ tests have been strongly recommended to researchers and health practitioners. However, there is a great variety of testing methods and devices, and the majority of them are expensive and nonportable. The present study examined the concurrent validity and test-retest reliability of My Jump 2 installed on an iPhone X compared to a validated Optojump instrument for measuring jump performance during SJ, CMJ, and CMJAS in recreationally active males and females. My Jump 2 was found to be highly valid and reliable in determining the jump height of an SJ, CMJ, and CMJAS in comparison with an Optojump. Moreover, CMJ and CMJAS tests showed to be practically useful to assess and monitor vertical jump performance in recreationally active adults. Furthermore, the data presented in Bland–Altman plots (Figures 2–4), show that most of the values are close to the mean of the differences between instruments, thereby representing a high level of agreement [27]. The plot shows a systematic bias (Figures 2–4) such that, across all jump heights, values derived from the Optojump tended to be slightly higher than those from My Jump 2 app (resulting in positive difference scores). The mean bias between My Jump 2 and the Optojump for jump height was less than 0.9 cm. According to the authors knowledge, this is the first study to compare these two instruments. However, the low bias obtained in our study is in agreement with previous studies (mean bias: 0.2–1.1 cm) that compared My Jump app with force platform [15,28,29]. Higher bias (1.37 cm) was found only in females for CMJAS, which could be due to higher variability influenced by the lack of proper technique among females.

Our test-retest design in the group of recreationally active males and females revealed that SJ, CMJ, and CMJAS appear as reliable assessment outcomes (ICC > 0.90), with slightly greater variability (CV > 5%) for SJ outcomes between two sessions. The current results showed mean differences of 0.3–2.3 cm in all jumps for both males and females. This is in line with a mean difference of 0.43 cm for CMJ reported in recreationally active adults on My Jump app [22].

The concurrent validity of SJ, CMJ, and CMJAS was assessed by comparing outcome measures to the Optojump, which is already validated for estimating vertical jump. Very large correlations were observed between My Jump 2 app and Optojump in both, the male ($r = 0.95-0.98$) and female ($r = 0.94-0.97$), recreationally active adults. Most studies have compared My Jump app with force platform on several different jumps [8,15,28]. The abovementioned studies showed nearly perfect correlation ($r = 0.97-0.99$) for CMJ and SJ in trained athletes [15,28], but also for drop jumps ($r = 0.94-0.97$) in sport science students [8]. The mean differences found in previous validity studies for CMJ performance that compared portable measurement devices with force plates were between −1.06 cm and 11.7 cm [18,30,31]. Regarding the My Jump app, Gallardo-Fuentes et al. [28] found a small mean difference between devices (0.1 cm) when testing CMJ and SJ jump in both male and female athletes. In one recent study [22] on recreationally active males and females, the mean difference in CMJ between devices was 0.21 cm, which is slightly lower than the mean difference found in our study for SJ and CMJ (0.4–0.9 cm). As mentioned earlier, concurrent validity studies have compared My Jump to force plate data. However, it was also important to examine the validity of My Jump compared to a more frequently used field measurement tool. Optojump has also been found to be a valid and reliable vertical jump measurement tool [18], that is amenable to multiple testing locations and, thus, is more commonly used in different vertical jump test settings.

From a practical perspective, the use of healthy recreational adults from across the general population, iPhone X with a 240 Hz high-speed camera, the relatively large number of participants, and field-testing conditions rather than a precise laboratory space all signify strengths of the current research. However, the main limitation was that we did not use force plate, which is considered as the "gold standard" in measuring vertical jump in various populations. Nevertheless, comparing My Jump app with Optojump is more appropriate because both use the flight time to measure jump height. Additionally, different methods for determining the height of the vertical jump exist, which can also impact the validity of instruments [32]. Most of the research has compared methods that calculate jump height to methods that calculate flight distance. Struzik and Zawadzki [33] mention a method based on a force–displacement curve. The method used to calculate jump height should be determined by the equipment available and the definition of jump height used by the practitioner [34].

Furthermore, a possible limitation of our study was that some participants might not have been familiar with the SJ jump style and the usage of hands in CMJAS test, especially among female participants. Relatively high variability obtained in SJ may be due to a lack of proper technique among recreational athletes, while previous research was conducted on elite athletes [28] with greater experience performing these jumps.

Additionally, in comparison to male participants, females have a little difference in achieved jump height between CMJ and CMJAS. We can speculate that females did not swing with their arms correctly and use them to enhance their jump performance. During this jump, the arms reduce the pressure on the ground by moving downward toward the ground, which creates a negative effect, and later the arm swing creates a positive effect by moving upward and increasing the pressure on the ground [35]. Optimal jump is performed when the arms move in the jumping movement direction [36]. Additionally, female athletes show the trend for the increased differences in jump height between the two devices with increasing jumping height, which was confirmed by Attia et al. [37].

Furthermore, another limitation was that we did not check for the inter-rater reliability because some factors could contribute to differences in scores (i.e., the experience of the tester, the different variability of scores, testers' seat position, and assessment view angle) [38]. Therefore, future study should include a larger number of observers to compare results and to account for probable human error. Nevertheless, our results support the usage of smartphone apps in measuring vertical jump in recreationally active males and females. Due to its advanced technology, popularity, low cost, and portability, smartphone apps will soon be commonplace for measuring variables associated with physical fitness and health with great precision [39].

5. Conclusions

The results of present research suggest that smartphone app My Jump 2 is a valid, reliable, and useful tool for measuring jump height in recreationally active adults. Therefore, in addition to its affordable price compared with several available reference methods and given its simplicity and practicality, it can be used by practitioners, coaches, and recreationally-active adults to evaluate physical fitness with a robust and simple test as SJ, CMJ, and CMJAS.

Author Contributions: Conceptualization, Š.B. and N.T.; methodology, N.T.; software, S.A.; validation, M.P., S.A. and N.T.; formal analysis, M.P.; investigation, S.A.; resources, S.A.; writing—original draft preparation, Š.B.; writing—review and editing, N.T.; visualization, Š.B.; supervision, M.P. All authors have read and agreed to the published version of the manuscript.

Funding: This research received no external funding.

Conflicts of Interest: The authors declare no conflict of interest.

References

1. WHO. *Global Recommendations on Physical Activity for Health*; WHO: Geneva, Switzerland, 2015.
2. Watkins, C.M.; Barillas, S.R.; Wong, M.A.; Archer, D.C.; Dobbs, I.J.; Lockie, R.G.; Coburn, J.W.; Tran, T.T.; Brown, L.E. Determination of Vertical Jump as a Measure of Neuromuscular Readiness and Fatigue. *J. Strength Cond. Res.* **2017**, *31*, 3305–3310. [CrossRef] [PubMed]
3. Spiteri, T.; Binetti, M.; Scanlan, A.T.; Dalbo, V.J.; Dolci, F.; Specos, C. Physical Determinants of Division 1 Collegiate Basketball, Women's National Basketball League, and Women's National Basketball Association Athletes: With Reference to Lower-Body Sidedness. *J. Strength Cond. Res.* **2019**, *33*, 159–166. [CrossRef] [PubMed]
4. Yingling, V.R.; Castro, D.A.; Duong, J.T.; Malpartida, F.J.; Usher, J.R.; Jenny, O. The reliability of vertical jump tests between the Vertec and My Jump phone application. *PeerJ* **2018**, *2018*, e4669. [CrossRef] [PubMed]
5. Aragón, L.F. Evaluation of Four Vertical Jump Tests: Methodology, Reliability, Validity, and Accuracy. *Meas. Phys. Educ. Exerc. Sci.* **2000**, *4*, 215–228. [CrossRef]
6. Gathercole, R.J.; Stellingwerff, T.; Sporer, B.C. Effect of acute fatigue and training adaptation on countermovement jump performance in elite snowboard cross athletes. *J. Strength Cond. Res.* **2015**, *29*, 37–46. [CrossRef] [PubMed]

7. Castagna, C.; Ganzetti, M.; Ditroilo, M.; Giovannelli, M.; Rocchetti, A.; Manzi, V. Concurrent validity of vertical jump performance assessment systems. *J. Strength Cond. Res.* **2013**, *27*, 761–768. [CrossRef]
8. Haynes, T.; Bishop, C.; Antrobus, M.; Brazier, J. The validity and reliability of the My Jump 2 app for measuring the reactive strength index and drop jump performance. *J. Sports Med. Phys. Fit.* **2019**, *59*, 253–258. [CrossRef]
9. Whitmer, T.D.; Fry, A.C.; Forsythe, C.M.; Andre, M.J.; Lane, M.T.; Hudy, A.; Honnold, D.E. Accuracy of a vertical jump contact mat for determining jump height and flight time. *J. Strength Cond. Res.* **2015**, *29*, 877–881. [CrossRef]
10. Pueo, B.; Lipinska, P.; Jiménez-Olmedo, J.M.; Zmijewski, P.; Hopkins, W.G. Accuracy of jump-mat systems for measuring jump height. *Int. J. Sports Physiol. Perform.* **2017**, *12*, 959–963. [CrossRef]
11. Carlos-Vivas, J.; Martin-Martinez, J.P.; Hernandez-Mocholi, M.A.; Perez-Gomez, J. Validation of the iPhone app using the force platform to estimate vertical jump height. *J. Sports Med. Phys. Fit.* **2018**, *58*, 227–232.
12. Bosquet, L.; Berryman, N.; Dupuy, O. A comparison of 2 optical timing systems designed to measure flight time and contact time during jumping and hopping. *J. Strength Cond. Res.* **2009**, *23*, 2660–2665. [CrossRef] [PubMed]
13. Cruvinel-Cabral, R.M.; Oliveira-Silva, I.; Medeiros, A.R.; Claudino, J.G.; Jiménez-Reyes, P.; Boullosa, D.A. The validity and reliability of the "my Jump App" for measuring jump height of the elderly. *PeerJ* **2018**, *2018*. [CrossRef] [PubMed]
14. Coswig, V.; Silva, A.D.A.C.E.; Barbalho, M.; de Faria, F.R.; Nogueira, C.D.; Borges, M.; Buratti, J.R.; Vieira, I.B.; Román, F.J.L.; Gorla, J.I. Assessing the validity of the MyJUMP2 app for measuring different jumps in professional cerebral palsy football players: An experimental study. *JMIR mHealth uHealth* **2019**, *7*, e11099. [CrossRef] [PubMed]
15. Balsalobre-Fernández, C.; Glaister, M.; Lockey, R.A. The validity and reliability of an iPhone app for measuring vertical jump performance. *J. Sports Sci.* **2015**, *33*, 1574–1579. [CrossRef] [PubMed]
16. Hopkins, W.G.; Schabort, E.J.; Hawley, J.A. Reliability of power in physical performance tests. *Sport. Med.* **2001**, *31*, 211–234. [CrossRef]
17. Brooks, E.R.; Benson, A.C.; Bruce, L.M. Novel Technologies Found to be Valid and Reliable for the Measurement of Vertical Jump Height With Jump-and-Reach Testing. *J. Strength Cond. Res.* **2018**, *32*, 2838–2845. [CrossRef]
18. Glatthorn, J.F.; Gouge, S.; Nussbaumer, S.; Stauffacher, S.; Impellizzeri, F.M.; Maffiuletti, N.A. Validity and reliability of optojump photoelectric cells for estimating vertical jump height. *J. Strength Cond. Res.* **2011**, *25*, 556–560. [CrossRef]
19. Samozino, P.; Morin, J.B.; Hintzy, F.; Belli, A. A simple method for measuring force, velocity and power output during squat jump. *J. Biomech.* **2008**, *41*, 2940–2945. [CrossRef]
20. Holsgaard Larsen, A.; Caserotti, P.; Puggaard, L.; Aagaard, P. Reproducibility and relationship of single-joint strength vs multi-joint strength and power in aging individuals. *Scand. J. Med. Sci. Sport.* **2007**, *17*, 43–53. [CrossRef]
21. Bosco, C.; Luhtanen, P.; Komi, P.V. A simple method for measurement of mechanical power in jumping. *Eur. J. Appl. Physiol. Occup. Physiol.* **1983**, *50*, 273–282. [CrossRef]
22. Stanton, R.; Wintour, S.A.; Kean, C.O. Validity and intra-rater reliability of MyJump app on iPhone 6s in jump performance. *J. Sci. Med. Sport* **2017**, *20*, 518–523. [CrossRef] [PubMed]
23. Hopkins, W. Reliability from consecutive pairs of trials (Excel spreadsheet). A new view of statistics. sportsci.org: Internet Society for Sport Science.—Open Access Library. *Internet Soc. Sport Sci.* **2007**, *11*, 23–36.
24. Koo, T.K.; Li, M.Y. A Guideline of Selecting and Reporting Intraclass Correlation Coefficients for Reliability Research. *J. Chiropr. Med.* **2016**, *15*, 155–163. [CrossRef] [PubMed]
25. Buchheit, M.; Lefebvre, B.; Laursen, P.B.; Ahmaidi, S. Reliability, usefulness, and validity of the 30–15 Intermittent Ice Test in young elite ice hockey players. *J. Strength Cond. Res.* **2011**, *25*, 1457–1464. [CrossRef] [PubMed]
26. Hopkins, W. How to Interpret Changes in an Athletic Performance Test. *Sportscience* **2004**, *8*, 1–7.
27. Bland, M.J.; Altman, D. Statistical Methods for Assessing Agreement Between Two Methods of Clinical Measurement. *Lancet* **1986**, *327*, 307–310. [CrossRef]
28. Gallardo-Fuentes, F.; Gallardo-Fuentes, J.; Ramírez-Campillo, R.; Balsalobre-Fernández, C.; Martínez, C.; Caniuqueo, A.; Cañas, R.; Banzer, W.; Loturco, I.; Nakamura, F.Y.; et al. Intersession and intrasession reliability

and validity of the my jump app for measuring different jump actions in trained male and female athletes. *J. Strength Cond. Res.* **2016**, *30*, 2049–2056. [CrossRef]
29. Driller, M.; Tavares, F.; McMaster, D.; O'Donnell, S. Assessing a smartphone application to measure counter-movement jumps in recreational athletes. *Int. J. Sports Sci. Coach.* **2017**, *12*, 661–664. [CrossRef]
30. Choukou, M.A.; Laffaye, G.; Taiar, R. Reliability and validity of an accele-rometric system for assessing vertical jumping performance. *Biol. Sport* **2014**, *31*, 55–62. [CrossRef]
31. Buckthorpe, M.; Morris, J.; Folland, J.P. Validity of vertical jump measurement devices. *J. Sports Sci.* **2012**, *30*, 63–69. [CrossRef]
32. Wade, L.; Lichtwark, G.A.; Farris, D.J. Comparisons of laboratory-based methods to calculate jump height and improvements to the field-based flight-time method. *Scand. J. Med. Sci. Sport.* **2020**, *30*, 31–37. [CrossRef] [PubMed]
33. Struzik, A.; Zawadzki, J. Estimation of potential elastic energy during the countermovement phase of a vertical jump based on the force-displacement curve. *Acta Bioeng. Biomech.* **2019**, *21*, 153–160.
34. Moir, G.L. Three Different Methods of Calculating Vertical Jump Height from Force Platform Data in Men and Women. *Meas. Phys. Educ. Exerc. Sci.* **2008**, *12*, 207–218. [CrossRef]
35. Lees, A.; Barton, G. The interpretation of relative momentum data to assess the contribution of the free limbs to the generation of vertical velocity in sports activities. *J. Sports Sci.* **1996**, *14*, 503–511. [CrossRef] [PubMed]
36. Hara, M.; Shibayama, A.; Arakawa, H.; Fukashiro, S. Effect of arm swing direction on forward and backward jump performance. *J. Biomech.* **2008**, *41*, 2806–2815. [CrossRef] [PubMed]
37. Attia, A.; Dhahbi, W.; Chaouachi, A.; Padulo, J.; Wong, D.P.; Chamari, K. Measurement errors when estimating the vertical jump height with flight time using photocell devices: The example of Optojump. *Biol. Sport* **2017**, *34*, 63–70. [CrossRef]
38. Bučar, M.; Čuk, I.; Pajek, J.; Karacsony, I.; Leskošek, B. Reliability and validity of judging in women's artistic gymnastics at University Games 2009. *Eur. J. Sport Sci.* **2012**, *12*, 207–215. [CrossRef]
39. Bort-Roig, J.; Gilson, N.D.; Puig-Ribera, A.; Contreras, R.S.; Trost, S.G. Measuring and influencing physical activity with smartphone technology: A systematic review. *Sport. Med.* **2014**, *44*, 671–686. [CrossRef]

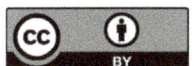

© 2020 by the authors. Licensee MDPI, Basel, Switzerland. This article is an open access article distributed under the terms and conditions of the Creative Commons Attribution (CC BY) license (http://creativecommons.org/licenses/by/4.0/).

MDPI
St. Alban-Anlage 66
4052 Basel
Switzerland
Tel. +41 61 683 77 34
Fax +41 61 302 89 18
www.mdpi.com

Applied Sciences Editorial Office
E-mail: applsci@mdpi.com
www.mdpi.com/journal/applsci

www.ingramcontent.com/pod-product-compliance
Lightning Source LLC
LaVergne TN
LVHW070443100526
838202LV00014B/1656